T0348810

Critical Care in the Emergency Department

Editors

JOHN C. GREENWOOD
TSUYOSHI MITARAI

EMERGENCY MEDICINE CLINICS OF NORTH AMERICA

www.emed.theclinics.com

Consulting Editor
AMAL MATTU

August 2019 • Volume 37 • Number 3

ELSEVIER

1600 John F. Kennedy Boulevard • Suite 1800 • Philadelphia, Pennsylvania, 19103-2899

http://www.theclinics.com

EMERGENCY MEDICINE CLINICS OF NORTH AMERICA Volume 37, Number 3
August 2019 ISSN 0733-8627, ISBN-13: 978-0-323-68217-6

Editor: Colleen Dietzler
Developmental Editor: Casey Potter

Emergency Medicine Clinics of North America (ISSN 0733-8627) is published quarterly by Elsevier Inc., 360 Park Avenue South, New York, NY, 10010-1710. Months of issue are February, May, August, and November. Business and Editorial Offices: 1600 John F. Kennedy Boulevard, Suite 1800, Philadelphia, PA 19103-2899. Customer Service Office: 6277 Sea Harbor Drive, Orlando, FL 32887-4800. Periodicals postage paid at New York, NY, and additional mailing offices. Subscription prices are $100.00 per year (US students), $349.00 per year (US individuals), $679.00 per year (US institutions), $220.00 per year (international students), $462.00 per year (international individuals), $836.00 per year (international institutions), $220.00 per year (Canadian students), $411.00 per year (Canadian individuals), and $836.00 per year (Canadian institutions). International air speed delivery is included in all *Clinics'* subscription prices. All prices are subject to change without notice. **POSTMASTER:** Send address changes to *Emergency Medicine Clinics of North America*, Elsevier Periodicals Customer Service, 11830 Westline Industrial Drive, St. Louis, MO 63146. Customer Service (orders, claims, online, change of address): Elsevier Periodicals **Customer Service, 11830 Westline Industrial Drive, St. Louis, MO 63146. Tel: 1-800-654-2452 (U.S. and Canada); 314-453-7041 (outside U.S. and Canada). Fax: 314-453-5170. E-mail: journalscustomerservice-usa@elsevier.com (for print support); journalsonlinesupport-usa@elsevier.com (for online support).**

Reprints. For copies of 100 or more of articles in this publication, please contact the Commercial Reprints Department, Elsevier Inc., 360 Park Avenue South, New York, NY 10010-1710. Tel.: 212-633-3874; Fax: 212-633-3820; E-mail: reprints@elsevier.com.

Emergency Medicine Clinics of North America is covered in *MEDLINE/PubMed (Index Medicus), Current Contents/Clinical Medicine, EMBASE/Excerpta Medica, BIOSIS, SciSearch, CINAHL, ISI/BIOMED,* and *Research Alert.*

Contributors

CONSULTING EDITOR

AMAL MATTU, MD
Professor and Vice Chair, Department of Emergency Medicine, University of Maryland, School of Medicine, Baltimore, Maryland

EDITORS

JOHN C. GREENWOOD, MD
Assistant Professor, Departments of Emergency Medicine, and Anesthesiology and Critical Care, Perelman School of Medicine, University of Pennsylvania, Philadelphia, Pennsylvania

TSUYOSHI MITARAI, MD, FACEP, FAAEM
Clinical Associate Professor, Director of Emergency Critical Care Program, Director of Critical Care Section, Department of Emergency Medicine, Stanford University School of Medicine, Stanford, California

AUTHORS

PAULOMI BHALLA, MD
Clinical Assistant Professor of Neurology and Neurocritical Care, Director of Tele-Neurology, Stanford Health Care - ValleyCare, Department of Neurology, Stanford University, Palo Alto, California

IVAN CO, MD
Assistant Professor, Departments of Emergency Medicine and Internal Medicine, Division of Pulmonary Critical Care, University of Michigan Health System, Ann Arbor, Michigan

SARA CRAGER, MD
Assistant Professor, Department of Emergency Medicine, Division of Critical Care, Department of Anesthesia, University of California, Los Angeles, David Geffen School of Medicine, Los Angeles, California

KYLE M. DeWITT, PharmD
Department of Pharmacy, University of Vermont Medical Center, Burlington, Vermont

JOHN C. GREENWOOD, MD
Assistant Professor, Departments of Emergency Medicine, and Anesthesiology and Critical Care, Perelman School of Medicine, University of Pennsylvania, Philadelphia, Pennsylvania

KYLE GUNNERSON, MD, FCCM
Associate Professor, Departments of Emergency Medicine, Anesthesiology, and Internal Medicine, Chief, Division of Emergency Critical Care, Medical Director, Massey Family Foundation Emergency Critical Center (EC3), University of Michigan Health System, Ann Arbor, Michigan

STEPHEN D. HALLISEY, MD
Department of Emergency Medicine, Hospital of the University of Pennsylvania, Philadelphia, Pennsylvania

CAMERON D. HYPES, MD, MPH, FACEP
Assistant Professor, Departments of Emergency Medicine and Medicine, Division of Pulmonary, Allergy, Critical Care and Sleep, University of Arizona College of Medicine, The University of Arizona, Tucson, Arizona

NICHOLAS J. JOHNSON, MD
Department of Emergency Medicine, Division of Pulmonary, Critical Care, and Sleep Medicine, University of Washington, Seattle, Washington

SHIKHA KAPIL, MD
Department of Anesthesia, Critical Care Fellow, Stanford University School of Medicine, Palo Alto, California

DANYA KHOUJAH, MBBS
Assistant Professor, Department of Emergency Medicine, University of Maryland School of Medicine, Baltimore, Maryland

HANEY MALLEMAT, MD
Associate Professor of Emergency Medicine and Critical Care Medicine, Cooper University Hospital, Camden, New Jersey

EVIE MARCOLINI, MD
Department of Surgery, Division of Emergency Medicine, Department of Neurology, Division of Neurocritical Care, The Robert Larner, M.D. College of Medicine, University of Vermont, Burlington, Vermont

ASHLEY N. MARTINELLI, PharmD, BCCCP
Clinical Pharmacy Specialist, Emergency Medicine, University of Maryland Medical Center, Baltimore, Maryland

KELSEY A. MILLER, MD
Fellow in Pediatric Emergency Medicine, Division of Emergency Medicine, Boston Children's Hospital, Clinical Fellow of Pediatrics, Harvard Medical School, Boston, Massachusetts

JARROD M. MOSIER, MD, FACEP, FCCM
Associate Professor, Departments of Emergency Medicine and Medicine, Division of Pulmonary, Allergy, Critical Care and Sleep, The University of Arizona College of Medicine, Tucson, Arizona

JOSHUA NAGLER, MD, MHPEd
Associate Division Chief, Director of Medical Education, Division of Emergency Medicine, Boston Children's Hospital, Associate Professor of Pediatrics and Emergency Medicine, Harvard Medical School, Boston, Massachusetts

CHRISTOPHER NOEL, MD
Fellow, Critical Care Medicine, Cooper University Hospital, Camden, New Jersey

CHIDINMA C. NWAKANMA, MD
Assistant Professor of Clinical Emergency Medicine, Perelman School of Medicine, Hospital of the University of Pennsylvania, Philadelphia, Pennsylvania

CHRISTOPH STRETZ, MD
Division of Vascular Neurology, Yale School of Medicine, New Haven, Connecticut

FELIPE TERAN, MD, MSCE
Division of Emergency Ultrasound, Department of Emergency Medicine, Center for Resuscitation Science, Hospital of the University of Pennsylvania, Philadelphia, Pennsylvania

ALFREDO E. URDANETA, MD
Clinical Assistant Professor of Emergency Medicine and Critical Care, Department of Emergency Medicine, Stanford University, Palo Alto, California

AMY C. WALKER, MD
Department of Emergency Medicine, University of Washington, Seattle, Washington

SUSAN R. WILCOX, MD, FACEP, FCCM
Chief, Division of Critical Care, Department of Emergency Medicine, Massachusetts General Hospital, Boston, Massachusetts

JENNIFER G. WILSON, MD, MS
Department of Emergency Medicine, Clinical Assistant Professor, Stanford University School of Medicine, Palo Alto, California

MICHAEL E. WINTERS, MD, MBA
Professor of Emergency Medicine and Medicine, University of Maryland School of Medicine, Baltimore, Maryland

BRIAN JOSEPH WRIGHT, MD, MPH
Associate Professor, Departments of Emergency Medicine and Neurosurgery, Renaissance School of Medicine, Stony Brook University, Stony Brook, New York

Contents

> Acute ischemic stroke (AIS) is a medical emergency that requires prompt recognition and streamlined work-up to ensure that time-dependent therapies are initiated to achieve the best outcomes. This article discusses frequently missed AIS in the emergency department, the role of various imagining modalities in the work-up of AIS, updates on the use of intravenous thrombolytics and endovascular therapy for AIS, pearls on supportive care management of AIS, and prehospital and hospital process improvements to shorten door-to-needle time.

> Despite recent advances, care of the post–cardiac arrest patient remains a challenge. In this article, the authors discuss an approach to the initial care of post–cardiac arrest patients with particular focus on targeted temperature management (TTM). The article starts with history, physiologic rationale, and the major randomized controlled trials that have shaped guidelines for post–cardiac arrest care. It also reviews controversial topics, including TTM for nonshockable rhythms, TTM dose, and surface versus endovascular cooling. The article concludes with a brief review of other key aspects of post–arrest care: coronary angiography, hemodynamic optimization, ventilator management, and prognostication.

> Patients in shock present frequently to the emergency department. The emergency physician must be skilled in the resuscitation of both differentiated and undifferentiated shock. Early, aggressive resuscitation of patients in shock is essential, using macrocirculatory, microcirculatory, and clinical end points to guide interventions. Therapy should focus on the restoration of oxygen delivery to match tissue demand. This article reviews

Video content accompanies this article at http://www.emed.
theclinics.com.

Airway management is the cornerstone to resuscitation efforts for many critically ill pediatric patients presenting for emergency care. Pediatric endotracheal intubation is uncommon in emergency medicine, making it challenging to maintain comfort with this critical procedure. This article offers strategies to facilitate pediatric airway management by addressing predictable anatomic and physiologic differences in children. Also reviewed are alternative approaches to airway management (eg, noninvasive ventilation and videolaryngoscopy) that might be used in cases of recognized difficult airways. Finally, recommendations for maintaining procedural skills in providers who may have limited clinical exposure to critically ill children requiring airway interventions are provided.

Although cardiogenic shock is uncommon in the emergency department, it is associated with high mortality. Most cardiogenic shock is caused by ischemia, but nonischemic etiologies are essential to recognize. Clinicians should optimize preload, contractility, and afterload. Volume-responsive patients should be resuscitated in small aliquots, although some patients may require diuresis to improve cardiac output. Vasopressors are important to restore end-organ perfusion, and inotropes improve contractility. Intubation and positive pressure ventilation impact hemodynamics, which, depending on volume status, may be beneficial or deleterious. Knowing indications for mechanical circulatory support is important for timely consultation or transfer as indicated.

Patients with end-stage liver disease (ESLD) who require intensive care unit admission have high rates of mortality. This article reviews the pathophysiology and emergency department assessment and management of the most frequent conditions and complications encountered in critically ill ESLD patients including hepatic encephalopathy, gastrointestinal bleeding, sepsis and bacterial peritonitis, hepatorenal syndrome, severe coagulopathy, and hepatic hydrothorax.

Central nervous system hemorrhage has multiple pathophysiologic etiologies, including intracerebral hemorrhage (ICH), subarachnoid hemorrhage (SAH), and traumatic brain injury (TBI). Given the nuances intrinsic to each of these etiologies and pathophysiologic processes, optimal blood pressure varies significantly and depends on type of hemorrhage and individual characteristics. This article reviews the most current evidence

EMERGENCY MEDICINE
CLINICS OF NORTH AMERICA

SERIES OF RELATED INTEREST

Critical Care Clinics
https://www.criticalcare.theclinics.com/

THE CLINICS ARE NOW AVAILABLE ONLINE!
Access your subscription at:
www.theclinics.com

Foreword

Beyond Triage and Resuscitation: Optimizing Care for the Critically Ill Emergency Department Patient

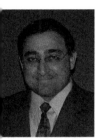

Amal Mattu, MD
Consulting Editor

During my last shift in the emergency department (ED), I assumed care at sign-out of an intubated patient with an acute asthma exacerbation as well as a patient with cardiogenic pulmonary edema who was receiving noninvasive ventilation. Shortly thereafter, prehospital personnel brought us a patient with respiratory failure due to emphysema who needed to be intubated, followed by a patient having an acute stroke who would receive thrombolytics, followed by a patient with hypotension who would later require pressors for septic shock. This latter patient received a central line and an arterial line in the ED. All five of these critically ill patients spent the majority of my shift boarding in the ED awaiting intensive care unit beds. All five of these patients required ongoing, active critical care management by our ED staff, and fortunately, all five had good outcomes.

During a brief lull in caring for these patients, I thought back to my days in residency training in the early 1990s and recalled that all five of these patients back then would have been transferred to an intensive care unit within an hour of their arrival. My care of these patients 25 years ago would therefore largely have been limited to the initial diagnosis and a short period of resuscitation. Such is not the case any longer. Nowadays, we diagnose these patients and continue aggressive care of these patients for many hours, sometimes for more than a day, before they are transferred upstairs. As a result, the distinction between the duties of an emergency physician and an intensive care physician has largely been blurred.

In the year 2019, it is no longer sufficient for an emergency physician to simply know the A-B-Cs of resuscitating critically ill patients. Because of rising ED acuity and volumes, we must know the entire alphabet of resuscitation. Furthermore, our skill set must go beyond just medical intensive care. We must also have surgical and neurologic intensive care skills. Emergency medicine residency programs have responded

Emerg Med Clin N Am 37 (2019) xiii–xiv
https://doi.org/10.1016/j.emc.2019.05.002
0733-8627/19/© 2019 Published by Elsevier Inc.

by incorporating more training months in intensive care units than ever before, and every major emergency medicine conference includes plenty of didactic sessions or workshops focused on critical care topics and procedures. Many emergency physicians are enrolling in critical care fellowships to increase their knowledge even further, and these physicians are helping to train the rest of us in what will undoubtedly become even more important in the coming years.

In this issue of *Emergency Medicine Clinics of North America*, 2 such emergency physicians with critical care fellowship training, Drs John Greenwood and Tsuyoshi Mitarai, have stepped forward as guest editors to provide us with further skills that will help us to care for the critically ill patients in the ED. They have assembled a group of national experts who have written an outstanding curriculum in critical care emergencies for us all.

The authors of this issue of *Emergency Medicine Clinics of North America* address many "hot topics," such as management of acute ischemic and hemorrhagic stroke, postarrest management, sepsis, mechanical ventilation, and cardiogenic shock. They also include articles that address specific, challenging patient populations, such as patients with liver disease, patients with kidney disease, and patients at the extremes of age. Articles are also provided that address a few key procedures, such as intubation, extubation, sedation, and analgesia, and the use of ultrasound in critically ill patients.

This issue of *Emergency Medicine Clinics of North America* should be considered must reading not only for practicing emergency physicians but also for emergency medicine trainees and for any other health care providers that are responsible for caring for critically ill patients. Knowledge and practice of the concepts that are discussed in the following pages are certain to save lives. Kudos to the guest editors and authors for providing us with this valuable addition to our specialty.

Amal Mattu, MD
Department of Emergency Medicine
University of Maryland School of Medicine
110 South Paca Street
6th Floor, Suite 200
Baltimore, MD 21201, USA

E-mail address:
amalmattu@comcast.net

Preface

Beyond Triage and Resuscitation: Optimizing Care for the Critically Ill Emergency Department Patient

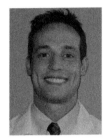
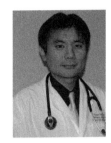

John C. Greenwood, MD   Tsuyoshi Mitarai, MD, FACEP, FAAEM
Editors

Since the last critical care issue of *Emergency Medicine Clinics of North America* published in 2014, emergency departments (ED) across the country have continued to experience an increase in critically ill patient volumes, intensive care unit (ICU) boarding times, clinical complexity, and expectations for care. Appropriate management of these patients by emergency medicine (EM) physicians is critical as the trajectory of the critically ill patient is often defined by the early and effective interventions delivered in the ED. Although EM physicians are well trained in the initial management of a broad spectrum of critical illness, longer ICU boarding times demand EM providers gain a deeper understanding and increased comfort in the management of the complex patient with high acuity beyond the initial resuscitation.

As EM-trained intensivists, we understand the time and resource limitations EM physicians face on a daily basis. We are excited to provide a series of cutting-edge and comprehensive clinical reviews, filled with clinical pearls that can be used during your next shift to save a patient's life.

In this issue of the *Emergency Medicine Clinics of North America*, our authors review cutting-edge resuscitation practice along with evidence-based interventions that can minimize morbidity, mortality, and complications associated with a number of commonly encountered critical illnesses. These articles are written by a talented group of EM intensivists and EM physician experts, who are regarded as the national leaders in this new and expanding field of emergency critical care. Based on recent literature, our authors review significant updates in acute stroke, post cardiac arrest care, and pediatric airway management. We address updates in protective and effective strategies in mechanical ventilation, including mechanical ventilation for hypoxemic respiratory failure and the obstructive lung disease patient, sedation strategies for the

Emerg Med Clin N Am 37 (2019) xv–xvi
https://doi.org/10.1016/j.emc.2019.05.001
0733-8627/19/© 2019 Published by Elsevier Inc.   emed.theclinics.com

intubated patient, and extubation in ED. Two articles are dedicated to state-of-the-art resuscitation practices, including goal-directed shock resuscitation and the integration of point-of-care ultrasound. Finally, this issue includes comprehensive reviews of the critical care management for high-risk patients with end-stage liver disease, acute renal failure, cardiogenic shock from nonischemic causes, and the critically ill geriatric patient.

John C. Greenwood, MD
Department of Emergency Medicine
Department of Anesthesiology and
Critical Care
Perelman School of Medicine
University of Pennsylvania
Ground Ravdin
3400 Spruce Street
Philadelphia, PA 19104, USA

Tsuyoshi Mitarai, MD, FACEP, FAAEM
Department of Emergency Medicine
Stanford University School of Medicine
Stanford, CA 94305, USA

900 Welch Road, Suite 350
Palo Alto, CA 94304, USA

E-mail addresses:
john.greenwood@pennmedicine.upenn.edu (J.C. Greenwood)
tmitarai@stanford.edu (T. Mitarai)

Cutting Edge Acute Ischemic Stroke Management

Alfredo E. Urdaneta, MD[a],*, Paulomi Bhalla, MD[b]

KEYWORDS

- Endovascular mechanical thrombectomy • Acute ischemic stroke
- Stroke management • Stroke window • Stroke imaging • System improvement
- Process improvement

KEY POINTS

- Tissue plasminogen activator (tPA) for ischemic stroke within 4.5 hours of symptom onset is broadly accepted and should not be withheld for those on antiplatelet agents or older than 80 years old.
- Endovascular therapy should be considered for any patient with stroke symptoms within 24 hours of symptom onset by utilizing clinical suspicion for large vessel occlusion and advanced neuroimaging.
- Medical management of stroke is not limited to the decision to administer tPA or endovascular treatments but includes blood pressure, glucose, temperature, and oxygen management.
- Efficient organized workflows in all stages of acute care from the prehospital setting to the interventional radiology suite and critical care unit are necessary to optimize patient outcomes.

INTRODUCTION

Acute ischemic stroke (AIS) is a significant medical event affecting 79,5000 people each year,[1] with substantial implications for the affected patients, their families, and society. Rapid recognition of stroke symptoms by the emergency medicine (EM) physician is key, because time-dependent treatments can drastically alter the neurologic sequalae of an AIS. The saying, "time is brain," should be on every EM physician's mind when evaluating and treating a patient with possible AIS.

Many articles and guidelines for the evaluation and treatment of AIS have been previously published.[2–7] Key parts of the work-up include a National Institutes of Health Stroke

Disclosure Statement: No disclosures to report.
[a] Department of Emergency Medicine, Stanford University, 900 Welch Road, Suite 350, Palo Alto, CA 94305, USA; [b] Department of Neurology, Stanford Health Care - Valley Care, Stanford University, 300 Pasteur Drive, Palo Alto, CA 94304, USA
* Corresponding author.
E-mail address: alfredou@stanford.edu

Emerg Med Clin N Am 37 (2019) 365–379
https://doi.org/10.1016/j.emc.2019.03.001
0733-8627/19/© 2019 Elsevier Inc. All rights reserved.

Scale (NIHSS) score and noncontrast head CT. An NIHSS score calculation is critical for all patients suspected of AIS and before any therapy is started, but EM physicians should not replace a comprehensive neurologic examination with the NIHSS. Intravenous thrombolytic (IVT) therapy with a tissue plasminogen activator (tPA), given within 4.5 hours of AIS onset, is the mainstay therapy. Endovascular therapy is a recent addition to the treatment armamentarium that is safe and improves neurologic outcomes.

DIAGNOSIS

Correct and timely identification of an AIS allows for appropriate time-dependent therapies to be initiated, providing the best opportunity for improved functional outcomes. Common stroke signs and symptoms are discussed in **Table 1**.

Stroke symptoms can be subtle, and the 2 most commonly missed strokes are posterior circulation strokes and those with low NIHSS scores[8]; 35% of patients presenting with dizziness were misdiagnosed as not having an AIS,[9] and patients with an emergency department (ED) discharge diagnosis of benign dizziness were at a 50-

Table 1 Common stroke symptoms	
Vascular Territory	**Physical Examination Findings**
Anterior cerebral artery	Contralateral motor deficits Contralateral sensory deficits Gait apraxia
MCA	Aphasia (expressive and receptive) Contralateral motor deficits Contralateral sensory deficits Homonymous hemianopia Neglect
Posterior cerebral artery	Alexia (inability to read) Choreoathetosis Cranial nerve III palsy Motor deficits Sensory deficits Visual disturbances
Vertebrobasilar artery	Ataxia Cranial nerve palsies Coma Dizziness with nausea and vomiting Dysarthria Dysphagia Motor deficits with contralateral sensory deficits
Posterior inferior cerebellar artery	Ataxia—ipsilateral Contralateral limb with ipsilateral face pain Cranial nerve IX and X palsy Dysmetria Ipsilateral Horner syndrome Nystagmus Vertigo
Anterior inferior cerebellar artery	Cranial nerves V and VII palsy Ipsilateral Horner syndrome Motor deficit of the face Nystagmus Vertigo

fold increase in stroke admission within the next 7 days.[10] Thus, having a good understanding of signs and symptoms of posterior circulation stroke is essential for an EM physician. Key to this is being able to differentiate peripheral from central causes of dizziness. In their review, Kerber and Newman-Toker[9] identified the eye movement examination as the best discriminator between peripheral and central causes of dizziness. The eye examination may be the only clue of a posterior circulation stroke, because the general neurologic examination can be normal in 80% of these stroke patients.[11] **Table 2** compares common abnormal eye movement features of a central versus a peripheral cause of dizziness.

Although the distinction of AIS secondary to large vessel occlusion (LVO) versus other causes (ie, lacunar stroke) does not affect the decision of IVT therapy, recognition of symptoms from LVO can help clinicians with the decision of advanced neuroimaging study (discussed later). LVO is defined as an occlusion of the anterior cerebral artery, basilar artery, carotid terminus, middle cerebral artery (MCA), and/or posterior cerebral artery. A left-sided LVO can present with right sided deficits and aphasia, whereas a right-sided LVO can present with left-sided deficits and neglect. A basilar artery occlusion can lead to a locked-in state where the patient is conscious and able to feel touch but unable to move anything except the eyes in the vertical plane; branches of the basilar artery occlusion can present with nausea vomiting and dizziness.

IMAGING
Computed Tomography/CT Angiography

Rapid neuroimaging plays an integral component in AIS management because it provides information on both stroke subtypes and eligibility for therapy. A current target time to imaging is 20 minutes from ED arrival for candidates for IVT or endovascular therapy. Noncontrast head CT is the preferred imaging modality for speed of acquisition, availability, cost-effectiveness, and high sensitivity for ruling out hemorrhage.[12] Other CT findings, such as early infarct signs and evidence of mass lesions, also may help guide early diagnosis and therapy.[13] If there is any suspicion of an LVO, CT angiogram (CTA) of head and neck should be obtained as long as last known normal is less than 24 hours. By using iodinated radiocontrast media to image intracranial and extracranial blood vessels, the location of the occlusive thrombus can be determined, and other features, such as tandem lesions, can be identified to facilitate preprocedural planning.[14] Additionally, CTA of head may provide information on collateral supply to the ischemic territory, with good collateral supply distal to the occlusion associated with positive clinical outcomes.[15] Inclusion of aortic arch in CTA of neck can identify atherosclerosis as well as rare but devastating type A aortic dissection as a potential cause of AIS.

Table 2 Comparison of central versus peripheral cause of dizziness	
Peripheral	**Central**
Transient (lasting <30 s) vertical-torsional nystagmus triggered by positional testing	Persistent spontaneous or gaze evoked vertical or torsional nystagmus
Unidirectional horizontal nystagmus during gaze testing that never changes direction with gaze direction shifts or head shaking, but changes velocity with gaze direction shift	Persistent horizontal gaze-evoked direction- changing nystagmus
	Nonfatiguing downbeat nystagmus triggered by positional testing

MRI/MR Angiography

MRI can provide a wealth of information in AIS but may be difficult to obtain without increasing door-to-needle (DTN) time.[16] Diffusion-weighted imaging (DWI) provides the most accurate measure of infarct core volume, shows early ischemic changes within minutes, and is the optimal study to evaluate posterior circulation infarcts.[15] Susceptibility-weighted imaging (SWI) can be used to assess for hemorrhage and cerebral microbleeds unseen on head CT, whereas fluid-attenuated inversion recovery (FLAIR) sequences can be used to assess brain parenchyma. An absence of hyperintensity in the region of infarct on FLAIR indicates that the stroke is less than 4.5 hours.[17] Time-of-flight or contrast-enhanced MR angiogram can be used to assess the intracranial and extracranial vasculature analogous to CTA (**Fig. 1**).

Perfusion Imaging

After vascular occlusion, the 3-compartment theory differentiates brain parenchyma into 3 categories: (1) the infarct core, which represents nonviable brain tissue, which cannot be salvaged; (2) the penumbra, which represents tissue that has reduced blood flow, but the potential for survival if blood flow is restored; and (3) the outer zone, which survives regardless of treatment. Recent endovascular therapy trials utilized perfusion imaging techniques to identify patients with a mismatch between the volume of hypoperfused tissue and the volume of nonsalvageable infarct core.

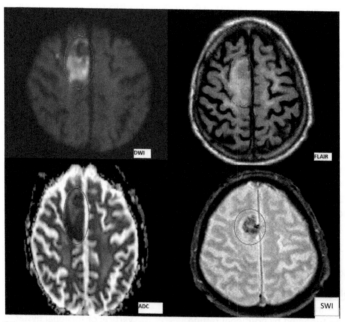

Fig. 1. An 85-year-old man with a history of multiple strokes and history of left-sided weakness presented with worsening weakness of his left side. Upper left panel shows MRI image with a hyperintense region on the DWI sequence with lower left panel showing the corresponding dark region on the apparent diffusion coefficient (ADC). The upper right panel shows the FLAIR sequence with a hyperintense area in the same region indicating the stroke is older than 4.5 hours. Finally, the lower right panel shows the SWI image with a hyperdense area within the stroke indicative of hemorrhage into the stroke.

Perfusion imaging can be performed by CT or MRI, and both use the same basic concepts to measure the time it takes for blood to reach brain tissue (time to peak of the residual function [Tmax] and mean transit time [MTT]) and the amount of blood flowing through the brain vasculature, including capillary and venular flow (cerebral blood volume [CBV] and cerebral blood flow [CBF]). Tmax is the time it takes the contrast to reach maximum enhancement in the selected region of interest. MTT reflects the time between the arterial inflow and the venous outflow. CBV is the volume of blood available per unit of brain tissue (**Fig. 2**). To simplify interpretation, recent endovascular trials used software (Rapid, iSchemaView, Menlo Park, California) for postprocessing of the images. This software defined a relative CBF less than 30% of normal brain as a marker of irreversible injury (infarct core) and defined the penumbral volume as tissue with a Tmax greater than 6 seconds (**Fig. 3**).[18,19] CT perfusion uses iodinated contrast whereas magnetic resonance perfusion uses gadolinium to achieve these measurements. The acquisition and processing of perfusion images take time and expose patients to additional iodinated contrast and radiation; an algorithm for obtaining different studies are outlined in **Fig. 4**.

STROKE MANAGEMENT
Tissue Plasminogen Activator Updates and Controversies

Currently, the only Food and Drug Administration (FDA)-approved therapy for AIS is alteplase, at a dose of 0.9 mg/kg. The inclusion and exclusion criteria for administration of alteplase are reviewed elsewhere.[5,7] This dose of tPA has been shown to increase the chance of having independent function 3 months after AIS by greater than 30%,[5] yet there remains skepticism within the EM community of the benefits versus harm of alteplase.

A meta-analysis looking at the standard dose of alteplase demonstrated that alteplase was associated with a 1.5% greater absolute risk of clinically significant intracranial hemorrhage (ICH) in patients with NIHSS scores between 0 and 4 and with a 3.7% greater absolute risk in patients with NIHSS score greater than 22 strokes compared with those not treated with alteplase. This increase in ICH was associated with a 2.3% absolute increase in deaths within 7 days.[20] These numbers present a real concern for the administration of alteplase but are outweighed by the benefits of alteplase administration. In patients with NIHSS score 0 to 4 stroke, alteplase had an absolute increase in excellent outcome by 8%, and for all strokes had an absolute increase in

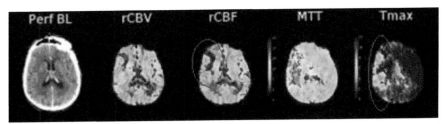

Fig. 2. CT perfusion maps of an 87-year-old man who presented with an NIHSS of 20 approximately 13.5 hours after last known well. In the figure, the first image is the Perf BL, second image is rCBV, third image is rCBF, fourth image is MTT, and fifth image is Tmax., In the third image, the dark blue area (*circled in red*) demonstrates tissue with low CBF (infarct core), whereas the circled area on the fifth image indicates areas where the blood is taking a longer time to reach maximum Hounsfield units (salvageable tissue). MTT, mean transit time; Perf BL, perfusion; rCBF, relative cerberal blood flow; rCBV, relative cerebral blood volume; Tmax, time to peak of the residual function.

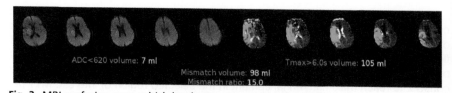

ADC<620 volume: 7 ml   Tmax>6.0s volume: 105 ml
Mismatch volume: 98 ml
Mismatch ratio: 15.0

Fig. 3. MRI perfusion scan, which has been processed by the RAPID software. A 64-year-old man presented 7 hours after the last known well with a NIHSS of 16. The processed image shows an infarct core volume of 7 mL (pink), and a penumbal volume of 105 mL (green).

the chance of an excellent outcome by 6.8%.[20] Patients and family should be informed of the risks of alteplase administration, but the EM physician should not withhold, or dissuade the decision maker against, the administration of alteplase.

An additional concern that is cited regarding tPA administration is its administration to patients on antiplatelet therapy (APT). Although tPA administration to a patient on APT is associated with an absolute increase in ICH of 4.5%, this increase in ICH is not associated with an increase in fatal ICH within 7 days or an increase in 30-day mortality.[21] Additionally, tPA administration to those on APT demonstrated a slight trend toward improved functional outcome compared with those on APT who were not treated with tPA.[21,22] These findings also were found for patients taking dual APT.[23] Given these data, tPA should not be withheld for those on APT or dual APT.

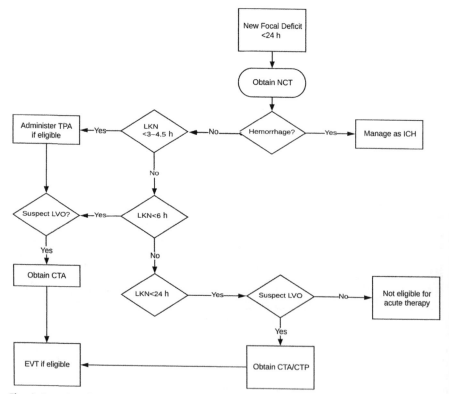

Fig. 4. Imaging decision algorithm. CTP, CT perfusion; EVT, endovascular therapy; LKN, last known normal; NCT, noncontrast CT; TPA, tissue plasminogen activator.

In the United States, tPA is recommended for patients greater than 80 years of age with AIS onset within 3 hours. There are no current recommendations for those greater than 80 years of age in the 3-hour to 4.5-hour onset window. The only study of patients greater than 80 years of age looked at the outcomes for patients who were given tPA in the less than 3-hour window compared with those who were given tPA in the 3-hour to 4.5-hour window. There was a 1.7% increase in ICH rate in the 3-hour to 4.5-hour treatment group compared with the 3-hour treatment group, but no difference in mortality or functional outcome at 3 months between the 2 groups.[24] Although there is a paucity of data on the subject, tPA should not be withheld in AIS for patients greater than 80 year old as long as it is within the 4.5-hour onset window.

Given the risk of ICH with administration of alteplase, several studies have attempted to examine if lower doses of alteplase would produce lower rates of ICH. The ENCHANTED was a noninferiority trial that looked at standard-dose alteplase (0.9 mg/kg) compared with low-dose alteplase (0.6 mg/kg). Because the studies were unable to demonstrate noninferiority of low-dose alteplase,[25,26] standard-dose alteplase at 0.9 mg/kg should be continued to be administered until further research demonstrates otherwise.

Tenecteplase

Alteplase is the current standard tPA for AIS. A potential alternative agent is tenecteplase, a bioengineered tPA that has a longer half-life than alteplase, allowing it to be delivered as a bolus, and has more specificity for fibrin and greater resistance against the plasminogen activator inhibitor.[27–30] Although some studies have shown tenecteplase to have superior recanalization rates and functional outcomes,[27,30,31] others have failed to demonstrate such differences.[28,29] Further research is needed before tenecteplase is considered for AIS.

Extended Window Intravenous Thrombolytic Therapy

In the WAKE-UP trial, MRI was utilized to identify patients who qualify for intravenous (IV) alteplase in patients with neurologic deficits on waking from sleep.[32] Patients who had a lesion on DWI without a corresponding lesion on the FLAIR sequence were treated with IV alteplase. The trial was stopped due to a lack of funding, but interim analysis showed treatment with IV alteplase was associated with a higher likelihood of an outcome with no or minimal neurologic deficit at 90 days compared with placebo. The rates of symptomatic intracerebral hemorrhage and death at 90 days, however, were higher with IV alteplase than with placebo. Although it is a promising study, further studies are needed before MRI-guided thrombolysis is recommended.

ENDOVASCULAR MECHANICAL THROMBECTOMY
Background

Since 2015, endovascular therapy has revolutionized AIS management in patients with LVO. Historically, treatment options were limited to IVT therapy, which only achieves recanalization in less than 30% and good clinical outcome in 25% of patients with LVO.[33] For patients who presented greater than 4.5 hours after the stroke symptoms, treatment options were limited even more.

Early investigations with intra-arterial therapies utilized local thrombolytic[34,35] and subsequently clot removal devices.[36,37] In 2015, the Multicenter Randomized Clinical Trial of Endovascular Treatment for Acute Ischemic Stroke in the

Netherlands (MR CLEAN), comparing thrombectomy to standard of care, demonstrated improved outcome at 90 days without an increase in symptomatic ICH or mortality.[38] After this study, several other studies (Extend-IA, ESCAPE, SWIFT PRIME, and REVASCAPT) [18,39–41] were terminated early after interim analysis demonstrated overwhelming efficacy of thrombectomy. Based on evidence from these trials, practice guidelines were updated recommending that endovascular therapy should be provided to patients within 6 hours of symptom onset plus occlusion of the internal carotid artery or proximal MCA regardless of the use of IVT therapy.

Extended Window Trials

In 2018, 2 large multicenter trials were published, which extended the time window for endovascular therapy: the DAWN and DEFUSE3 trials.[19,42] The DAWN trial enrolled patients up to 24 hours from symptom onset and restricted thrombectomy to the use of the Trevo device (STRYKER, Kalamazoo, MI), whereas DEFUSE3 allowed all FDA-approved devices and enrolled patients who presented within 16 hours of last known normal. Both trials required the use of advanced neuroimaging to capture patients who had a significant mismatch between infarcted core and hypoperfused tissue, with both trials showing better functional outcomes at 90 days.[19,42] **Table 3** demonstrates the key difference between the 2 studies. Based on these 2 studies, the American Heart Association (AHA) updated their stroke guidelines. **Box 1** lists the updated AHA recommendations for endovascular therapy.

Table 3 Characteristics of DAWN and DEFUSE-3 trials	
DAWN	**DEFUSE-3**

Clinical inclusion criteria
  Age $\geq$18
  Baseline NIHSS score $\geq$10
  Prestroke mRS <2
  Anticipated life expectancy
    $\geq$6 mo
  Ineligible for IV tPA
	Clinical inclusion criteria
	  Age 18–90 y
	  Baseline NIHSS score $\geq$6
	  Prestroke mRS $\leq$2

Eligible 6–24 h after last seen well	Eligible 6–16 h after last seen well

Occlusion of intracranial
  ICA or proximal MCA
	Occlusion of extracranial or intracranial
	  ICA or proximal MCA

Group A: >80 y, NIHSS $\geq$10;
  infarct volume <21 mL
Group B: <80 y; NIHSS $\geq$10;
  infarct volume <31 mL
Group C: <80 y; NIHSS $\geq$20;
  infarct volume 31 mL to <51 mL
	Infarct volume <70 mL
	+ ratio of volume of ischemic tissue to initial
	  infarct volume of $\geq$1.8

CT or magnetic resonance–based imaging	CT or magnetic resonance–based imaging
Rapid software for image analysis	Rapid software for image analysis

Only Trevo (Stryker,
  Kalamazoo, MI) device allowed
  for recanalization
	All FDA-approved devices for recanalization allowed

Sponsored by Stryker (Kalamazoo, MI)	Sponsored by National Institutes of Health

---

Box 1
Summary of American Heart Association acute ischemic stroke guidelines related to endovascular therapy

IVT should not be withheld regardless of whether EVT is considered, and EVT should not be delayed assessing for a clinical response to IVT.

EVT therapy with a stent retriever device should be performed if
1. The procedure can begin within 6 hours of symptom onset
2. Baseline functional status of mRS 0 to 1
3. M1 or ICA occlusion on CTA
4. Age ≥18 years old, ASPECTS ≥ 6 and NIHSS ≥6

Patients with an LVO in the anterior circulation maybe a candidate for EVT if
1. LKN 6 hours to 16 hours and they meet eligibility criteria for DAWN[38] or DEFUSE 3[39]
2. LKN 16 hours to 24 hours and they meet eligibility criteria for DAWN[38]

It also can provide an estimate of ischemic tissue by applying the ASPECTS, a 10-point score that subtracts a point for each predefined region of parenchymal hypoattenuation within the anterior circulation. [14]

Abbreviations: ASPECTS, Alberta Stroke Program Early CT Score; EVT, endovascular therapy; LKN, last known normal; mRS, modified Rankin score; M1, 1st segment of middle cerebral artery.

Data from Powers WJ, Rabinstein AA, Ackerson T, et al. 2018 Guidelines for the early management of patients with acute ischemic stroke: a guideline for healthcare professionals from the American Heart Association/American Stroke Association. Stroke 2018;49(3): p. e46–110.

OTHER MEDICAL MANAGEMENT AND MONITORING

As with all acutely ill patients, the ABCs need to be assessed and addressed. All patients with AIS who undergo an intervention need to be admitted and monitored in a dedicated stroke unit. More specific management recommendations are discussed.

Blood Pressure

Approximately 75% of patients who present to the ED with AIS have an elevated systolic blood pressure (SBP) greater than 140 mm Hg. There are strict blood pressure (BP) recommendations for patients with AIS who are to undergo tPA administration or endovascular therapy. Prior to any therapy, the SBP should be lowered to less than 185 mm Hg and diastolic BP (DBP) less than 110 mm Hg. Once therapy has started, the BP should be maintained less than 180/105 mm Hg for the following 24 hours. During tPA administration, the BP must be measured every 15 minutes for 2 hours, every 30 minutes for 6 hours, and then every hour for the next 16 hours.[13] Short-acting titratable agents, such as labetalol, nicardipine, and clevidipine, should be used to achieve the BP goals.

The current AHA guidelines do not address SBP goals in patients with AIS not eligible for tPA or endovascular therapy.[13] Studies looking at aggressive BP control have not demonstrated a mortality or functional outcome benefit.[43] Excessive reduction of BP in AIS can lead to hypoperfusion of at-risk brain tissue due to loss of cerebral autoregulation and further enlarge the ischemic territory. Thus, in patients who do not receive tPA or endovascular therapy, it is reasonable to attempt a 15% reduction in BP over the first 24 hours when the SBP is greater than 220 mm Hg or DBP is greater than 120 mm Hg. [44]

Hypotension should be corrected with volume repletion and then vasopressors, but no recommendation for a lower limit of SBP goal exists in the literature. Given that no recommendation exists, it is reasonable to aim for a mean arterial pressure goal greater than 65 mm Hg, as is done with other patients in shock, and adjust as needed based on the adequacy of end-organ perfusion.

Temperature Management

Hyperthermia has been associated with an increased mortality and worse neurologic outcomes in AIS.[15] Measures should be taken to treat hyperthermia, but there are no specific guidelines to dictate how to achieve this goal. Reasonable options include the use of antipyretics and active cooling to normothermia. The use of therapeutic hypothermia for AIS has not been established and the current 2018 AHA guidelines state that therapeutic hypothermia should be conducted on a research basis only. [13]

Blood Glucose

Measurement of blood glucose is an absolute requirement before the administration of tPA because hypoglycemia can mimic the examination findings in AIS.[13] Hypoglycemia also can worsen functional outcomes in AIS. Conversely, hyperglycemia has been shown to increase neuronal apoptosis and cerebral edema, resulting in worse functional outcome.[45] Therefore, an emphasis should be placed on prevention of hypoglycemia while correcting hyperglycemia. The 2018 AHA guidelines recommend aiming for blood glucose between 140 mg/dL and 180 mg/dL for all patients with ischemic stroke. [13]

Oxygen

Hypoxemia is believed to lead to further injury of ischemic tissue in the penumbral region of the stroke and should be avoided; on the other hand, there is no role for the administration of prophylactic oxygen administration in AIS patients without hypoxia.[46] Thus, supplemental oxygen should be administered only to AIS patients whose pulse -oximetry is less than or equal to 94%.

Tissue Plasminogen Activator Complications

The 2 most common life-threatening complications of tPA administration are ICH and angioedema. Angioedema is found to affect primarily the orolingual region and is more strongly associated with patients taking angiotensin-converting enzyme inhibitor. Signs and symptoms of ICH from tPA administration are listed in **Box 2**. Once ICH is suspected, tPA should be stopped and immediate noncontrast head CT should be performed. Treatment of tPA-associated ICH includes stopping the tPA administration, close monitoring of the airway, and supportive care. Although there are no quality studies to support the use of cryoprecipitates and antifibrinolytics to reverse the effects of tPA, several societies recommend these agents[47] and, based on these recommendations, reversal should be considered.

Box 2
Signs/symptoms of intracranial hemorrhage associated with tissue plasminogen activator administration

Change in level of consciousness

Change in pupil size and reactivity

New-onset nausea and vomiting

New-onset severe headache

Worsening hypertension

SYSTEMS OF CARE AND PROCESS IMPROVEMENT

With the success of recent extended window trials, the number of patients eligible for endovascular therapy is expected to increase. Despite the extended time windows, it is still evident that faster treatment times are beneficial for both IVT and endovascular therapy.[48,49] Quality-improvement initiatives should be implemented in each hospital to decrease the DTN times. The Helsinki model achieved a median DTN time of 20 minutes without an increase in complications.[50,51] Some key components of this model are (1) EMS prenotification with patient details activating a stroke team to meet the patient on arrival, (2) direct transfer of patients from triage to the CT table on the ambulance stretcher, and (3) IVT administered in CT scanner after rapid reading of imaging by stroke neurologist.

Because many hospitals are not equipped with capabilities to perform endovascular therapy, a local protocol should be developed to achieve a prompt transfer of patients with potential eligibility for endovascular therapy. Thus, a crucial question is, What is the most time-efficient model for transfer for AIS patients eligible for endovascular therapy? Currently, there are 4 organizational models for intra-arterial treatment, which have been described: mother-ship, drip-and-ship, trip-and-treat, and mobile stroke unit model. [52]

In the mother-ship model, patients are transported directly to the nearest comprehensive stroke center (CSC), bypassing any primary stroke center (PSC), and thus is dependent on accurate identification of LVO by EMS to avoid overuse of resources as well as time delays in patients eligible for IVT but not endovascular therapy. A recent study evaluated 13 validated prehospital scales used to identify patients with LVO and determined that with the standard cutoffs there was high accuracy but greater than or equal to 20% of patients would be routed incorrectly away from a CSC. [53]

In the drip-and-ship model, patients are taken to the nearest PSC, treated with IVT if indicated, and transferred to a CSC if an LVO is identified on vessel imaging. In this model, the door-in to door-out time at the PSC has been identified as a significant component of total transfer time; thus, efficient workflows are crucial for patient outcomes. [29]

For both models, telemedicine is an accepted method for decision making. Experienced stroke neurologists can provide consultation to PSCs or prehospital care providers in the ambulance.[54] A recent study described a health care network that used a modified Helsinki protocol and a centralized telemedicine approach to improve both the DTN times and the amount of people treated with IVT. [55]

The trip-and-treat model was evaluated in New York City, where a mobile interventional stroke team traveled to 4 PSCs within the city to provide onsite interventional services. In this urban environment, there was shorter time-to-treatment for endovascular therapy compared with the drip-and-ship model[56]; however, it remains to be seen if this is reproducible in suburban or rural communities.

A mobile stroke unit is essentially an ambulance equipped with at least a CT scanner, telemedicine capabilities, and a point-of-care laboratory system to make hyperacute ischemic stroke decisions in the field. In Germany, where this model has been utilized the most, there has been an increase in IVT rates, with significantly shorter time to treatment compared with conventional care. [57]

Although there are ongoing studies evaluating these models, it is likely that the best model will be dependent on factors specific to the region, such as geography, local infrastructure, population density, transportation times, and distribution of centers.

SUMMARY

Prompt recognition of AIS symptoms is a critical step to ensuring the delivery of time-dependent therapies in the ED. Posterior circulation stroke presenting with dizziness may be mistaken for peripheral causes, and focused eye examination should be utilized to help distinguish the 2. Unless contraindicated, IV tPA should be considered in all patients within 4.5 hours of symptom onset, including in patients greater than 80 years or on APT. Eligibility of endovascular therapy should be evaluated for any patient with AIS presenting within 24 hours of symptom onset by utilizing clinical suspicion for LVO and advanced neuroimaging. Regardless of the eligibility of tPA and endovascular therapy, patients with AIS should receive appropriate supportive care to meet BP, glucose, temperature, and oxygen goals. Finally, each hospital should develop a protocol to improve DTN time and efficiency of the transfer process to a CSC for eligible patients.

REFERENCES

1. Benjamin EJ, Virani SS, Callaway CW, et al. Heart disease and stroke statistics-2018 update: a report from the American Heart Association. Circulation 2018; 137(12):e67–492.
2. American College of Emergency Physicians Clinical Policies Subcommittee (Writing Committee) on Use of Intravenous tPA for Ischemic Stroke, Brown MD, Burton JH, Nazarian DJ, et al. Clinical policy: use of intravenous tissue plasminogen activator for the management of acute ischemic stroke in the Emergency Department. Ann Emerg Med 2015;66(3):322–33.e31.
3. Jauch EC, Saver JL, Adams HP Jr, et al. Guidelines for the early management of patients with acute ischemic stroke: a guideline for healthcare professionals from the American Heart Association/American Stroke Association. Stroke 2013;44(3): 870–947.
4. Powers WJ, Derdeyn CP, Biller J, et al. 2015 American Heart Association/American Stroke Association focused update of the 2013 guidelines for the early management of patients with acute ischemic stroke regarding endovascular treatment: a guideline for healthcare professionals from the American Heart Association/American Stroke Association. Stroke 2015;46(10):3020–35.
5. Hasan TF, Rabinstein AA, Middlebrooks EH, et al. Diagnosis and management of acute ischemic stroke. Mayo Clin Proc 2018;93(4):523–38.
6. Nentwich LM. Diagnosis of acute ischemic stoke. Emerg Med Clin North Am 2016;34(4):837–59.
7. Cassella CR, Jagoda A. Ischemic stroke: advances in diagnosis and management. Emerg Med Clin North Am 2017;35(4):911–30.
8. Tarnutzer AA, Lee SH, Robinson KA, et al. ED misdiagnosis of cerebrovascular events in the era of modern neuroimaging: a meta-analysis. Neurology 2017; 88(15):1468–77.
9. Kerber KA, Newman-Toker DE. Misdiagnosing dizzy patients: common pitfalls in clinical practice. Neurol Clin 2015;33(3):565–75, viii.
10. Saber Tehrani AS, Kattah JC, Kerber KA, et al. Diagnosing stroke in acute dizziness and vertigo: pitfalls and pearls. Stroke 2018;49(3):788–95.
11. Kattah JC, Talkad AV, Wang DZ, et al. HINTS to diagnose stroke in the acute vestibular syndrome: three-step bedside oculomotor examination more sensitive than early MRI diffusion-weighted imaging. Stroke 2009;40(11):3504–10.
12. von Kummer R, Allen KL, Holle R, et al. Acute stroke: usefulness of early CT findings before thrombolytic therapy. Radiology 1997;205(2):327–33.

13. Powers WJ, Rabinstein AA, Ackerson T, et al. 2018 guidelines for the early man-agement of patients with acute ischemic stroke: a guideline for healthcare profes-sionals from the American Heart Association/American Stroke Association. Stroke 2018;49(3):e46–110.

14. Smith AG, Rowland Hill C. Imaging assessment of acute ischaemic stroke: a re-view of radiological methods. Br J Radiol 2018;91(1083):20170573.

15. Saxena M, Young P, Pilcher D, et al. Early temperature and mortality in critically ill patients with acute neurological diseases: trauma and stroke differ from infection. Intensive Care Med 2015;41(5):823–32.

16. Yoo SH, Kwon SU, Lee DH, et al. Comparison between MRI screening and CT-plus-MRI screening for thrombolysis within 3 h of ischemic stroke. J Neurol Sci 2010;294(1–2):119–23.

17. Thomalla G, Cheng B, Ebinger M, et al. DWI-FLAIR mismatch for the identification of patients with acute ischaemic stroke within 4.5 h of symptom onset (PRE-FLAIR): a multicentre observational study. Lancet Neurol 2011;10(11):978–86.

18. Campbell BC, Mitchell PJ, Kleinig TJ, et al. Endovascular therapy for ischemic stroke with perfusion-imaging selection. N Engl J Med 2015;372(11):1009–18.

19. Albers GW, Lansberg MG, Kemp S, et al. A multicenter randomized controlled trial of endovascular therapy following imaging evaluation for ischemic stroke (DEFUSE 3). Int J Stroke 2017;12(8):896–905.

20. Whiteley WN, Emberson J, Lees KR, et al. Risk of intracerebral haemorrhage with alteplase after acute ischaemic stroke: a secondary analysis of an individual pa-tient data meta-analysis. Lancet Neurol 2016;15(9):925–33.

21. Tsivgoulis G, Katsanos AH, Zand R, et al. Antiplatelet pretreatment and outcomes in intravenous thrombolysis for stroke: a systematic review and meta-analysis. J Neurol 2017;264(6):1227–35.

22. Robinson TG, Wang X, Arima H, et al. Low- versus standard-dose alteplase in pa-tients on prior antiplatelet therapy: the ENCHANTED Trial (Enhanced Control of Hypertension and Thrombolysis Stroke Study). Stroke 2017;48(7):1877–83.

23. Diedler J, Ahmed N, Sykora M, et al. Safety of intravenous thrombolysis for acute ischemic stroke in patients receiving antiplatelet therapy at stroke onset. Stroke 2010;41(2):288–94.

24. Ahmed N, Lees KR, Ringleb PA, et al. Outcome after stroke thrombolysis in pa-tients >80 years treated within 3 hours vs >3-4.5 hours. Neurology 2017; 89(15):1561–8.

25. Anderson CS, Robinson T, Lindley RI, et al. Low-dose versus standard-dose intra-venous alteplase in acute ischemic stroke. N Engl J Med 2016;374(24):2313–23.

26. Wang X, Robinson TG, Lee TH, et al. Low-dose vs standard-dose alteplase for patients with acute ischemic stroke: secondary analysis of the ENCHANTED ran-domized clinical trial. JAMA Neurol 2017;74(11):1328–35.

27. Campbell BCV, Mitchell PJ, Churilov L, et al. Tenecteplase versus alteplase before thrombectomy for ischemic stroke. N Engl J Med 2018;378(17):1573–82.

28. Huang X, Cheripelli BK, Lloyd SM, et al. Alteplase versus tenecteplase for throm-bolysis after ischaemic stroke (ATTEST): a phase 2, randomised, open-label, blinded endpoint study. Lancet Neurol 2015;14(4):368–76.

29. Logallo N, Novotny V, Assmus J, et al. Tenecteplase versus alteplase for manage-ment of acute ischaemic stroke (NOR-TEST): a phase 3, randomised, open-label, blinded endpoint trial. Lancet Neurol 2017;16(10):781–8.

30. Parsons M, Spratt N, Bivard A, et al. A randomized trial of tenecteplase versus alteplase for acute ischemic stroke. N Engl J Med 2012;366(12):1099–107.

31. Bivard A, Huang X, Levi CR, et al. Tenecteplase in ischemic stroke offers improved recanalization: analysis of 2 trials. Neurology 2017;89(1):62–7.

32. Thomalla G, Simonsen CZ, Boutitie F, et al. MRI-guided thrombolysis for stroke with unknown time of onset. N Engl J Med 2018;379(7):611–22.

33. Bhatia R, Hill MD, Shobha N, et al. Low rates of acute recanalization with intravenous recombinant tissue plasminogen activator in ischemic stroke: real-world experience and a call for action. Stroke 2010;41(10):2254–8.

34. del Zoppo GJ, Higashida RT, Furlan AJ, et al. PROACT: a phase II randomized trial of recombinant pro-urokinase by direct arterial delivery in acute middle cerebral artery stroke. PROACT Investigators. Prolyse in acute cerebral thromboembolism. Stroke 1998;29(1):4–11.

35. Furlan A, Higashida R, Wechsler L, et al. Intra-arterial prourokinase for acute ischemic stroke. The PROACT II study: a randomized controlled trial. Prolyse in Acute Cerebral Thromboembolism. JAMA 1999;282(21):2003–11.

36. Saver JL, Jahan R, Levy EI, et al. Solitaire flow restoration device versus the Merci Retriever in patients with acute ischaemic stroke (SWIFT): a randomised, parallel-group, non-inferiority trial. Lancet 2012;380(9849):1241–9.

37. Smith WS, Sung G, Starkman S, et al. Safety and efficacy of mechanical embolectomy in acute ischemic stroke: results of the MERCI trial. Stroke 2005;36(7):1432–8.

38. Berkhemer OA, Fransen PS, Beumer D, et al. A randomized trial of intraarterial treatment for acute ischemic stroke. N Engl J Med 2015;372(1):11–20.

39. Goyal M, Demchuk AM, Menon BK, et al. Randomized assessment of rapid endovascular treatment of ischemic stroke. N Engl J Med 2015;372(11):1019–30.

40. Saver JL, Goyal M, Bonafe A, et al. Solitaire with the intention for thrombectomy as primary endovascular treatment for acute ischemic stroke (SWIFT PRIME) trial: protocol for a randomized, controlled, multicenter study comparing the Solitaire revascularization device with IV tPA with IV tPA alone in acute ischemic stroke. Int J Stroke 2015;10(3):439–48.

41. Goyal M, Menon BK, van Zwam WH, et al. Endovascular thrombectomy after large-vessel ischaemic stroke: a meta-analysis of individual patient data from five randomised trials. Lancet 2016;387(10029):1723–31.

42. Nogueira RG, Jadhav AP, Haussen DC, et al. Thrombectomy 6 to 24 hours after stroke with a mismatch between deficit and infarct. N Engl J Med 2018;378(1):11–21.

43. Lobanova I, Qureshi AI. Blood pressure goals in acute stroke-how low do you go? Curr Hypertens Rep 2018;20(4):28.

44. AlSibai A, Qureshi AI. Management of acute hypertensive response in patients with ischemic stroke. Neurohospitalist 2016;6(3):122–9.

45. Li WA, Moore-Langston S, Chakraborty T, et al. Hyperglycemia in stroke and possible treatments. Neurol Res 2013;35(5):479–91.

46. Roffe C, Nevatte T, Sim J, et al. Effect of routine low-dose oxygen supplementation on death and disability in adults with acute stroke: the stroke oxygen study randomized clinical trial. JAMA 2017;318(12):1125–35.

47. Frontera JA, Lewin JJ 3rd, Rabinstein AA, et al. Guideline for reversal of antithrombotics in intracranial hemorrhage: executive summary. a statement for healthcare professionals from the Neurocritical Care Society and the Society of Critical Care Medicine. Crit Care Med 2016;44(12):2251–7.

48. Saver JL, Levine SR. Alteplase for ischaemic stroke–much sooner is much better. Lancet 2010;375(9727):1667–8.

49. Saver JL, Goyal M, van der Lugt A, et al. Time to treatment with endovascular thrombectomy and outcomes from ischemic stroke: a meta-analysis. JAMA 2016;316(12):1279–88.
50. Meretoja A, Weir L, Ugalde M, et al. Helsinki model cut stroke thrombolysis delays to 25 minutes in Melbourne in only 4 months. Neurology 2013;81(12):1071–6.
51. Meretoja A, Strbian D, Mustanoja S, et al. Reducing in-hospital delay to 20 minutes in stroke thrombolysis. Neurology 2012;79(4):306–13.
52. Ciccone A, Berge E, Fischer U. Systematic review of organizational models for intra-arterial treatment of acute ischemic stroke. Int J Stroke 2019;14(1):12–22.
53. Turc G, Maïer B, Naggara O, et al. Clinical scales do not reliably identify acute ischemic stroke patients with large-artery occlusion. Stroke 2016;47(6):1466–72.
54. Zerna C, Thomalla G, Campbell BCV, et al. Current practice and future directions in the diagnosis and acute treatment of ischaemic stroke. Lancet 2018; 392(10154):1247–56.
55. Nguyen-Huynh MN, Klingman JG, Avins AL, et al. Novel telestroke program improves thrombolysis for acute stroke across 21 hospitals of an integrated healthcare system. Stroke 2018;49(1):133–9.
56. Wei D, Oxley TJ, Nistal DA, et al. Mobile interventional stroke teams lead to faster treatment times for thrombectomy in large vessel occlusion. Stroke 2017;48(12): 3295–300.
57. John S, Stock S, Cerejo R, et al. Brain imaging using mobile CT: current status and future prospects. J Neuroimaging 2016;26(1):5–15.

Targeted Temperature Management and Postcardiac arrest Care

Check for updates

Amy C. Walker, MD[a],*, Nicholas J. Johnson, MD[a,b]

KEYWORDS

- Targeted temperature management • Cardiac arrest • Therapeutic hypothermia
- Shockable rhythm • Out-of-hospital cardiac arrest

KEY POINTS

- Targeted temperature management (TTM) has been shown to reduce neurologic injury after cardiac arrest and is a cornerstone of postarrest care.
- The optimal dose (defined as temperature achieved multiplied by duration) of TTM is controversial, but current evidence suggests targeting 32°C to 36°C for at least 24 hours in adults with initial shockable cardiac rhythms, and consideration in patients with non-shockable rhythms.
- There is currently no role for prehospital induction of TTM using cold intravenous fluid, and targeted normothermia is the preferred approach in pediatric cardiac arrest.
- Key aspects of postarrest care, in addition to TTM, include ventilator management, hemodynamic optimization, identifying and addressing precipitating pathologic condition, and prognostication.

INTRODUCTION

Sudden cardiac arrest affects more than 500,000 people in the United States each year. Although survival is improving, there remains significant regional variation in care and outcomes and opportunity for improvement.[1–3] Advances in postresuscitation care, such as targeted temperature management (TTM), have been demonstrated to improve outcome, but implementation has been challenging, and the ideal approach has not been defined.

In this article, the authors review the history, physiologic rationale, and evidence behind TTM and address controversies and practical considerations. They discuss

Funding Sources/Disclosures: The authors report no conflicts of interest. N.J. Johnson receives funding from the National Institutes of Health (U01HL123008-02) and Medic One Foundation.
[a] Department of Emergency Medicine, University of Washington, Seattle, WA, USA; [b] Division of Pulmonary, Critical Care, and Sleep Medicine, University of Washington, Seattle, WA, USA
* Corresponding author. Department of Emergency Medicine, University of Washington/Harborview Medical Center, 325 9th Avenue, Box 359702, Seattle, WA 98104.
E-mail address: acw20@uw.edu

other important facets of postarrest care, such as coronary angiography (CAG), ventilator management, and prognostication, and highlight emerging concepts.

TARGETED TEMPERATURE MANAGEMENT
History

The earliest clinical reports of TTM or induced hypothermia in resuscitation date back more than 200 years, when the "Russian method" of packing the bodies of cardiac arrest victims in snow was first described.[4] Numerous other case reports followed, leading to TTM being used during brain and cardiac surgery in the early twentieth century. In 1959, Benson and colleagues[5] described a series of resuscitated cardiac arrest victims treated with TTM who had favorable neurologic outcomes but a host of other complications, including cardiac arrhythmias and infections. In the 1960s, the legendary resuscitation scientist Dr. Peter Safar outlined his vision and clinical practice around using TTM for comatose survivors of cardiac arrest and brain injury of other causes.[6] Several subsequent reports of miraculous recoveries of cold water drowning victims in the 1970s and 1980s fueled interest in this topic, but it was not until the 1990s, after several large animal studies demonstrated efficacy, that rigorous human trials were considered.[6–8]

Physiologic Rationale

TTM is thought to mitigate brain injury by slowing cerebral metabolism and reducing consumption of oxygen and adenosine triphosphate, although this is likely not its only important effect.[9] Hypothermia has been shown to predictably decrease cerebral metabolism at an estimated rate of 6% to 7% per 1°C.[4,10] It also decreases cerebral blood flow and intracranial pressure. TTM inhibits excitatory cell death by reducing glutamate release, lowering concentrations of intracellular calcium, inducing antiapoptotic factors, and suppressing proapoptotic factors.[11–15] Oxidative injury is also reduced by TTM, as is global cerebral inflammation.[16,17] It is likely the cumulative effect of all of these pathways that leads to the beneficial effects demonstrated in several clinical trials. Some practical considerations and potential pitfalls are presented in **Box 1**.

Evidence

Current guidelines and evidence suggest that all adult comatose survivors with out-of-hospital cardiac arrest (OHCA) with an initial shockable cardiac rhythm should receive TTM with a goal temperature of 32°C to 36°C, and it should be considered even among patients with nonshockable initial rhythms.[18] This recommendation is based largely on 2 landmark randomized trials demonstrating improved neurologic outcome when these patients were cooled to 32°C to 34°C, and a subsequent trial demonstrating equivalence comparing this temperature range and 36°C[18–21] **(Table 1)**.

Prehospital induction of TTM via infusion of cold intravenous (IV) fluid cannot be recommended at this time. Two studies on prehospital induction of TTM via administration of 2-L boluses of cold IV fluid failed to demonstrate improved outcome.[22,23] Potential harm, possibly related to IV fluid administration, was demonstrated in both trials.

In children, targeted normothermia is the recommended approach. The Therapeutic Hypothermia After Pediatric Cardiac Arrest (out-of-hospital arrest) (THAPCA-OH) trial compared hypothermia (33°C) to targeted normothermia (36.8°C) in children with OHCA and found no statistically significant difference in neurobehavioral outcome at 12 months after arrest.[24] The THAPCA-IH (in-hospital cardiac arrest) trial was

Box 1
Summary of practical considerations and potential pitfalls in the application of targeted temperature management after cardiac arrest

Hemodynamics

- Decreases cardiac output and oxygen consumption

- Increased SVR and MAP[87]
  - Nielsen and colleagues[24] trial found increased SOFA cardiovascular scores (increased vasoactive requirement) in the 33°C group versus the 36°C group

The clinical importance of these hemodynamic changes remains unclear

Cold diuresis[87]

- May lead to hypovolemia and hypotension

- Careful monitoring of urine output and fluid repletion may be necessary

Cardiac rhythm[87]

- Bradycardia, widening of QRS, PR, QTc intervals; rarely requires intervention

- Malignant arrhythmias are not common until lower temperatures (28°C–30°C)

Impaired platelet function and coagulation[87]

- Usually not clinically important

- May consider Desmopressin and platelet transfusion if patient requires surgical intervention

Shivering

- May lead to increased cerebral metabolism, blood flow, and intracranial pressure[87,88]

- May be treated with acetaminophen, magnesium, analgesia, sedation, and neuromuscular blockade

Insulin resistance

- Most common during induction of TTM

- Target normoglycemia[41]

Electrolyte abnormalities

- Hypokalemia and hypomagnesemia common during rewarming phase[24]

Infection

- Possible increase in pneumonia and sepsis, but no increase in overall infection[20]

- Unclear overall effect on mortality

- No protective effect of prophylactic antibiotics over clinically driven antibiotic administration[78]

- Infection can be subtle and challenging to diagnose in comatose patients undergoing TTM; therefore, low threshold for infectious workup and antibiotics is recommended

Drug metabolism

- Hypothermia slows metabolism of certain medications[33,87]

- Recommend intermittent bolus dosing of medications over continuous infusions

Blood gas interpretation[33]

- May be affected by temperature

- May consider temperature-corrected blood gas calculations.

Abbreviations: SOFA, sequential organ failure assessment; SVR, systemic vascular resistance.

Table 1
Summary of targeted temperature management randomized trials in adults

Study	Temperatures	Arrest Rhythm	No. of Patients	Primary Outcome
Bernard et al,[88] 2002	33°C vs normal	VT/VF	77	Neurologically intact survival to discharge 49% vs 26%
HACA,[20] 2002	32°C–34°C vs normal	VT/VF	273	Neurologically intact survival at 6 mo 55% vs 39%*
Kim et al,[22] 2014	Prehospital cooling vs usual care	VT/VF PEA Asystole	1359	Survival & neurologic status at discharge No difference
Nielsen et al,[21] 2013	33°C vs 36°C	VT/VF PEA Asystole	939	All-cause mortality at 90 d 50% vs 48%
Bernard et al,[23] 2016	Prehospital intra-arrest cooling vs usual care	VT	1198	Survival to hospital discharge 10% vs 11%
Kirkegaard et al,[33] 2017	33°C × 24 h vs 33°C × 48 h	VT/VF PEA Asystole	355	Neurologically intact survival at 6 mo 69% vs 64%

Abbreviations: HACA, hypothermia after cardiac arrest study group; PEA, pulseless electrical activity; VF, ventricular fibrillation; VT, ventricular tachycardia.

Adapted from C, Johnson NJ. Critical care of the post-cardiac arrest patient. Cardiol Clin 2018;36(3):419–28. Review. PMID: 30293608.

stopped early for futility, with no difference in mortality, neurobehavioral outcome, or complication rates between the 2 groups.[25]

Controversies

Targeted temperature management dose

The optimal dose of TTM also remains a question. TTM dose is typically defined as achieved temperature multiplied by duration. The ideal target temperature during TTM remains controversial. Although the 2002 Bernard and colleagues[19] and HACA trials[20] both targeted 32°C to 34°C (see **Table 1**), numerous subsequent studies of TTM demonstrated mixed results, and controversy remained about the utility of this therapy. In particular, temperature was not tightly maintained in the control groups of either trial. In the HACA trial, hyperthermia developed in a substantial proportion of control patients.[20,26,27] Hyperthermia has been consistently demonstrated to be associated with poor outcome after cardiac arrest.[28–30] An even larger study by Nielsen and colleagues demonstrated no difference in mortality or neurologic outcome comparing TTM at 33°C and 36°C in nearly a thousand patients with OHCA of presumed cardiac cause.

Efficacy trials, such as that of Nielsen and colleagues,[21] describe whether an intervention (eg, TTM) produces the desired results under the ideal circumstances of a tightly controlled clinical trial. Since the Nielsen and colleagues trial,[21] retrospective studies have been performed to assess the effectiveness of 33°C versus 36°C in real-world conditions and have found a consistent theme: TTM at 36°C is often poorly implemented; adherence to a temperature management protocol is low; and a substantially increased risk of hyperthermia exists.[31,32] In addition to a higher incidence of hyperthermia, 1 large database study found that before the TTM trial, the in-hospital mortality was decreasing by 1.3% per year. After the TTM trial, the rate of improvement slowed to 0.6% per year. The investigators hypothesized that these findings may be due to less active temperature management at 36°C and higher incidence of fever, which, as mentioned above, has been demonstrated to be associated with worse outcome after cardiac arrest.[28–30]

In order to assess ideal duration, Kirkegaard and colleagues[33] conducted a randomized controlled trial (RCT) that compared 24 versus 48 hours of TTM (with a goal temperature of 32°C–34°C; see **Table 1**). A nearly 5% difference favoring the longer, 48-hour duration of TTM was found, but this did not reach significance. Some have contended that the study was underpowered because of overestimation of the expected effect size.[34] Although the trial was inconclusive for the primary outcome, the investigators did find that the 48-hour group had more adverse events, mainly hypotension, infection, and bleeding.[33]

Surface versus endovascular cooling

A variety of methods exist for modulating temperature after cardiac arrest. Surface cooling can be performed using direct placement of icepacks, cooling pads, and blankets. Endovascular cooling requires a specialized central venous catheter. Endovascular cooling may achieve target temperature more quickly as well as tighter temperature regulation, but when compared with surface cooling did not significantly improve mortality or neurologic outcome.[35] Endovascular cooling is not without risk, because specialized cooling catheters have been associated with a higher risk of venous thrombosis compared with standard central lines.[36]

Nonshockable rhythms

Application of TTM to patients with nonshockable rhythms (pulseless electrical activity and asystole as the initial cardiac arrest rhythm) is controversial, because no randomized trial has been performed to specifically address this population. The TTM and THAPCA trials did include a significant number of patients with nonshockable rhythms, but no difference in neurologic outcome or survival was found among these subgroups.

The remaining data are mixed. Several retrospective studies found no association between TTM and neurologic outcome or mortality among patients with nonshockable cardiac rhythms.[27,37–42] In contrast, several other retrospective cohort studies have found associations between therapeutic hypothermia and improved neurologic outcomes as well as decreased mortality in patients with nonshockable rhythms.[43–46]

These retrospective studies have significant potential for selection bias. In the absence of high-quality data, clinicians must weigh the unclear potential benefit and harm for each individual patient. Current guidelines encourage consideration of TTM for all resuscitated cardiac arrest patients, regardless of initial rhythm.[18]

Future Directions

Several important questions remain regarding TTM after cardiac arrest. First, several upcoming trials aim to address both optimal goal temperature (ClinicalTrials.gov identifiers: NCT02908308, NCT02011568) and duration of TTM. Second, controversy remains regarding application of TTM to patients with nonshockable rhythms and in-hospital cardiac arrest; a single-center trial is currently recruiting (NCT01994772). Third, the optimal method or device has not yet been defined. Finally, emerging techniques, such as extracorporeal life support, are increasingly being used during and after cardiac arrest for hemodynamic support, and the optimal approach to temperature management in these patients is unknown.

REVIEW OF KEY COMPONENTS OF POST–CARDIAC ARREST CARE
Coronary Angiography

An electrocardiogram (ECG) should be performed immediately after return of spontaneous circulation (ROSC) (**Fig. 1**). Immediate CAG is recommended for patients with ST-elevation myocardial infarction (STEMI).[18] Because the postarrest ECG is notoriously insensitive for ischemia in patients without STEMI, the ideal timing of CAG is less clear in such cases. A meta-analysis of 7 observational studies and 1 RCT found associations between urgent CAG and both improved survival and favorable neurologic outcome among postarrest patients without STEMI.[47] Urgent CAG was defined

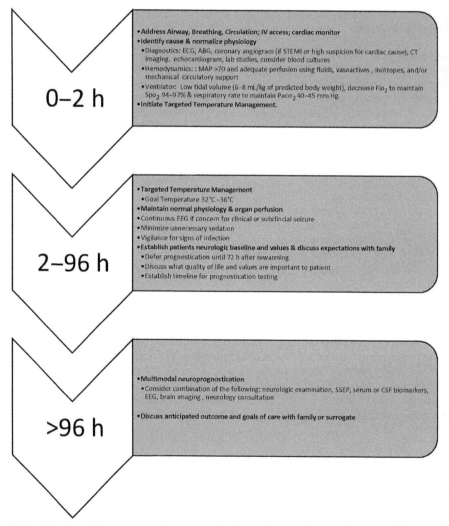

0–2 h
- Address Airway, Breathing, Circulation; IV access; cardiac monitor
- Identify cause & normalize physiology
  - Diagnostics: ECG, ABG, coronary angiogram (if STEMI or high suspicion for cardiac cause), CT imaging, echocardiogram, lab studies, consider blood cultures
  - Hemodynamics: : MAP >70 and adequate perfusion using fluids, vasoactives, inotropes, and/or mechanical circulatory support
  - Ventilator: Low tidal volume (6–8 mL/kg of predicted body weight), decrease Fio_2 to maintain Spo_2 94–97% & respiratory rate to maintain $Paco_2$ 40–45 mm Hg
- Initiate Targeted Temperature Management.

2–96 h
- Targeted Temperature Management
  - Goal Temperature 32°C–36°C
- Maintain normal physiology & organ perfusion
- Continuous EEG if concern for clinical or subclinical seizure
- Minimize unnecessary sedation
- Vigilance for signs of infection
- Establish patients neurologic baseline and values & discuss expectations with family
  - Defer prognostication until 72 h after rewarming
  - Discuss what quality of life and values are important to patient
  - Establish timeline for prognostication testing

>96 h
- Multimodal neuroprognostication
  - Consider combination of the following: neurologic examination, SSEP, serum or CSF biomarkers, EEG, brain imaging, neurology consultation
- Discuss anticipated outcome and goals of care with family or surrogate

Fig. 1. Timeline of key post–cardiac arrest critical care interventions. ABG, arterial-blood gas test; CSF, cerebrospinal fluid; CT, computed tomography; EEG, electroencephalogram; SSEP, somatosensory evoked potential. (*From* Walker AC, Johnson NJ. Critical care of the post-cardiac arrest patient. Cardiol Clin 2018;36(3):419–28. https://doi.org/10.1016/j.ccl.2018.03.009; with permission.)

differently across studies, ranging from immediate to within 12 hours of admission. There is potential for bias in these observational studies, because physicians may be less likely to perform CAG on patients with unfavorable cardiac arrest features. Although largely retrospective, data suggest benefit for early CAG in OHCA without STEMI and without other identifiable noncardiac cause of arrest.

Hemodynamic Optimization

After cardiac arrest, patients often have significant hemodynamic compromise, which is often the result of myocardial stunning and systemic inflammatory response leading to vasoplegia due to ischemic-reperfusion injury.[48] Careful hemodynamic monitoring is recommended. Many patients will likely need invasive monitoring with arterial and central venous catheters. It is reasonable to trend hemodynamic and perfusion parameters, including mean arterial pressure (MAP), lactate, measures of organ function, coagulation parameters, urine output, and central venous oxygen saturation. An echocardiogram may also be obtained to assess cardiac function and potentially to identify an underlying cause.

The optimal MAP goal after cardiac arrest remains unclear. Observational data suggest that higher MAP is associated with improved outcomes, regardless of vasopressor use, and hypotension has been shown to be an independent predictor of mortality.[49–51] Results are pending from NEUROPROTECT (NCT02541591), which compared goal-directed hemodynamic targets with MAP 65 mm Hg versus 85 to 100 mm Hg, looking specifically at brain injury as a primary outcome.

Oxygenation, Ventilation, and Lung Injury

Ventilator management, with attention to oxygenation, ventilation, and prevention of secondary lung injury, is an essential component of post–cardiac arrest care.[52] Multiple studies have demonstrated an association with poor clinical outcomes in postarrest patients with either hyperoxemia or hypoxemia.[53–63] Because of the potential risk posed by hyperoxemia, the authors suggest immediate titration of fraction of inspired oxygen to maintain SpO_2 94% to 97% as soon as feasible.

The authors also suggest maintenance of partial pressure of carbon dioxide ($PaCO_2$) in a high-normal range (40–50 mm Hg) when feasible. Numerous observational studies have examined the association between partial pressure of carbon dioxide ($PaCO_2$) and outcome, with variable findings.[56,57,64–72] Arterial hypocarbia has been associated with unfavorable neurologic outcome. Mild permissive hypercarbia is an experimental strategy that warrants further study, although it has been tested in several pilot trials.[73,74] Early blood gas analysis should be performed after ROSC, as prescribed minute ventilation and end-tidal CO_2 values correlate poorly with $PaCO_2$.[66,69,75]

Patients who suffer cardiac arrest are at increased risk of pulmonary infection and acute respiratory distress syndrome (ARDS).[76–79] The authors recommend vigilance for signs of infection and consideration of early sampling of the lower respiratory tract and empiric antimicrobial treatment.[80]

Several studies have demonstrated that nearly two-thirds of cardiac arrest patients meet criteria for ARDS.[79,81,82] Low-tidal volume ventilation applied to patients with ARDS led to a 9% absolute decrease in mortality, and observational data suggest that ventilation with lower-tidal volumes may be associated with fewer pulmonary complications in patients without ARDS.[83,84] A propensity-matched cohort study demonstrated an association between lower-tidal volumes (defined as ≤ 8 mL/kg of predicted body weight) and favorable neurologic status in 256 patients who suffered OHCA; this association was not found in a cohort of patients with in-hospital cardiac arrest.[85,86] A recent randomized trial, in which 25% of patients of the 961 patients experienced cardiac arrest, demonstrated no benefit to low-tidal volume ventilation among patients without ARDS.[87] Clinicians should treat postarrest patients who meet the definition of ARDS using a low-tidal volume strategy and consider such a strategy even in patients without ARDS.

Prognostication

Current guidelines recommend delaying prognostication until at least 72 hours after rewarming, or 72 hours after arrest in patients who did not undergo TTM.[18] Early clinical examination findings are notoriously unreliable for determining prognosis, particularly in the first 24 hours after cardiac arrest.[18] A multimodal approach to prognostication is recommended, including clinical examination, biomarkers, somatosensory-evoked potentials, electroencephalography, and imaging, with the goal of accurate prognostication and avoiding withdrawal of life-sustaining treatments in patients who may have a meaningful neurologic recovery.

SUMMARY

Patients who suffer cardiac arrest represent the extreme of critical illness. Meticulous attention to temperature management, identifying and reversing precipitating pathologic condition, mechanical ventilation, and hemodynamics are key components of postarrest care. Most patients who suffer OHCA should undergo TTM, although the ideal goal temperature and duration are not clear. Prognostication should generally not occur in the emergency department, and in most cases, should be deferred until 72 hours after rewarming.

REFERENCES

1. Callaway CW, Schmicker R, Kampmeyer M, et al. Receiving hospital characteristics associated with survival after out-of-hospital cardiac arrest. Resuscitation 2010;81(5):524–9.
2. Daya MR, Schmicker RH, Zive DM, et al, Resuscitation Outcomes Consortium Investigators. Out-of-hospital cardiac arrest survival improving over time: results from the Resuscitation Outcomes Consortium (ROC). Resuscitation 2015;91: 108–15.
3. Girotra S, Nallamothu BK, Spertus JA, et al. Trends in survival after in-hospital cardiac arrest. N Engl J Med 2012;367(20):1912–20.
4. Varon J, Acosta P. Therapeutic hypothermia: past, present, and future. Chest 2008;133(5):1267–74.
5. Benson DW, Williams GR, Spencer FC, et al. The use of hypothermia after cardiac arrest. Anesth Analg 1959;38:423–8.
6. Kochanek PM, Drabek T, Tisherman SA. Therapeutic hypothermia: the Safar vision. J Neurotrauma 2009;26(3):417–20.
7. Leonov Y, Sterz F, Safar P, et al. Mild cerebral hypothermia during and after cardiac arrest improves neurologic outcome in dogs. J Cereb Blood Flow Metab 1990;10(1):57–70.
8. Kuboyama K, Safar P, Radovsky A, et al. Delay in cooling negates the beneficial effect of mild resuscitative cerebral hypothermia after cardiac arrest in dogs: a prospective, randomized study. Crit Care Med 1993;21(9):1348–58 [see comment].
9. Holzer M. Targeted temperature management for comatose survivors of cardiac arrest. N Engl J Med 2010;363(13):1256–64.

10. Rosomoff HL, Holaday DA. Cerebral blood flow and cerebral oxygen consumption during hypothermia. Am J Physiol 1954;179(1):85–8.
11. Zeiner A, Holzer M, Sterz F, et al. Mild resuscitative hypothermia to improve neurological outcome after cardiac arrest. A clinical feasibility trial. Hypothermia After Cardiac Arrest (HACA) Study Group. Stroke 2000;31(1):86–94.
12. Hicks SD, DeFranco DB, Callaway CW. Hypothermia during reperfusion after asphyxial cardiac arrest improves functional recovery and selectively alters stress-induced protein expression. J Cereb Blood Flow Metab 2000;20(3):520–30.
13. Hicks SD, Parmele KT, DeFranco DB, et al. Hypothermia differentially increases extracellular signal-regulated kinase and stress-activated protein kinase/c-Jun terminal kinase activation in the hippocampus during reperfusion after asphyxial cardiac arrest. Neuroscience 2000;98(4):677–85.
14. D'Cruz BJ, Fertig KC, Filiano AJ, et al. Hypothermic reperfusion after cardiac arrest augments brain-derived neurotrophic factor activation. J Cereb Blood Flow Metab 2002;22(7):843–51.
15. Hachimi-Idrissi S, Van Hemelrijck A, Michotte A, et al. Postischemic mild hypothermia reduces neurotransmitter release and astroglial cell proliferation during reperfusion after asphyxial cardiac arrest in rats. Brain Res 2004;1019(1–2):217–25.
16. Webster CM, Kelly S, Koike MA, et al. Inflammation and NFkappaB activation is decreased by hypothermia following global cerebral ischemia. Neurobiol Dis 2009;33(2):301–12.
17. Maier CM, Sun GH, Cheng D, et al. Effects of mild hypothermia on superoxide anion production, superoxide dismutase expression, and activity following transient focal cerebral ischemia. Neurobiol Dis 2002;11(1):28–42.
18. Callaway CW, Donnino MW, Fink EL, et al. Part 8: post-cardiac arrest care: 2015 American Heart Association guidelines update for cardiopulmonary resuscitation and emergency cardiovascular care. Circulation 2015;132(18):S465–82.
19. Bernard SA, Gray TW, Buist MD, et al. Induced hypothermia after out-of-hospital cardiac arrest - treatment of comatose survivors of out-of-hospital cardiac arrest with therapeutic hypothermia. N Engl J Med 2002;346(8):557–63.
20. Hypothermia after Cardiac Arrest Study Group. Mild therapeutic hypothermia to improve the neurologic outcome after cardiac arrest. N Engl J Med 2002;346(8):549–56.
21. Nielsen N, Wetterslev J, Cronberg T, et al, TTM Trial Investigators. Targeted temperature management at 33°C versus 36°C after cardiac arrest. N Engl J Med 2013;369(23):2197–206.
22. Kim F, Nichol G, Maynard C, et al. Effect of prehospital induction of mild hypothermia on survival and neurological status among adults with cardiac arrest: a randomized clinical trial. JAMA 2014;311(1):45–52.
23. Bernard SA, Smith K, Finn J, et al. Induction of therapeutic hypothermia during out-of-hospital cardiac arrest using a rapid infusion of cold saline. Circulation 2016;134(11):797–805.
24. Moler FW, Silverstein FS, Holubkov R, et al. Therapeutic hypothermia after out-of-hospital cardiac arrest in children. N Engl J Med 2015;372(20):1898–908.
25. Moler FW, Silverstein FS, Holubkov R, et al. Therapeutic hypothermia after in-hospital cardiac arrest in children. N Engl J Med 2017;376(4):318–29.
26. Nielsen N, Friberg H, Gluud C, et al. Hypothermia after cardiac arrest should be further evaluated—a systematic review of randomised trials with meta-analysis and trial sequential analysis. Int J Cardiol 2011;151(3):333–41.

27. Mader TJ, Nathanson BH, Soares WE, et al. Comparative effectiveness of therapeutic hypothermia after out-of-hospital cardiac arrest: insight from a large data registry. Ther Hypothermia Temp Manag 2014;4(1):21–31.

28. Leary M, Grossestreuer AV, Iannacone S, et al. Pyrexia and neurologic outcomes after therapeutic hypothermia for cardiac arrest. Resuscitation 2013;84(8): 1056–61.

29. Bro-jeppesen J, Hassager C, Wanscher M, et al. Post-hypothermia fever is associated with increased mortality after out-of-hospital cardiac arrest. Resuscitation 2013;84(12):1734–40.

30. Zeiner A, Holzer M, Sterz F. Hyperthermia after cardiac arrest is associated with an unfavorable neurologic outcome. Arch Intern Med 2001;161:2007–12.

31. Bray JE, Stub D, Bloom JE, et al. Changing target temperature from 33C to 36C in the ICU management of out-of-hospital cardiac arrest: a before and after study. Resuscitation 2017;113:39–43.

32. Salter R, Bailey M, Bellomo R, et al. Changes in temperature management of cardiac arrest patients following publication of the target temperature management trial. Crit Care Med 2018;46(11):1722–30.

33. Kirkegaard H, Søreide E, de Haas I, et al. Targeted temperature management for 48 vs 24 hours and neurologic outcome after out-of-hospital cardiac arrest. JAMA 2017;318(4):341.

34. Callaway CW. Targeted temperature management after cardiac arrest. JAMA 2017;318(4):334.

35. Deye N, Cariou A, Girardie P, et al, Clinical and Economical Impact of Endovascular Cooling in the Management of Cardiac Arrest (ICEREA) Study Group. Endovascular versus external targeted temperature management for patients with out-of-hospital cardiac arrest: a randomized, controlled study. Circulation 2015; 132(3):182–93.

36. Andremont O, du Cheyron D, Terzi N, et al. Endovascular cooling versus standard femoral catheters and intravascular complications: a propensity-matched cohort study. Resuscitation 2018;124:1–6.

37. Dumas F, Grimaldi D, Zuber B, et al. Is hypothermia after cardiac arrest effective in both shockable and nonshockable patients?: insights from a large registry. Circulation 2011;123(8):877–86.

38. Frydland M, Kjaergaard J, Erlinge D, et al. Target temperature management of 33°C and 36°C in patients with out-of-hospital cardiac arrest with initial nonshockable rhythm - a TTM sub-study. Resuscitation 2015;89:142–8.

39. Doshi P, Patel K, Banuelos R, et al. Effect of therapeutic hypothermia on survival to hospital discharge in out-of-hospital cardiac arrest secondary to nonshockable rhythms. Acad Emerg Med 2016;23(1):15–20.

40. Don CW, Longstreth WT, Maynard C, et al. Active surface cooling protocol to induce mild therapeutic hypothermia after out-of-hospital cardiac arrest: a retrospective before-and-after comparison in a single hospital. Crit Care Med 2009; 37(12):3062–9.

41. Nichol G, Huszti E, Kim F, et al. Does induction of hypothermia improve outcomes after in-hospital cardiac arrest? Resuscitation 2013;84(5):620–5.

42. Kim YM, Yim HW, Jeong SH, et al. Does therapeutic hypothermia benefit adult cardiac arrest patients presenting with non-shockable initial rhythms?: a systematic review and meta-analysis of randomized and non-randomized studies. Resuscitation 2012;83(2):188–96.

43. Lundbye JB, Rai M, Ramu B, et al. Therapeutic hypothermia is associated with improved neurologic outcome and survival in cardiac arrest survivors of non-shockable rhythms. Resuscitation 2012;83(2):202–7.

44. Sung G, Bosson N, Kaji AH, et al. Therapeutic hypothermia after resuscitation from a non-shockable rhythm improves outcomes in a regionalized system of cardiac arrest care. Neurocrit Care 2016;24(1):90–6.

45. Testori C, Sterz F, Behringer W, et al. Mild therapeutic hypothermia is associated with favourable outcome in patients after cardiac arrest with non-shockable rhythms. Resuscitation 2011;82(9):1162–7.

46. Perman SM, Grossestreuer AV, Wiebe DJ, et al. The utility of therapeutic hypothermia for post-cardiac arrest syndrome patients with an initial nonshockable rhythm. Circulation 2015;132(22):2146–51.

47. Khan MS, Shah SMM, Mubashir A, et al. Early coronary angiography in patients resuscitated from out of hospital cardiac arrest without ST-segment elevation: a systematic review and meta-analysis. Resuscitation 2017;121:127–34.

48. Neumar RW, Nolan JP. Post-cardiac arrest syndrome. Circulation 2008;118: 2452–83.

49. Chiu YK, Lui CT, Tsui KL. Impact of hypotension after return of spontaneous circulation on survival in patients of out-of-hospital cardiac arrest. Am J Emerg Med 2018;36(1):79–83.

50. Kilgannon JH, Roberts BW, Reihl LR, et al. Early arterial hypotension is common in the post-cardiac arrest syndrome and associated with increased in-hospital mortality. Resuscitation 2008;79(3):410–6.

51. Trzeciak S, Jones AE, Kilgannon JH, et al. Significance of arterial hypotension after resuscitation from cardiac arrest. Crit Care Med 2009;37(11):2895–903 [quiz: 2904].

52. Johnson NJ, Carlbom DJ, Gaieski DF. Ventilator management and respiratory care after cardiac arrest: oxygenation, ventilation, infection, and injury. Chest 2018;153(6):1466–77.

53. Janz DR, Hollenbeck RD, Pollock JS, et al. Hyperoxia is associated with increased mortality in patients treated with mild therapeutic hypothermia after sudden cardiac arrest. Crit Care Med 2013;40(12):3135–9.

54. Ferguson LP, Durward A, Tibby SM. Relationship between arterial partial oxygen pressure after resuscitation from cardiac arrest and mortality in children. Circulation 2012;126:335–42.

55. Johnson NJ, Dodampahala K, Rosselot B, et al. The association between arterial oxygen tension and neurological outcome after cardiac arrest. Ther Hypothermia Temp Manag 2017;7(1):36–41.

56. Vaahersalo J, Bendel S, Reinikainen M, et al. Arterial blood gas tensions after resuscitation from out-of-hospital cardiac arrest: associations with long-term neurological outcome. Crit Care Med 2014;42(6):1–8.

57. Bennett KS, Clark AE, Meert KL, et al. Early oxygenation and ventilation measurements after pediatric cardiac arrest: lack of association with outcome. Crit Care Med 2013;41(6):1534–42.

58. Bellomo R, Bailey M, Eastwood GM, et al. Arterial hyperoxia and in-hospital mortality after resuscitation from cardiac arrest. Crit Care 2011;15(2):R90.

59. Balan IS, Fiskum G, Hazelton J, et al. Oximetry-guided reoxygenation improves neurological outcome after experimental cardiac arrest. Stroke 2006;37(12): 3008–13.

60. Vereczki V, Martin E, Rosenthal RE, et al. Normoxic resuscitation after cardiac arrest protects against hippocampal oxidative stress, metabolic dysfunction, and neuronal death. J Cereb Blood Flow Metab 2006;26(6):821–35.
61. Angelos MG, Yeh ST, Aune SE. Post-cardiac arrest hyperoxia and mitochondrial function. Resuscitation 2011;82:S48–51.
62. Kilgannon JH, Jones AE, Shapiro NI, et al. Association between arterial hyperoxia following resuscitation from cardiac arrest and in-hospital mortality. JAMA 2010; 303(21):2165–71.
63. Kilgannon JH, Jones AE, Parrillo JE, et al. Relationship between supranormal oxygen tension and outcome after resuscitation from cardiac arrest. Circulation 2011;123:2717–22.
64. Roberts BW, Kilgannon JH, Chansky ME, et al. Association between postresuscitation partial pressure of arterial carbon dioxide and neurological outcome in patients with post-cardiac arrest syndrome. Circulation 2013;127(21):2107–13.
65. Schneider AG, Eastwood GM, Bellomo R, et al. Arterial carbon dioxide tension and outcome in patients admitted to the intensive care unit after cardiac arrest. Resuscitation 2013;84(7):927–34.
66. Roberts BW, Kilgannon JH, Chansky ME, et al. Association between initial prescribed minute ventilation and post-resuscitation partial pressure of arterial carbon dioxide in patients with post-cardiac arrest syndrome. Ann Intensive Care 2014;4(9):1–9.
67. Lee BK, Jeung KW, Lee HY, et al. Association between mean arterial blood gas tension and outcome in cardiac arrest patients treated with therapeutic hypothermia. Am J Emerg Med 2014;32(1):55–60.
68. Helmerhorst HJF, Roos-Blom MJ, Van Westerloo DJ, et al. Associations of arterial carbon dioxide and arterial oxygen concentrations with hospital mortality after resuscitation from cardiac arrest. Crit Care 2015;19(1):348.
69. Tolins ML, Henning DJ, Gaieski DF, et al. Initial arterial carbon dioxide tension is associated with neurological outcome after resuscitation from cardiac arrest. Resuscitation 2017;114:53–8.
70. Wang C-H, Huang C-H, Chang W-T, et al. Association between early arterial blood gas tensions and neurological outcome in adult patients following in-hospital cardiac arrest. Resuscitation 2015;89:1–7.
71. McKenzie N, Williams TA, Tohira H, et al. A systematic review and meta-analysis of the association between arterial carbon dioxide tension and outcomes after cardiac arrest. Resuscitation 2017;111:116–26.
72. Kilgannon JH, Hunter BR, Puskarich MA, et al. Partial pressure of arterial carbon dioxide after resuscitation from cardiac arrest and neurological outcome: a prospective multi-center protocol-directed cohort study. Resuscitation 2019;135: 212–20.
73. Eastwood GM, Tanaka A, Bellomo R. Cerebral oxygenation in mechanically ventilated early cardiac arrest survivors: the impact of hypercapnia. Resuscitation 2016;102:11–6.
74. Eastwood GM, Schneider AG, Suzuki S, et al. Targeted therapeutic mild hypercapnia after cardiac arrest: a phase II multi-centre randomised controlled trial (the CCC trial). Resuscitation 2016;104:83–90.
75. Moon S-W, Lee S-W, Choi S-H, et al. Arterial minus end-tidal CO2 as a prognostic factor of hospital survival in patients resuscitated from cardiac arrest. Resuscitation 2007;72(2):219–25.

76. Mongardon N, Perbet S, Lemiale V, et al. Infectious complications in out-of-hospital cardiac arrest patients in the therapeutic hypothermia era. Crit Care Med 2011;39(6):1359–64.
77. Gaussorgues P, Gueugniaud PY, Vedrinne JM, et al. Bacteremia following cardiac arrest and cardiopulmonary resuscitation. Intensive Care Med 1988;14(5):575–7.
78. Tsai MS, Chiang WC, Lee CC, et al. Infections in the survivors of out-of-hospital cardiac arrest in the first 7 days. Intensive Care Med 2005;31(5):621–6.
79. Johnson NJ, Rea T, Caldwell E, et al. ARDS and low tidal volume ventilation after out-of-hospital cardiac arrest. Crit Care Med 2018;46:136.
80. Ribaric SF, Turel M, Knafelj R, et al. Prophylactic versus clinically-driven antibiotics in comatose survivors of out-of-hospital cardiac arrest-a randomized pilot study. Resuscitation 2017;111:103–9.
81. Elmer J, Wang B, Melhem S, et al. Exposure to high concentrations of inspired oxygen does not worsen lung injury after cardiac arrest. Crit Care 2015;19:105.
82. Sutherasan Y, Peñuelas O, Muriel A, et al. Management and outcome of mechanically ventilated patients after cardiac arrest. Crit Care 2015;19:215.
83. Acute Respiratory Distress Syndrome Network, Brower RG, Matthay MA, Morris A, et al. Ventilation with lower tidal volumes as compared with traditional tidal volumes for acute lung injury and the acute respiratory distress syndrome. N Engl J Med 2000;342:1301–8.
84. Serpa Neto A, Nagtzaam L, Schultz MJ. Ventilation with lower tidal volumes for critically ill patients without the acute respiratory distress syndrome: a systematic translational review and meta-analysis. Curr Opin Crit Care 2014;20(1):25–32.
85. Beitler JR, Ghafouri TB, Joshua J. Favorable neurocognitive outcome with low tidal volume ventilation after cardiac arrest. Am J Respir Crit Care Med 2017; 195(9):1198–206.
86. Moskowitz A, Grossestreuer AV, Berg KM, et al. The association between tidal volume and neurological outcome following in-hospital cardiac arrest. Resuscitation 2018;124:106–11.
87. Simonis FD, Serpa Neto A, Binnekade JM, et al. Effect of a low vs intermediate tidal volume strategy on ventilator-free days in intensive care unit patients without ARDS. JAMA 2018;320(18):1872.
88. Bernard SA, Gray TW, Buist MD, et al. Treatment of comatose survivors of out-of-hospital cardiac arrest with induced hypothermia. N Engl J Med 2002;346(8): 557–63.

Beyond Mean Arterial Pressure and Lactate: Perfusion End Points for Managing the Shocked Patient

Stephen D. Hallisey, MD[a],*, John C. Greenwood, MD[a,b]

KEYWORDS

- Resuscitation end points • Resuscitation • Sepsis • Cardiogenic shock
- Critical care • Lactate • Capillary refill time

KEY POINTS

- Resuscitation of shock should focus on the restoration of oxygen delivery at the level of the tissues.
- Macrocirculatory end points, such as blood pressure and cardiac output, should be the initial focus of resuscitation.
- Restoration of hemodynamic indices does not guarantee tissue-level oxygen delivery, and microcirculatory and metabolic end points should guide further interventions.
- Capillary refill time and urine output are important clinical markers of perfusion that should continue to have a role in resuscitation of the shocked patient.
- Resuscitation and resuscitation end points should be adjusted based on the best available evidence for specific shock phenotypes and patient response.

INTRODUCTION

Circulatory shock is a clinical state in which blood flow and oxygen supply is inadequate for cellular demands.[1] Generally, shock can be classified into 4 macrocirculatory types: distributive, cardiogenic, obstructive, and hypovolemic. Patients may present with clinical findings of inadequate perfusion, such as hypotension, delayed capillary refill time (CRT), decreased urine output (UOP), and altered mental status.

Funding Sources: Nothing to disclose.
Conflict of Interest: Nothing to disclose.
[a] Department of Emergency Medicine, University of Pennsylvania - Perelman School of Medicine, 3400 Spruce Street, Ground Ravdin, Philadelphia, PA 19104, USA; [b] Department of Anesthesiology and Critical Care, University of Pennsylvania - Perelman School of Medicine, 3400 Spruce Street, Ground Ravdin, Philadelphia, PA 19014, USA
* Corresponding author.
E-mail address: stephen.hallisey@uphs.upenn.edu

Emerg Med Clin N Am 37 (2019) 395–408
https://doi.org/10.1016/j.emc.2019.03.005
0733-8627/19/© 2019 Elsevier Inc. All rights reserved.

However, these mechanisms are not exclusive, and it is common for patients to present with multiple phenotypes of shock.

In general, the clinician's primary goal is to restore adequate tissue oxygen delivery (DO_2) to match the metabolic demand. There are multiple macrocirculatory, microcirculatory, and clinical targets that can be used as end points of resuscitation in the emergency department. Specific targets for each end point remain controversial.

MACROCIRCULATORY END POINTS
Blood Pressure

Restoration of the macrocirculation is one of the most important initial goals of a resuscitation. The mean arterial pressure (MAP) is calculated as (MAP) = [1/3] *([2*diastolic blood pressure] + [systolic blood pressure]) and is a common target to restore end-organ perfusion. Arterial hypotension is defined as a MAP of less than 70 mm Hg, but inadequate organ perfusion can occur with an abnormal systolic, diastolic, mean, or acute relative change in blood pressure.

Sepsis

Sepsis is defined by an acute infection that leads to a dysregulated host response and life-threatening organ dysfunction.[2] The hallmark of sepsis-induced circulatory dysfunction is diffuse vasodilation, often caused by bacterial endotoxin exposure. The Surviving Sepsis Campaign defines sepsis-related hypotension as a systolic blood pressure of less than 100 mm Hg, a 40-mm Hg decrease from baseline, or a MAP of less than 70 mm Hg.[2] An initial MAP target of 65 mm Hg is recommended, with personalized titration after stabilization.[3] The 65-mm Hg threshold is based on small set of prospective, retrospective, and observational studies that showed adequate perfusion measures and mortality benefit above this target.[4,5] Higher MAP targets have not been found to routinely improve outcomes. The SEPSISPAM trial, a randomized, controlled trial with 776 patients randomized to MAPs of 80 to 85 mm Hg versus 65 to 70 mm Hg showed no significant difference in mortality at 28 or 90 days.[6]

For most patients with sepsis and hemodynamic instability, current guidelines recommend an empiric crystalloid fluid bolus of 30 mL/kg to increase intravascular filling pressures and cardiac output, guided by dynamic measures of volume responsiveness if possible.[3] Vasopressor therapy should be promptly initiated for fluid-refractory hypotension.[7] Every 1-hour delay in vasopressor initiation during the first 6 hours of septic shock is associated with a 5.3% increase in mortality risk.[8] Norepinephrine initiation should not be delayed for central venous access, because evidence suggests that the complications of peripheral vasopressor use are rare if proximal, large-bore peripheral access is used.[9]

In some patients, early volume resuscitation and administration of norepinephrine may not provide enough support to achieve an adequate MAP. In these patients, fixed-dose vasopressin or a titrated epinephrine infusion is recommended as a second-line vasopressor.[10] The role of steroids remains controversial, yet most guidelines still recommend empiric hydrocortisone therapy in patients requiring escalating catecholamine doses. The recent APROCCHSS and ADRENAL trials add to the current literature base of the use of steroids in septic shock; however, both studies reported conflicting results on patient mortality.[11,12]

Hemorrhagic shock

Hemorrhagic shock is commonly the result of trauma, gastrointestinal bleeding, gynecologic pathology, and vascular pathology. Resuscitation should focus on hemorrhage control combined with rapid volume reexpansion. In trauma patients without brain injury, damage control resuscitation is a commonly implemented strategy that tolerates moderate hypotension to prevent excessive hemorrhage and the need for fluid administration until definitive hemorrhage control is provided.[13] Current European guidelines recommend a target systolic blood pressure of 80 to 90 mm Hg until major bleeding has been controlled.[14] Human trial data are conflicting; however, and there is no definitive evidence to support a specific MAP-based strategy.[15–17] Resuscitation of the patient in hemorrhagic shock should aim to restore perfusion, prevent hypothermia, and correct acidosis. Resuscitation with balanced blood product administration, either a 1:1:1 ratio or whole blood over intravenous crystalloid therapy, is preferred.[18]

Postcardiac arrest

Postcardiac arrest syndrome is often encountered after a return of spontaneous circulation from a cardiac arrest. The common features of postcardiac arrest syndrome include significant brain injury owing to impaired autoregulation of cerebral blood flow, myocardial dysfunction, and a systemic ischemia/reperfusion injury causing a vasoplegic shock state.[19] Meticulous attention must be made to avoid even a single episode of hypotension (MAP of <70 mm Hg), which can cause secondary brain injury and worse neurologic outcomes.[20,21] Owing to a lack of data from large, randomized trials, current guidelines recommend targeting a MAP of greater than 65 mm Hg and an systolic blood pressure of greater than 90 mm Hg.[22]

Unfortunately, a uniform MAP target fails to recognize one of the most critical pathophysiologic phenomena present in the postarrest patient. Cerebral autoregulation is a protective mechanism by which cerebral blood flow is maintained over a wide range of MAPs. After the return of spontaneous circulation, cerebral perfusion is heterogeneous and characterized by an early hyperemic phase, followed by a period of hypoperfusion, then restoration of normal blood flow.[23] Throughout each phase, cerebral blood flow autoregulation is often shifted, so that patients need a higher and tighter MAP target (80–100 mm Hg) to achieve adequate cerebral blood flow (**Fig. 1**). Targeting a higher MAP may result in improved neurologic outcomes.[24]

Neurogenic shock

Neurogenic shock occurs when the sympathetic chain is interrupted, leading to unopposed vagal tone and hypotension owing to vasodilation. Patients with acute spinal cord injury or ischemia without concomitant traumatic brain injury, may benefit from a higher MAP target (85–90 mm Hg) for the first 7 days to optimize spinal cord perfusion.[25–27] First-line therapy includes volume resuscitation to ensure euvolemia followed by vasopressors or inotropes if necessary. There is no currently accepted first-line vasoactive agent. Norepinephrine has alpha- and beta-adrenergic activity that may improve both hypotension and bradycardia (**Box 1**).

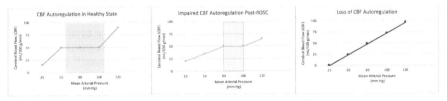

Fig. 1. Phases of cerebral blood flow autoregulation. ROSC, return of spontaneous circulation.

Box 1
Resuscitation end point pearls: Blood pressure

Measurement

- Arterial catheter
- Noninvasive cuff

Initial target

- MAP of >65 mm Hg followed by titration to individual patient response and etiology of shock

Pearls and pitfalls

- Vasopressor initiation should not be delayed for central venous access; delays in pressor initiation are associated with increased in mortality in patients with sepsis.
- Patient with postcardiac arrest syndrome, spinal cord injury, or chronic hypertension may benefit from a higher MAP target (80–100 mm Hg).
- Higher MAP has not been shown to improve outcomes in all comers with septic shock.

Cardiac Output

Cardiac output is defined as heart rate times the stroke volume and is an additional important macrocirculatory end point. Cardiac index, often interchanged with cardiac output, is defined as cardiac output/body surface area. Normal cardiac output is 4 to 8 L/min, and normal cardiac index is 2.5 to 4 L/min/m^2. Volume responsiveness is a concept closely intertwined with cardiac output/cardiac index, and is defined as an increase in stroke volume of 10% to 15% with a 500-mL fluid challenge. If the patient is on the ascending portion of their cardiac starling curve, a fluid challenge will increase the patient's stroke volume and consequently increase the cardiac output and blood pressure. Cardiac output/cardiac index is frequently impaired in all etiologies of shock and has been associated with poor outcomes in patients with cardiogenic shock, sepsis, and trauma.[28–33]

Cardiac output can be measured at the bedside through a variety of noninvasive and invasive methods. The pulmonary artery catheter was once commonly used in patients with shock, but routine use has been shown to lack a significant benefit and its use has fallen out of favor.[34] Noninvasive methods include bedside echocardiography, bioreactance measurement systems, and pulse wave contour analysis. Bedside echocardiography requires equipment available in most emergency departments, and cardiac output can be easily calculated by measurement of the left ventricular outflow tract velocity-time integral and aortic valve area. These measurements require minimal additional training, are simple to calculate, and can be easily repeated to assess response to resuscitation.

Despite the poor outcomes associated with decreased cardiac output, end points remain poorly defined and there is limited evidence to guide standard practice. Inotropic support should be considered in a shocked patient with a cardiac index of less than 2.2 L/min/m^2 who has adequate intravascular volume, poor systolic function, and evidence of poor perfusion. A supratherapeutic cardiac index target of greater than 2.5 L/min/m^2 has not been shown to improve clinical outcomes.[35] Dobutamine is often the inotrope of choice in most emergency department settings. Inodilator therapy (dobutamine, milrinone, etc) must be used with caution because these agents can cause significant hypotension. In the patient with cardiogenic shock, it is imperative to start vasopressor therapy first, to avoid developing further hypotension and subsequent coronary malperfusion. Dopamine should be avoided owing to its association with arrhythmias[36] (**Box 2**).

MICROCIRCULATORY AND METABOLIC END POINTS

The restoration of hemodynamic indices, although important, does not guarantee end-organ perfusion. For perfusion to be adequate, the DO_2 must meet the demands of cellular oxygen consumption.[1] In many shock states, there is a loss of hemodynamic coherence where an improvement in systemic hemodynamics occurs without similar improvement in microcirculatory blood flow and end-organ perfusion.[37]

New technologies such as incident dark field microscopy allow for the direct visualization and measurement of microcirculatory blood flow, but are not widely available or ready for clinical use. Instead, commonly available laboratory markers such as lactate, mixed venous oxygen saturation/central venous oxygen saturation (ScvO2), and central venous-to-arterial carbon dioxide gap (PvaCO2) can be used as surrogates for microcirculatory blood flow with some limitations.

Lactate

Lactate is an end product of glycolysis during anaerobic conditions and is produced by most tissues in the body. Serum lactate levels are quickly measured in the clinical setting with a venous or arterial blood gas. Normal levels in resting healthy individuals 0.5 to 2 mmol/L. Generally, there is a good correlation between arterial and venous lactate levels, although this may vary with extreme elevations.[38]

A number of mechanisms can lead to lactate production in the critically ill (**Fig. 2**). In circulatory shock, lactate generation is often the result of inadequate DO_2 relative to local tissue demand.[39] Despite the limitations of confounders, a high lactate level should prompt a rapid clinical evaluation. Elevated lactate has been consistently associated with increased mortality, regardless of hypotension, and is a powerful risk stratification tool.[40,41]

Lactate normalization within the first 6 hours of resuscitation is the strongest independent predictor of survival in patients with septic shock.[42] Cryptic shock, defined

---

Box 2
Resuscitation end point pearls: Cardiac output

Measurement

- Pulmonary artery catheter
- Echocardiography
- Bioreactance measurement systems
- Pulse wave contour analysis

Normal values

- Cardiac index: 2.5–4 L/min/m²
- Cardiac output: 4–8 L/min

Pearls and pitfalls

- Inaccurate aortic valve area measurements can significantly affect the accuracy of cardiac output calculation.
- Inotropes should be used cautiously, in patients whose shock is not from systolic heart failure.
- Supranormal cardiac index has not been shown to improve outcomes.

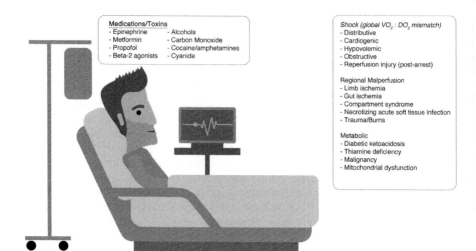

Medications/Toxins
- Epinephrine   - Alcohols
- Metformin   - Carbon Monoxide
- Propofol   - Cocaine/amphetamines
- Beta-2 agonists - Cyanide

Shock (global $VO_2 : DO_2$ mismatch)
- Distributive
- Cardiogenic
- Hypovolemic
- Obstructive
- Reperfusion injury (post-arrest)

Regional Malperfusion
- Limb ischemia
- Gut ischemia
- Compartment syndrome
- Necrotizing acute soft tissue infection
- Trauma/Burns

Metabolic
- Diabetic ketoacidosis
- Thiamine deficiency
- Malignancy
- Mitochondrial dysfunction

Fig. 2. Mechanisms leading to lactate production in the critically ill.

as a lactate level of more than 4 mmol/L without hypotension, is associated with a similar mortality rate as those in overt shock.[43] Prolonged lactate clearance is particularly worrisome and should also prompt further investigation.[44] Lactate levels remain the most important target for early resuscitation in patients with septic shock.[45,46]

A strong correlation between outcomes and hyperlactatemia have been found in other shock states as well. In hemorrhagic shock, blood loss leads to increased oxygen debt, anaerobic metabolism, and lactic acidosis. The stress response may also further increase patient lactate levels. A failure to normalize lactate is a strong predictor of mortality, and resuscitation should focus on early blood product administration to avoid coagulopathy and restore DO_2.[47,48]

In cardiogenic shock, impaired DO_2, increased adrenergic tone, and decreased clearance can all lead to increased lactate.[49] Lactic acidosis in cardiogenic shock is associated with mortality and its clearance with improved mortality.[50–52] Interventions should focus on identifying the etiology of cardiogenic shock (**Box 3**). Lactate levels may remain elevated after adequate resuscitation, particularly in the setting of epinephrine administration or significant hepatic congestion (**Box 4**).

Box 3
Common causes of cardiogenic shock in the emergency department

1. Acute coronary syndrome, coronary hypoperfusion

2. Valvular insufficiency

3. Acute on chronic left ventricular disease

4. Acute on chronic right ventricular disease

5. Ventricular outflow obstruction (aortic stenosis, systolic anterior motion of the mitral valve, etc)

6. Arrhythmias

7. Myocarditis

> **Box 4**
> **Resuscitation end point pearls: Lactate**
>
> *Measurement*
> - Arterial or venous blood gas
>
> *Normal levels*
> - 0.5 – 2 mmol/L
>
> *Pearls and pitfalls*
> - Alternate etiologies of lactate elevation such as medications, adrenergic surge, and delayed clearance can cause hyperlactatemia.
> - Lactate elevation without hypotension (cryptic shock) is associated with similar mortality outcomes as in those patients with overt hypotension.

Mixed and Central Venous Oxygen Saturation

Achieving adequate tissue oxygenation is essential to prevent cell injury, oxygen debt, organ dysfunction, and death. Mixed venous oxygen saturation and $ScvO_2$ are global measures of tissue oxygen extraction and DO_2/oxygen consumption balance.[53] $ScvO_2$ can be easily obtained using a venous blood gas sample from the distal port of a central venous catheter where the tip lies ideally within the junction of the superior vena cava and right atrium. Given the anatomic importance of $ScvO_2$ sampling, values drawn from femoral central venous catheters are useless.[54]

The normal range for $ScvO_2$ is 65% to 75%. Unfortunately, normal and supranormal values do not guarantee adequate tissue oxygenation.[55,56] Many conditions can influence the DO_2/oxygen consumption balance (**Table 1**).

Sepsis

Based on the work of Rivers and colleagues,[57] an $ScvO_2$ target of greater than 70% would suggest adequate DO_2 in patients with septic shock. Interpreting $ScvO_2$ values can be challenging in hyperdynamic states like sepsis. Despite increased cardiac output and a decrease in systemic vascular resistance, abnormal mitochondrial respiration and microcirculatory blood flow lead to decreased oxygen consumption.[58] Thus, a normal $ScvO_2$ may not reflect the degree of tissue dysoxia present. $ScvO_2$ levels of greater than 90% should raise concern for peripheral arteriovenous shunting and are particularly ominous.[55]

Table 1
Clinical factors that impact central and mixed venous O_2 saturation

Factors that Increase Vo_2	Factors that Decrease Vo_2
Trauma, burns	Sedation/analgesia
Sepsis	Paralysis
Inflammation	Shock
Hyperthyroidism	Mechanical ventilation
Pyrexia	Hypothermia/cooling
Shivering	Antipyretics
Agitation/anxiety/pain	Hypovolemia
Adrenergic drugs	Mitochondrial dysfunction, toxins

Cardiogenic shock

Patients in cardiogenic shock are unable to increase cardiac output to meet circulatory demands. As the circulating blood volume remains in the periphery for prolonged periods of time, tissue oxygen extraction increases, leading to low venous oxygen saturations. Therapy should target increasing cardiac output with a goal $ScvO_2$ of greater than 60%. A low $ScvO_2$ is often present in both overt and occult cardiogenic shock.[59] An $ScvO_2$ of less than 60% has been associated with major adverse cardiac events in patients with acute decompensated heart failure requiring inotropes[60] (**Box 5**).

Central Venous-Arterial Carbon Dioxide Gap

Recognizing the limitations of $ScvO_2$ in detecting adequate end-organ perfusion, the central venous-to-arterial carbon dioxide gap ($PvaCO_2$) may provide valuable clinical information to determine the adequacy of both perfusion and cardiac output. Carbon dioxide is much more soluble in the blood and less easily manipulated than O_2 concentration.[61] The $PvaCO_2$ is calculated by subtracting the arterial blood gas' P_{CO_2} from the P_{CO_2} obtained from a central venous blood gas. In sepsis, a $PvaCO_2$ of less than 6 mm Hg is associated with lactate normalization, a higher cardiac index, and improved tissue perfusion.[61–63] Patients with septic shock and a $PvaCO_2$ gap of greater than 6 mm Hg likely need additional fluid resuscitation or inotropic therapy[64] (**Box 6**).

CLINICAL MARKERS OF PERFUSION

Beyond hemodynamic and laboratory resuscitation parameters, frequent clinical assessments are critical to determine resuscitation progress. UOP and CRT both provide feedback regarding end-organ perfusion and are an easy, cost-effective method to assess response to interventions. The clinician must remain aware of limitations of these end points and potential pitfalls.

Urine Output

Acute kidney injury is a rapid decrease in the glomerular filtration rate, leading to an increase in serum creatinine or decrease in UOP.[65] A UOP of less than 0.5 mL/kg/h for 6 hours is an early sign of poor renal perfusion owing to hypovolemia and other shock states. Early interventions should focus on intravascular volume optimization and the avoidance of hypotension. Decreased UOP in hemorrhagic shock is a marker of inadequate volume resuscitation and may be one of the earliest signs

---

Box 5
Resuscitation end point pearls: Central venous oxygen saturation

Measurement

- Obtain from the central venous catheter at the junction of the superior vena cava and right atrium.

Normal values

- 60% to 70%

Pearls and pitfalls

- Normal $ScvO_2$ may not reflect tissue dysoxia in sepsis.
- $ScvO_2$ levels of >90% should raise concern for peripheral arteriovenous shunting.

Box 6
Resuscitation end point pearls: central venous-to-arterial carbon dioxide gap (PvaCO$_2$)

Measurement

- Subtract Pco$_2$ obtained from arterial blood gas from Pco$_2$ from central venous blood gas.

Normal values

- <6 mm Hg

Pearls and pitfalls

- Patients with septic shock and a PvaCO$_2$ gap of >6 mm Hg likely need ongoing resuscitation.

---

of shock.[66–68] In patients with sepsis, multiple mechanisms cause impaired renal perfusion, which may impair the clinician's ability to rely on UOP as a clinical monitor of resuscitation.[69] Attempts at increasing renal blood flow to decrease acute kidney injury with dopamine have not been effective and should be avoided.[70]

A low UOP in cardiogenic shock can also be challenging to differentiate. An acute reduction in cardiac output can lead to an impaired afferent blood flow, whereas an acute decompensated heart failure patient may have a significant efferent pathology (excessive central venous pressure). Even modest increases in central venous pressure can have a profound impact on renal perfusion and the glomerular filtration rate.[71] In patients with cardiogenic shock who are volume overloaded, loop diuretics may be appropriate, but should be used with caution in the acute resuscitative phase (**Box 7**).

Capillary Refill Time

Assessment of CRT is a simple examination finding that can be used to assess microvascular perfusion in peripheral vascular beds. Patients in shock will shunt blood flow to their vital organs preferentially, away from the skin. A normal CRT is less than 3.5 seconds, and values greater than 5 seconds despite hemodynamic optimization suggest a significant risk of progressive organ failure.[72] Other factors can affect CRT, such as skin temperature and vasodilatory medications like nitroglycerin. CRT does not require any technology, making it especially useful in resource-poor settings. Further, studies of interrater reliability have shown 80% concordance at the finger, and 95% at the knee cap.[73]

Box 7
Resuscitation end point pearls: UOP

Measurement

- Consider Foley catheter placement for accurate measurement.

Normal values

- >0.5 mL/kg/h

Pearls and pitfalls

- Dopamine has not been shown to decrease the incidence of acute kidney injury.
- UOP may be a good marker of renal malperfusion in early hypovolemic states, but is a confounded end point in hyperinflammatory states like sepsis.

Box 8
Resuscitation end point pearls: CRT

Measurement
- Fingertip
- Knee cap

Normal values
- <3.5 seconds

Pitfalls
- Skin temperature and vasodilatory medications can affect CRT.
- Failure to normalize at 6 hours is predictive of worsening shock.
- >5 s despite resuscitation suggests risk of organ failure

In patients with septic shock, recent literature suggests that CRT may be a useful tool to assess global perfusion during resuscitation.[74,75] Normalization of CRT at 6 hours is associated with successful resuscitation, whereas failure to normalize may be predictive of worsening shock.[72,76] The upcoming ANDROMEDA-SHOCK trial comparing peripheral perfusion versus lactate-guided resuscitation will provide valuable guidance on the value of CRT in the management of patients with septic shock[77] (**Box 8**).

SUMMARY

Patients in shock frequently present to the emergency department and the emergency physician must be facile in rapid diagnosis and aggressive resuscitation using well-defined end points. Resuscitation efforts should focus on rapid correction of macrocirculatory derangements such as MAP and cardiac output with specific goals dependent on the type of shock and individual patient response. After the correction of macrocirculatory derangements, microcirculatory end points such as peripheral lactate, mixed venous oxygen saturation or $ScvO_2$, and $PvaCO_2$ should guide resuscitation optimization. Finally, clinical end points such as CRT and UOP still provide valuable information at the bedside and should continue to be incorporated into a comprehensive resuscitation plan for monitoring and to assist in guiding further intervention.

REFERENCES

1. Vincent J-L, Ince C, Bakker J. Clinical review: circulatory shock–an update: a tribute to Professor Max Harry Weil. Crit Care 2012;16(6):239.
2. Singer M, Deutschman CS, Seymour CW, et al. The third international consensus definitions for sepsis and septic shock (Sepsis-3). JAMA 2016;315(8):801.
3. Dellinger RP, Levy MM, Rhodes A, et al. Surviving Sepsis Campaign: international guidelines for management of severe sepsis and septic shock. Crit Care Med 2013;41(2):580–637.
4. Varpula M, Tallgren M, Saukkonen K, et al. Hemodynamic variables related to outcome in septic shock. Intensive Care Med 2005;31(8):1066–71.
5. LeDoux D, Astiz ME, Carpati CM, et al. Effects of perfusion pressure on tissue perfusion in septic shock. Crit Care Med 2000;28(8):2729–32.

6. Asfar P, Meziani F, Hamel J-F, et al. High versus low blood-pressure target in patients with septic shock. N Engl J Med 2014;370(17):1583–93.
7. De Backer D, Aldecoa C, Njimi H, et al. Dopamine versus norepinephrine in the treatment of septic shock: a meta-analysis*. Crit Care Med 2012;40(3): 725–30.
8. Bai X, Yu W, Ji W, et al. Early versus delayed administration of norepinephrine in patients with septic shock. Crit Care 2014;18(5):532.
9. Cardenas-Garcia J, Schaub KF, Belchikov YG, et al. Safety of peripheral intravenous administration of vasoactive medication: peripheral administration of VM. J Hosp Med 2015;10(9):581–5.
10. Russell JA, Walley KR, Singer J, et al. Vasopressin versus norepinephrine infusion in patients with septic shock. N Engl J Med 2008;358(9):877–87.
11. Venkatesh B, Finfer S, Cohen J, et al. Adjunctive glucocorticoid therapy in patients with septic shock. N Engl J Med 2018;378(9):797–808.
12. Annane D, Renault A, Brun-Buisson C, et al. Hydrocortisone plus Fludrocortisone for adults with septic shock. N Engl J Med 2018;378(9):809–18.
13. Mizobata Y. Damage control resuscitation: a practical approach for severely hemorrhagic patients and its effects on trauma surgery. J Intensive Care 2017;5(1):4.
14. Rossaint R, Bouillon B, Cerny V, et al. The European guideline on management of major bleeding and coagulopathy following trauma: fourth edition. Crit Care 2016;20(1):100.
15. Dutton RP, Mackenzie CF, Scalea TM. Hypotensive resuscitation during active hemorrhage: impact on in-hospital mortality. J Trauma 2002;52(6):1141–6.
16. Bickell WH, Wall MJ, Pepe PE, et al. Immediate versus delayed fluid resuscitation for hypotensive patients with penetrating torso injuries. N Engl J Med 1994; 331(17):1105–9.
17. Hasler RM, Nuesch E, Jüni P, et al. Systolic blood pressure below 110mmHg is associated with increased mortality in blunt major trauma patients: multicentre cohort study. Resuscitation 2011;82(9):1202–7.
18. Holcomb JB, Tilley BC, Baraniuk S, et al. Transfusion of plasma, platelets, and red blood cells in a 1:1:1 vs a 1:1:2 ratio and mortality in patients with severe trauma: the PROPPR randomized clinical trial. JAMA 2015;313(5):471.
19. Neumar RW, Nolan JP, Adrie C, et al. Post-cardiac arrest syndrome: epidemiology, pathophysiology, treatment, and prognostication. A consensus statement from the International Liaison Committee on Resuscitation (American Heart Association, Australian and New Zealand Council on Resuscitation, European Resuscitation Council, Heart and Stroke Foundation of Canada, InterAmerican Heart Foundation, Resuscitation Council of Asia, and the Resuscitation Council of Southern Africa); the American Heart Association Emergency Cardiovascular Care Committee; the Council on Cardiovascular Surgery and Anesthesia; the Council on Cardiopulmonary, Perioperative, and Critical Care; the Council on Clinical Cardiology; and the Stroke Council. Circulation 2008;118(23):2452–83.
20. Laurikkala J, Wilkman E, Pettilä V, et al. Mean arterial pressure and vasopressor load after out-of-hospital cardiac arrest: associations with one-year neurologic outcome. Resuscitation 2016;105:116–22.
21. Müllner M, Sterz F, Binder M, et al. Arterial blood pressure after human cardiac arrest and neurological recovery. Stroke 1996;27(1):59–62.
22. Trzeciak S, Jones AE, Kilgannon JH, et al. Significance of arterial hypotension after resuscitation from cardiac arrest. Crit Care Med 2009;37(11):2895–903 [quiz: 2904].

23. Hossmann KA. Reperfusion of the brain after global ischemia: hemodynamic disturbances. Shock 1997;8(2):95–101 [discussion: 102–3].

24. Roberts BW, Kilgannon JH, Hunter BR, et al. Association between elevated mean arterial blood pressure and neurologic outcome after resuscitation from cardiac arrest: results from a multicenter prospective cohort study. Crit Care Med 2019; 47(1):93–100.

25. Walters BC, Hadley MN, Hurlbert RJ, et al. Guidelines for the management of acute cervical spine and spinal cord injuries: 2013 update. Neurosurgery 2013; 60:82–91.

26. Hawryluk G, Whetstone W, Saigal R, et al. Mean arterial blood pressure correlates with neurological recovery after human spinal cord injury: analysis of high frequency physiologic data. J Neurotrauma 2015;32(24):1958–67.

27. Levi L, Wolf A, Belzberg H. Hemodynamic parameters in patients with acute cervical cord trauma: description, intervention, and prediction of outcome. Neurosurgery 1993;33(6):1007–16 [discussion: 1016–17].

28. Parker MM, Shelhamer JH, Natanson C, et al. Serial cardiovascular variables in survivors and nonsurvivors of human septic shock: heart rate as an early predictor of prognosis. Crit Care Med 1987;15(10):923–9.

29. Hasdai D, Holmes DR, Califf RM, et al. Cardiogenic shock complicating acute myocardial infarction: predictors of death. Am Heart J 1999;138(1):21–31.

30. Torgersen C, Schmittinger CA, Wagner S, et al. Hemodynamic variables and mortality in cardiogenic shock: a retrospective cohort study. Crit Care 2009;13(5): R157.

31. Bishop MH, Shoemaker WC, Appel PL, et al. Prospective, randomized trial of survivor values of cardiac index, oxygen delivery, and oxygen consumption as resuscitation endpoints in severe trauma. J Trauma 1995;38(5):780–7.

32. Rady MY, Edwards JD, Nightingale P. Early cardiorespiratory findings after severe blunt thoracic trauma and their relation to outcome. Br J Surg 1992;79(1): 65–8.

33. Fincke R, Hochman JS, Lowe AM, et al. Cardiac power is the strongest hemodynamic correlate of mortality in cardiogenic shock: a report from the SHOCK trial registry. J Am Coll Cardiol 2004;44(2):340–8.

34. Harvey S, Harrison DA, Singer M, et al. Assessment of the clinical effectiveness of pulmonary artery catheters in management of patients in intensive care (PAC-Man): a randomised controlled trial. Lancet 2005;366(9484):472–7.

35. Hayes MA, Timmins AC, Yau E, et al. Elevation of systemic oxygen delivery in the treatment of critically ill patients. N Engl J Med 1994;330(24):1717–22.

36. De Backer D, Biston P, Devriendt J, et al. Comparison of dopamine and norepinephrine in the treatment of shock. N Engl J Med 2010;362(9):779–89.

37. Ince C. Hemodynamic coherence and the rationale for monitoring the microcirculation. Crit Care 2015;19(Suppl 3):S8.

38. Middleton P, Kelly A-M, Brown J, et al. Agreement between arterial and central venous values for pH, bicarbonate, base excess, and lactate. Emerg Med J 2006;23(8):622–4.

39. Friedman G, De Backer D, Shahla M, et al. Oxygen supply dependency can characterize septic shock. Intensive Care Med 1998;24(2):118–23.

40. Shapiro NI, Howell MD, Talmor D, et al. Serum lactate as a predictor of mortality in emergency department patients with infection. Ann Emerg Med 2005;45(5): 524–8.

41. Mikkelsen ME, Miltiades AN, Gaieski DF, et al. Serum lactate is associated with mortality in severe sepsis independent of organ failure and shock. Crit Care Med 2009;37(5):1670–7.
42. Puskarich MA, Trzeciak S, Shapiro NI, et al. Whole blood lactate kinetics in patients undergoing quantitative resuscitation for severe sepsis and septic shock. Chest 2013;143(6):1548–53.
43. Puskarich MA, Trzeciak S, Shapiro NI, et al. Outcomes of patients undergoing early sepsis resuscitation for cryptic shock compared with overt shock. Resuscitation 2011;82(10):1289–93.
44. McNelis J, Marini CP, Jurkiewicz A, et al. Prolonged lactate clearance is associated with increased mortality in the surgical intensive care unit. Am J Surg 2001; 182(5):481–5.
45. Jansen TC, van Bommel J, Schoonderbeek FJ, et al. Early lactate-guided therapy in intensive care unit patients: a multicenter, open-label, randomized controlled trial. Am J Respir Crit Care Med 2010;182(6):752–61.
46. Hernandez G, Boerma EC, Dubin A, et al. Severe abnormalities in microvascular perfused vessel density are associated to organ dysfunctions and mortality and can be predicted by hyperlactatemia and norepinephrine requirements in septic shock patients. J Crit Care 2013;28(4):538.e9-14.
47. Dezman ZDW, Comer AC, Smith GS, et al. Failure to clear elevated lactate predicts 24-hour mortality in trauma patients. J Trauma Acute Care Surg 2015; 79(4):580–5.
48. Abramson D, Scalea TM, Hitchcock R, et al. Lactate clearance and survival following injury. J Trauma 1993;35(4):584–8 [discussion: 588–9].
49. Lazzeri C, Valente S, Chiostri M, et al. Clinical significance of Lactate in acute cardiac patients. World J Cardiol 2015;7(8):483.
50. Valente S, Lazzeri C, Vecchio S, et al. Predictors of in-hospital mortality after percutaneous coronary intervention for cardiogenic shock. Int J Cardiol 2007; 114(2):176–82.
51. Attanà P, Lazzeri C, Chiostri M, et al. Strong-ion gap approach in patients with cardiogenic shock following ST-elevation myocardial infarction. Acute Card Care 2013;15(3):58–62.
52. Attaná P, Lazzeri C, Chiostri M, et al. Lactate clearance in cardiogenic shock following ST elevation myocardial infarction: a pilot study. Acute Card Care 2012;14(1):20–6.
53. Kandel G. Mixed venous oxygen saturation. Its role in the assessment of the critically ill patient. Arch Intern Med 1983;143(7):1400–2.
54. Davison DL, Chawla LS, Selassie L, et al. Femoral-based central venous oxygen saturation is not a reliable substitute for subclavian/internal jugular-based central venous oxygen saturation in patients who are critically ill. Chest 2010;138(1): 76–83.
55. Pope JV, Jones AE, Gaieski DF, et al. Multicenter study of central venous oxygen saturation (ScvO2) as a predictor of mortality in patients with sepsis. Ann Emerg Med 2010;55(1):40–6.e1.
56. Perz S, Uhlig T, Kohl M, et al. Low and "supranormal" central venous oxygen saturation and markers of tissue hypoxia in cardiac surgery patients: a prospective observational study. Intensive Care Med 2011;37(1):52–9.
57. Rivers E, Nguyen B, Havstad S, et al. Early goal-directed therapy in the treatment of severe sepsis and septic shock. N Engl J Med 2001;345(19):1368–77.
58. Walley KR. Heterogeneity of oxygen delivery impairs oxygen extraction by peripheral tissues: theory. J Appl Physiol 1996;81(2):885–94.

59. Ander DS, Jaggi M, Rivers E, et al. Undetected cardiogenic shock in patients with congestive heart failure presenting to the emergency department. Am J Cardiol 1998;82(7):888–91.
60. Gallet R, Lellouche N, Mitchell-Heggs L, et al. Prognosis value of central venous oxygen saturation in acute decompensated heart failure. Arch Cardiovasc Dis 2012;105(1):5–12.
61. Vallée F, Vallet B, Mathe O, et al. Central venous-to-arterial carbon dioxide difference: an additional target for goal-directed therapy in septic shock? Intensive Care Med 2008;34(12):2218–25.
62. Bakker J, Vincent J-L, Gris P, et al. Veno-arterial carbon dioxide gradient in human septic shock. Chest 1992;101(2):509–15.
63. Ospina-Tascón GA, Umaña M, Bermúdez WF, et al. Can venous-to-arterial carbon dioxide differences reflect microcirculatory alterations in patients with septic shock? Intensive Care Med 2016;42(2):211–21.
64. Zhang H, Vincent J-L. Arteriovenous differences in P_{CO_2} and pH are good indicators of critical hypoperfusion. Am Rev Respir Dis 1993;148(4_pt_1):867–71.
65. Summary of recommendation statements. Kidney Int Suppl (2011) 2012;2(1): 8–12.
66. American College of Surgeons, Committee on Trauma. Advanced trauma life support: student course manual. Chicago: American College of Surgeons; 2018.
67. Gutierrez G, Reines HD, Wulf-Gutierrez ME. Clinical review: hemorrhagic shock. Crit Care 2004;8(5):373–81.
68. Porter JM, Ivatury RR. In search of the optimal end points of resuscitation in trauma patients: a review. J Trauma 1998;44(5):908–14.
69. Uchino S. Acute renal failure in critically ill patients: a multinational, multicenter study. JAMA 2005;294(7):813.
70. Bellomo R, Chapman M, Finfer S, et al. Low-dose dopamine in patients with early renal dysfunction: a placebo-controlled randomised trial. Australian and New Zealand Intensive Care Society (ANZICS) Clinical Trials Group. Lancet 2000; 356(9248):2139–43.
71. Damman K, van Deursen VM, Navis G, et al. Increased central venous pressure is associated with impaired renal function and mortality in a broad spectrum of patients with cardiovascular disease. J Am Coll Cardiol 2009;53(7):582–8.
72. Lima A, Jansen TC, van Bommel J, et al. The prognostic value of the subjective assessment of peripheral perfusion in critically ill patients. Crit Care Med 2009; 37(3):934–8.
73. Ait-Oufella H, Bige N, Boelle PY, et al. Capillary refill time exploration during septic shock. Intensive Care Med 2014;40(7):958–64.
74. van Genderen ME, Engels N, van der Valk RJP, et al. Early peripheral perfusion-guided fluid therapy in patients with septic shock. Am J Respir Crit Care Med 2015;191(4):477–80.
75. Ait-Oufella H, Lemoinne S, Boelle PY, et al. Mottling score predicts survival in septic shock. Intensive Care Med 2011;37(5):801–7.
76. Hernandez G, Pedreros C, Veas E, et al. Evolution of peripheral vs metabolic perfusion parameters during septic shock resuscitation. A clinical-physiologic study. J Crit Care 2012;27(3):283–8.
77. Hernández G, Cavalcanti AB, Ospina-Tascón G, et al, The ANDROMEDA-SHOCK Study Investigators. Early goal-directed therapy using a physiological holistic view: the ANDROMEDA-SHOCK—a randomized controlled trial. Ann Intensive Care 2018;8(1):52.

Resuscitative Cardiopulmonary Ultrasound and Transesophageal Echocardiography in the Emergency Department

Felipe Teran, MD, MSCE

KEYWORDS

- Ultrasound • Echocardiography • Point-of-care ultrasound • Resuscitation • Shock
- Critical care • Transesophageal echocardiography

KEY POINTS

- The use of point-of-care ultrasound is the standard of care in the evaluation of patients with shock, hypotension, or acute hemodynamic decompensation in the emergency department.
- The scope of focused cardiopulmonary ultrasound has expanded to include some advanced techniques that tailor therapeutic interventions to a patient's underlying physiology.
- Qualitative and quantitative evaluation of left and right ventricular function, identification of pericardial effusion and tamponade, evaluation of preload and fluid responsiveness, and hemodynamic monitoring are key ultrasound applications during the resuscitation phase of critical care.

INTRODUCTION

The scope of focused cardiopulmonary ultrasound (FOCUS), resuscitative ultrasound, and transesophageal echocardiography (TEE) has evolved rapidly over the past 2 decades in critical care and emergency environments. The concept of "resuscitative ultrasound" is used to describe specific applications of FOCUS for diagnostic assessment, monitoring, therapy titration, and procedural guidance in critically ill patients. There are several distinctive qualities of resuscitative ultrasound, compared with comprehensive ultrasound or echocardiography:

1. Aims to answer specific clinical questions
2. Can be performed multiple times during the patient's clinical course

Division of Emergency Ultrasound and Center for Resuscitation Science, Department of Emergency Medicine, Hospital of the University of Pennsylvania, 3400 Spruce Street, Ground Ravdin, Philadelphia, PA 19104, USA
E-mail addresses: felipeteran@gmail.com; felipe.teran-merino@uphs.upenn.edu

Emerg Med Clin N Am 37 (2019) 409–430
https://doi.org/10.1016/j.emc.2019.03.003   emed.theclinics.com

3. Is a scalable diagnostic tool that can be tailored to fit both the patient's complexity (ie, number or sophistication of questions asked) and the experience of the clinician.

The increase of emergency ultrasound (EUS) and emergency medicine–critical care trained physicians has contributed to the expansion of EUS, beyond the traditional core applications.[1] This review provides a description of the fundamentals and main clinical applications of resuscitative ultrasound that can be helpful in the emergency department (ED) setting.

RESUSCITATIVE CARDIOPULMONARY ULTRASOUND

Resuscitative cardiopulmonary ultrasound can allow the emergency physician (EP) to characterize the predominant physiology of a patient with shock, establish the cause of acute hypoxemia, and assess the effect of therapeutic interventions, such as administration of vasoactive drugs or intravenous fluids.

Although a core set of 5 parasternal and subcostal views is often described in FOCUS, with some additional knowledge, practice, and views, the care provider can improve his or her clinical decision making. A description of the probe location, visualized anatomy, and clinical applications of 9 resuscitative cardiac ultrasound views is provided in **Table 1**.

Evaluation of Left Ventricular Systolic Function

The evaluation of left ventricular (LV) systolic function and ejection fraction (LVEF), is the most common echocardiographic evaluation performed in the ED. Differentiating between a normal and depressed LVEF has a number of clinical implications, including the risk of cardiogenic shock, cardiac versus pulmonary cause of dyspnea, and the need for resuscitative fluids or vasoactive drugs. Quantitative methods, traditionally used in comprehensive echocardiography,[2] are technically challenging, time-consuming, and not suitable for use at the point of care.

Simplified qualitative and semiquantitative methods to assess LV systolic function have been described and validated in the ED setting. These include visual estimation of LVEF[3] and E-point septal separation (EPSS).[4] Both of these methods have good correlation with LVEF using volumetric methods. When used by ED physicians in real time, these methods have shown to accurately categorize patients among normal, reduced, and severely reduced LVEF.[3,5–7]

The visual assessment of LV systolic function can be performed using 3 elements: (1) systolic excursion of the endocardium toward the center of the LV (*endocardial excursion*), (2) systolic thickening of the myocardium (*myocardial thickening*), and (3) excursion of the anterior leaflet of the mitral valve (MV) toward the septum during early diastole (*EPSS*).

The first 2 elements are the foundation of the assessment of ventricular contractility. The third, EPSS, is a semiquantitative parameter that represents the closest distance between the anterior leaflet of the MV and the septum obtained by M-mode. Multiple cutoff values have been used to accurately identify patients with reduced LVEF.[4,8,9] An EPSS >7 mm has been found to have 100% sensitivity for identifying patients with an LVEF less than 30%.[4] The accuracy of visual estimation of LVEF appears to be more dependent on experience compared with EPSS (**Fig. 1**).

Clinicians must be aware of the limitations when estimating LV systolic function. Mitral stenosis and aortic regurgitation will both affect the distance between the MV and septum during diastole.[8,10] If present, EPSS should not be used to estimate LVEF. LVEF estimation also may not be useful in patients with LV hypertrophy,

Table 1
Description of the probe location, visualized anatomy and clinical applications of 9 resuscitative cardiac ultrasound views

View	Probe Position	Ultrasound Anatomy	Clinical Applications
Parasternal long axis (PLAX)			LV systolic function E-point septal separation RV dilation Chamber dimensions Pericardial effusion
Parasternal short axis (PSAX)			LV systolic function RV dilation Septal kinetics Wall motion abnormalities Pericardial effusion
Apical 4 chamber (A4C)			LV systolic function Chamber dimensions RV function (TAPSE) Pericardial effusion Wall motion abnormalities MV/TV pathology Left atrial pressures

(continued on next page)

Table 1
(continued)

View	Probe Position	Ultrasound Anatomy	Clinical Applications
Apical 5 chamber (A5C)			Quantitative LV function (LVOT-VTI)
Apical 2 chamber (A2C)			LV systolic function Wall motion abnormalities (inferior/anterior) MV pathology Mitral inflow velocities Left atrial pressures
Parasternal short of aortic valve (AV SAX)			Chamber dimensions Clot in transit IAS defects AV pathology Procedural guidance

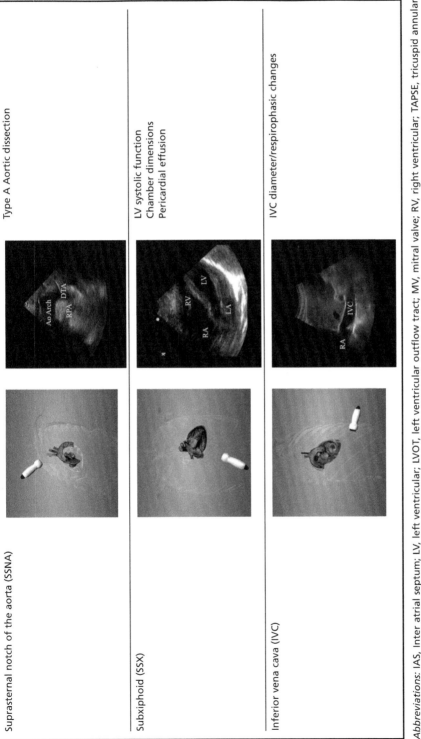

Suprasternal notch of the aorta (SSNA)		Type A Aortic dissection
Subxiphoid (SSX)		LV systolic function Chamber dimensions Pericardial effusion
Inferior vena cava (IVC)		IVC diameter/respirophasic changes

Abbreviations: IAS, Inter atrial septum; LV, left ventricular; LVOT, left ventricular outflow tract; MV, mitral valve; RV, right ventricular; TAPSE, tricuspid annular plane systolic excursion; TV, tricuspid valve; VTI, velocity-time integral.

3D Graphics Courtesy of Heartworks, Intelligent Ultrasound, Ltd, Abingdon, United Kingdom.

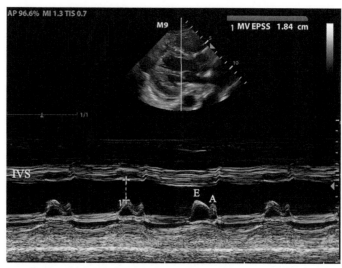

Fig. 1. Evaluation of LV systolic function with EPSS. Parasternal long view with M-mode through the anterior leaflet of the MV. In this example, EPSS is 1.8 cm, which suggests severe systolic dysfunction. IVS, intraventricular septum; E, early diastole; A, late diastole.

hypovolemia, and right ventricular (RV) dysfunction. Stroke volume (SV) assessment is likely more useful in these patients.

Qualitative Evaluation of Right Ventricular Function

The importance of RV function has been increasingly recognized over the past decade. Identification of acute RV failure is essential during a resuscitation. Identifying acute RV dysfunction at the point of care can significantly alter patient management, and is an independent predictor of mortality in patients with acute pulmonary embolism (PE), acute respiratory distress syndrome (ARDS), and acute myocardial infarction.[11–13] A summary of echocardiographic findings of RV dysfunction is listed in **Table 2**.

Table 2	
Summary of basic and advanced applications of resuscitative cardiopulmonary ultrasound	
Basic Resuscitative Cardiopulmonary Ultrasound	**Advanced Resuscitative Cardiopulmonary Ultrasound**
Qualitative LV function	Quantitative LV function: SV and CO estimation
Qualitative RV function	Quantitative RV function
Identification of pericardial effusion	Evaluation of tamponade physiology
Evaluation of IVC diameter/respirophasic changes	Resuscitative TEE
Identification of pneumothorax	Evaluation fluid tolerance (IVC, SVC, LA pressures)
Identification of pulmonary edema	Hemodynamic monitoring
Identification of pleural effusion	

Abbreviations: CO, cardiac output; IVC, inferior vena cava; LA, left atrial; LV, left ventricular; RV, right ventricular; SV, stroke volume; SVC, superior vena cava; TEE, transesophageal echocardiography; US, ultrasound.

RV function can be evaluated with qualitative or quantitative assessments. RV dilation and septal kinetics are the main qualitative screening tools that can be easily and reliably performed by ED physicians.[14–16] Weekes and colleagues[14] prospectively demonstrated 100% sensitivity and 99% specificity for identifying RV dysfunction in normotensive patients with PE, and that FOCUS had better diagnostic accuracy identifying RV dysfunction than troponin or brain natriuretic peptide alone.

Qualitative assessment of the RV relies on understudying its key anatomic features. The RV has a characteristic crescent shape, normally is approximately two-thirds the size of the LV, and has a thinner myocardial free wall. Dilation of the RV with an RV/LV ratio greater than 0.6 and deviation of the septum toward the LV (leading the LV to adopt a D-shape) indicates right ventricular dysfunction.[2] An RV free wall thickness <5 mm, can further help distinguish acute pathology, as patients with chronically elevated RV pressures develop RV hypertrophy.

Regional hypokinesia or akinesia of the RV free wall with preserved function at the apex, known as the McConnell sign, has a high specificity but low sensitivity for acute PE or acute RV infarct.[17,18] The McConnell sign also may be found in patients with acute chest syndrome.[19] **Table 3** summarizes the main echocardiographic findings of RV dysfunction.

The main challenge of qualitative RV is obtaining adequate in-plane images that accurately reflect the RV size (the RV is normally located under the sternum). Clinicians should be careful with underestimating RV size, particularly in the apical 4 and subxiphoid chamber views.

Evaluation of Pericardial Effusion

Identification of pericardial effusion is one of the original elements of the FOCUS examination,[1] and several studies have shown that ED physicians can accurately and reliably detect pericardial effusions compared with comprehensive echocardiography.[20]

The pericardial space is normally minimal, with only 10 mL of fluid that normally does not separate the pericardium from the myocardial wall. As the volume increases, pericardial effusion can be seen as an anechoic (black) stripe posterior to the LV in parasternal views, whereas in the subxiphoid view it can be seen between the pericardium and RV free wall (**Fig. 2**). The amount of fluid should be measured during diastole, and can be classified as a small, moderate, or large effusion.[21]

Clinicians must be familiar with pericardial fluid mimics. Epicardial fat pads can mimic a small anterior effusion. Small, nonloculated effusions will follow gravity and will accumulate posteriorly. Larger, simple effusions will eventually become circumferential. Epicardial fat is often hypoechoic (shade of gray) as opposed to simple

Table 3 Summary of some of the main echocardiographic findings seeing in presence of RV dysfunction	
Echocardiography Findings of RV Dysfunction	
RV dilation	RV/LV diameter ratio >0.6
Septal flattening	D-shape of LV due to increased RV pressure
Moderate/Severe TR	Dilation of tricuspid annulus due to increased RV volume
McConnell sign	Akinesia of the RV free wall with preservation of the apex
TAPSE <17 mm	Longitudinal excursion of the lateral tricuspid annulus

Abbreviations: LV, left ventricle; RV, right ventricle; TAPSE, tricuspid annular plane systolic excursion; TR, tricuspid regurgitation.

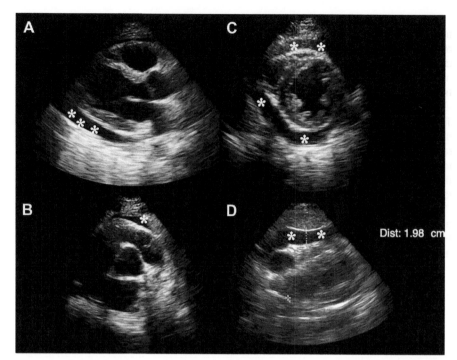

Fig. 2. Visualization of pericardial effusion (*asterisk*) in different views. (*A*) Parasternal long view. (*B*) Parasternal short aortic valve. (*C*) Parasternal short midpapillary. (*D*) Subxiphoid view with a measured pericardial effusion of 1.98 cm (moderate) between the pericardium and RV free wall.

effusions that are anechoic (black). Pleural effusions can mimic pericardial effusions, but track posterior to the descending thoracic aorta (DTA), whereas pericardial effusion will be anterior to the DTA (**Fig. 3**).

Evaluation Preload Using the Inferior Vena Cava

The evaluation of the inferior vena cava (IVC) represents a noninvasive parameter of preload with several clinically relevant applications. It has been widely used in

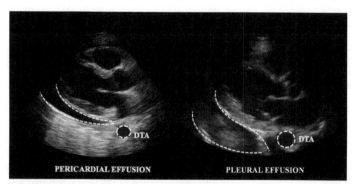

Fig. 3. Echocardiographic appearance of pericardial effusion versus pleural effusion in parasternal long axis view. Pericardial effusion follows a plane that is anterior to the DTA, whereas pleural effusion is posterior.

emergency medicine and critical care point-of-care ultrasonography because it is often easy to visualize, but has significant limitations.

IVC diameter and variation provide a noninvasive estimate of central venous and right atrial pressures. The IVC is best visualized through the subcostal window in short or long axis. In long axis view, the IVC is visualized entering the right atrium (RA). Using M-mode, the maximum and minimum diameters are measured and the percentage of collapse estimated. Diameter measurements should be made just distal to the hepatic vein, approximately 2 to 3 cm distal to the RA (**Fig. 4**).

The use of IVC variation to predict volume responsiveness has been extensively studied in both spontaneously breathing (SB) and mechanically ventilated patients.[22–24] Despite widespread use of IVC ultrasound to guide volume resuscitation, the heterogeneity of populations and measurement techniques has made the interpretation of the evidence challenging.

The use of IVC diameter and collapsibility to predict volume responsiveness has many limitations **Table 4** Via and colleagues[25] provided a comprehensive review of the multiple physiologic mechanisms that affect the reliability of using IVC a measure of preload.

Recent systematic reviews and meta-analyses, including studies conducted in the intensive care unit (ICU) and ED over the past 2 decades, suggest that IVC diameter evaluation as a predictor of fluid responsiveness is most reliable in the following[23,24]:

1. Non-SB patients, receiving mechanical ventilation
2. Prescribed tidal volume (TV) $\geq$8 mL/kg and positive end-expiratory pressure (PEEP) $\leq$5 cm H_2O
3. In sinus rhythm, without evidence of RV dysfunction

In SB patients, IVC should be used with caution and in conjunction with other parameters, such as LV systolic function and lung ultrasound profile. Recently, Corl and colleagues[26] conducted the largest ICU study assessing the predictive value of IVC in SB patients and found that an IVC collapsibility cutoff $\geq$25% identified fluid responsive patients with sensitivity and specificity of 87% and 81%, respectively, with a positive likelihood ratio of 4.5. As in prior studies, the lack of respiratory effort standardization during IVC measurements likely explains the misclassification of patients as fluid responsive (16%), and limits the generalizability of these findings.

For the EP, the clinical scenario in which IVC evaluation can be most helpful is in managing the hypotensive patient whose IVC is plethoric, without tamponade, and

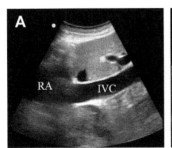 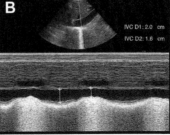

Fig. 4. (A) Long axis view of the IVC. (B) M-mode image of the IVC depicting maximum (IVC D1) and minimum (IVC D2) diameters in an SB patient. Inspiration lowers the intrathoracic pressure, which augments the venous return. This method allows determination of the IVC collapsibility index.

Table 4
Conditions affecting the reliability of IVC assessment as a predictor of fluid responsiveness in spontaneously breathing (SB) and mechanically ventilated (MV) patients

False Positives	False Negatives	Type of Ventilation
Significant inspiratory effort leading to exaggerated intrathoracic pressures	Weak inspiratory effort leading to small intrathoracic pressures	SB
Patients with COPD/asthma: forced expiration (ie, "abdominal breathing") leading to expiratory collapse of IVC	Patients with COPD/asthma: lung hyperinflation and auto-PEEP leading to reduced venous return	SB
Off-plane imagine during longitudinal measurement in M-mode (false collapse of IVC)	Chronic RV dysfunction: increased RA pressures and chronic dilation of IVC	SB or MV
Extrinsic compression of the IVC by masses	Increased abdominal pressure: IVC collapsibility reduced by external pressure over IVC	SB or MV
	High levels of PEEP: increased RA pressures with reduced venous return	MV
	Small tidal volume (<8 mL/kg): smaller variations in IVC in response to lung-heart interactions	MV

Abbreviations: COPD, chronic obstructive pulmonary disease; IVC, inferior vena cava; PEEP, positive end-expiratory pressure; RA, right atrium; RV, right ventricle.

Adapted from Via G, Tavazzi G, Price S. Ten situations where inferior vena cava ultrasound may fail to accurately predict fluid responsiveness: a physiologically based point of view. Intensive Care Med 2016;42(7):1164–7. https://doi.org/10.1007/s00134-016-4357-9; with permission.

minimal respiratory collapse. In this case, the patient is unlikely to benefit from intravenous fluids and vasoactive therapy should be considered instead. In light of the available evidence, additional methods to establish the patient's preload and fluid tolerance should be used.[27]

Focused Lung Ultrasound

Combined with FOCUS, lung ultrasound (LUS) can provide critical diagnostic information to narrow the differential diagnosis and guide management in critically ill patients with respiratory distress.[28,29] Lung ultrasound can identify pulmonary edema, pleural effusion, and pneumothorax with greater diagnostic accuracy compared with clinical examination and chest radiography.[30–32] Lung ultrasound relies on the presence or absence of specific ultrasound artifacts. An in-depth review of these artifacts (and the LUS technique) is beyond the scope of this article, but is well described in Dietrich and colleagues[33] and Bianco and colleagues.[34]

The first step of focused LUS is the evaluation of pleural sliding by visualizing the pleural line moving during respirations with a high-frequency (ie, linear) probe in the anterior chest. The absence of lung sliding suggests the possibility of pneumothorax, but is not the only possible diagnosis. M-mode in the same location can distinguish between a normal pattern or nonventilated lung parenchyma known as the stratosphere sign (**Fig. 5**). The diagnosis of pneumothorax can be made with reported specificity of 100% if there is no lung sliding, no stratosphere sign, or the presence of a lung point.[35]

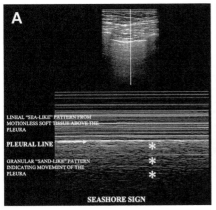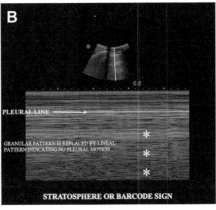

Fig. 5. Evaluation pleural sliding for the assessment of pneumothorax using LUS. (*A*) The interface between the lineal "sealike" pattern of the motionless tissues above the pleural line, with the granular "sandlike" pattern of the subpleural space indicating normal sliding forms the "seashore sign." (*asterisk*) (*B*) A continuous, smooth pattern is seen in presence of lung that is not being ventilated. This is known as the "stratosphere sign" (*asterisk*) and is suggestive of pneumothorax.

The second part of focused LUS is the evaluation of lung parenchyma using a low-frequency (ie, curvilinear or phased array) probe set at a depth of 18 cm. A 6-window protocol (3 in each hemithorax) can provide similar diagnostic accuracy to a traditional 8-view examination.[30,36] Patients can be classified into 4 main ultrasonographic lung patterns, each suggesting different diagnostic entities: A-line pattern, B-line pattern, effusion, or consolidation.

A-lines are horizontal linear artifacts, representing reverberation (mirror effect) of the pleural line, with normal lung. The presence of A-lines in a patient with dyspnea should orient to noninterstitial pathology (ie, consider chronic obstructive pulmonary disease [COPD], PE, or acute coronary syndrome).

B-lines are vertical lines resulting from increased interstitial tissue density. The presence of more than 3 B-lines per lung zone suggests the presence interstitial fluid, which can suggest pulmonary edema (diffuse and bilateral), ARDS (bilateral with areas of sparing), or focal interstitial syndrome (unilateral, often with patchy appearance) such as pneumonia (**Fig. 6**).[37,38]

ADVANCED FOCUSED CARDIAC ULTRASOUND TECHNIQUES

Although the basic applications of FOCUS are sufficient in most cases, the management of complex critically ill patients often requires additional information to understand the patient's cardiovascular physiology and hemodynamics.

Examples of these scenarios include cases in which LVEF does not accurately represent the SV, when quantitative assessment of the cardiac output is needed to titrate vasoactive drugs, suspected acute RV failure, and in the evaluation of tamponade. By understanding additional principles, clinicians can extend their scope of resuscitative ultrasound and better guide management in these clinical situations.

Principles of Doppler

Doppler allows a measurement of frequency shift in moving elements, which in the case of echocardiography enables the detection of blood flow velocities. Pulse

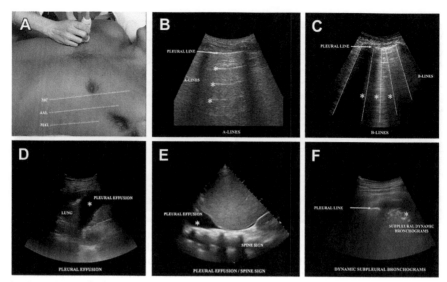

Fig. 6. Main LUS findings. (*A*) Six zone scanning protocol for LUS. The left and right sides of chest wall are divided following 3 lines: mid-clavicular (MC), anterior axillary line (AAL) and mid-axillary line (MAL). (*B*) A-line pattern, indicating normal parenchyma (*asterisk*). (*C*) B-line pattern (*asterisk*) indicating increased extravascular lung water and interstitial lung syndrome. (*D*) Left-sided pleural effusion (*asterisk*). (*E*) Right-sided pleural effusion (*asterisk*). The thoracic spine vertebral bodies are seen due to enhanced transmission of ultrasound by pleural effusion.[59] (*F*) Subpleural bronchograms (*asterisk*) indicating lung consolidation from pneumonia. ([A] *Adapted from* [A] Pivetta E, Goffi A, Lupia E, et al. Lung ultrasound-implemented diagnosis of acute decompensated heart failure in the ED: A SIMEU multicenter study. Chest 2015;148(1):202–10; with permission.)

Wave (PW) Doppler uses pulsed wave ultrasound signals to determine the depth of a measurement. Continuous Wave Doppler uses continuous signals that are simultaneously emitted and received, yielding measurement of velocities throughout the entire ultrasound beam.

Doppler velocity is reliable only if the ultrasound beam is less than 15° from the parallel position of blood flow. As this angle increases, velocity will be progressively underestimated, reaching no detected signal (no flow) when the beam is perpendicular to flow. This concept has important clinical implications, as obtaining acceptable alignment between ultrasound signal and blood flow is often difficult and represents an important source of error.

Quantitative Evaluation of Systolic Left Ventricular Function

EPs can incorporate PW Doppler to perform quantitative assessment of LV function, including estimation of SV and cardiac output (CO). SV is estimated by calculating the product of the area patient's LV outflow tract velocity-time integral (LVOT-VTI) and aortic valve area (AVA).

From the parasternal long axis (PSL) view, the LVOT diameter is measured during early systole from intima to intima to calculate the AVA. To measure the LVOT-VTI, the PW Doppler gate should be placed proximal to the aortic valve leaflets in an apical 5-chamber window. The image is then captured to trace the contour of the Doppler velocity profile to obtain the VTI (**Fig. 7**). This measurement should be averaged over 3 consecutive waveforms to account for beat-to-beat SV variation due to respiration.

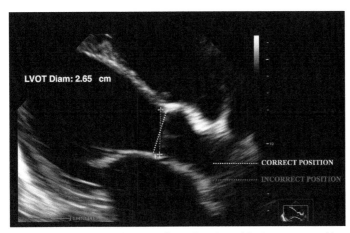

Fig. 7. Measurement of the LVOT diameter for estimation of SV. In parasternal long view, the LVOT should be measured placing caliper perpendicular to the direction of flow (*yellow dotted line*). Note that measurement is being made with image zoomed to increase accuracy.

There are a few important sources of error the clinician should be aware of when estimating SV using VTI. First, because the LVOT diameter is squared in the AVA calculation, small errors in the measurement will lead to significant error in the final product. Zooming in to the LVOT allows for the most accurate measurement possible (**Fig. 8**). The caliper

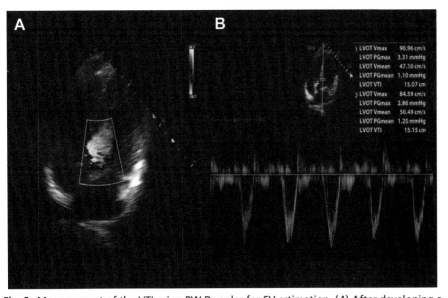

Fig. 8. Measurement of the VTI using PW Doppler for SV estimation. (*A*) After developing a 5-chamber view, CF Doppler is used to visualize the center of laminar flow into the LVOT. Blue denotes flow away from the probe. (*B*) The sample volume of PW Doppler is positioned at the LVOT aiming for an angle of insonation of less than 15 degrees to avoid underestimation of velocity. At least two or three envelopes are traced to improve accuracy, and the average calculated VTI is used to estimate the SV. Once the LVOT diameter and VTI are known with these methods, the SV can be estimated using the formula: SV = π [LVOT diameter/2]^2 × [LVOT-VTI]. CF, color flow.

should be positioned perpendicular to the direction of blood flow and not following a vertical line. Second, adequate positioning of the PW sample volume, approximately 5 mm proximal to the aortic valve, is key for reliable measurements. If the sample volume is too close to the valve, velocities will be overestimated due to higher flow through the valve, while measuring too far from the valve will underestimate the velocities.

Quantitative Evaluation of Right Ventricular Function

Unlike assessment of the LV, the qualitative evaluation of RV systolic function is much less reliable.[39] Chamber dimensions and septal deviation may be sufficient to make the diagnosis of RV dysfunction in many cases, but a quantitative approach can improve the accuracy and reliability of the RV function. There are several quantitative methods used to assess RV function, including fractional area of change, myocardial performance index, tricuspid annular velocity, and tricuspid annular plane systolic excursion (TAPSE). Although there is no universal agreement, TAPSE has been the most studied parameter in ED and ICU settings.[40]

TAPSE can be measured using M-mode in an apical 4-chamber view to measure the maximum longitudinal excursion of the lateral tricuspid annulus, between the end of systole and the end of diastole. A TAPSE ≥ 17 mm has been shown to have good correlation with normal RV function[2,41,42] Abnormal TAPSE has been established as a marker of poor clinical outcome in several pathologies, including ARDS, PE, and septic cardiomyopathy.[40]

One important ED application is the risk stratification of patients with suspected or diagnosed PE. A recent prospective study of TAPSE in patients with suspected PE found that a TAPSE less than 15.2 mm was able to identify ED patients with clinically significant acute PE (specificity of 100% but a low sensitivity of 53%).[43] A similar study showed that a TAPSE ≤ 17 mm had 90% sensitivity for centrally located PE and that when combined with lower extremity ultrasound for deep vein thrombosis, sensitivity was 100%.[44]

Although quick and relatively easy to perform, TAPSE has some limitations due to its single dimensional measurement. First, it measures only longitudinal excursion, which is one component of RV function. Some patients with frank RV dysfunction, due to pulmonary hypertension, for example, may have a preserved TAPSE. Second, it is angle dependent. If the beam is not parallel to the RV free wall, the longitudinal excursion will be underestimated.

Evaluation of Pericardial Tamponade Physiology

EPs can assess for echocardiographic signs of tamponade physiology in the patient with a pericardial effusion. The hallmark of pericardial tamponade is impaired diastolic filling of right-sided chambers, leading to a decrease of LV SV and hemodynamic compromise.[21]

The first step is evaluation of IVC diameter and respiratory variation. Due to the increased intrapericardial pressures during tamponade, the RA cannot receive venous return, causing distension of the IVC throughout the respiratory cycle. A plethoric IVC, with no or minimal respiratory variation, is highly sensitive for tamponade physiology (>95%). In the absence of this finding, the presence of tamponade physiology is extremely unlikely.[21,45]

The second step is evaluation of RV diastolic collapse. When intrapericardial pressure exceeds the intracardiac filling pressure, the RV free wall collapses. This can be measured using M-mode in PSL view, aligning the beam through the RV free wall and the anterior leaflet of the MV. Diastolic collapse of the RV has a specificity between 75% and 90% and a relatively low sensitivity of 48% to 60%.[21]

Last, using PW Doppler in A4C view, pathologic inflow velocity variation through the mitral or tricuspid valves can be evaluated. Respirophasic variation of the peak inflow velocities greater than 30% at the MV and greater than 60% at the TV suggest increased ventricular interdependence and is highly specific for tamponade.[21,46]

Integrating Resuscitative Ultrasound for Hemodynamic Monitoring

Hemodynamic monitoring has an important role in the management of critically ill patients guiding therapeutic decisions and providing endpoints of resuscitation. There has been an increasing use of ultrasound for hemodynamic monitoring in recent years, likely because it meets many of the proprieties of an "ideal" hemodynamic monitor.[47,48]

A number of echocardiographic parameters can be used to tailor interventions to meet an individual patient's physiologic needs. For instance, serial VTI measurements with transthoracic echocardiogram (TTE) or TEE to estimate SV and CO can monitor fluid responsiveness and response to vasoactive therapy. Systemic vascular resistance (SVR) can be estimated using the formula: SVR = 80*(MAP − RA pressure [mm Hg])/CO (L/min). These quantitative data can be helpful when differentiating a patient's macro circulatory shock phenotype and choosing a therapeutic intervention.

TEE has the unique advantage that allows visualization of the superior vena cava (SVC), which can be used to predict fluid responsiveness, avoiding confounders such as abnormal intra-abdominal pressure. In mechanically ventilated patients, SVC collapsibility greater than 36% has been found to predict fluid responsiveness with sensitivity and specificity of 90% and 100%, respectively.[49]

Last, although the assessment of diastolic function has been traditionally beyond the scope of FOCUS, mitral inflow velocities and Tissue Doppler Imaging of the mitral annulus using TTE or TEE can provide valuable information during resuscitation.[50] A ratio E/A ≥2 in patients with decreased LV function (ejection fraction <40%) or E/e' ≥14 with normal LV systolic function, has been shown to predict elevated left atrial pressure (LAP), indicating severe LV diastolic dysfunction. Although the exact values of LAP do not correlate with preload sensitivity,[51] this binary assessment (ie, normal vs elevated) can help to identify patients at high risk for developing hydrostatic pulmonary edema from fluid therapy, and differentiate cardiogenic pulmonary edema from ARDS.

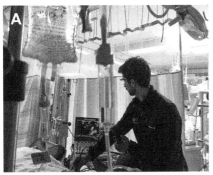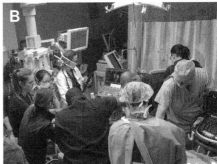

Fig. 9. Common applications of resuscitative TEE in the ED. (*A*) Physician performing assessment of undifferentiated shock in a mechanically ventilated patient. (*B*) Performance of resuscitative TEE for the guidance of cannula placement, with ongoing cardiopulmonary resuscitation during a case of ECPR. ECPR, extracorporeal cardiopulmonary resuscitation; ED, emergency department.

Table 5
TEE probe graphics courtesy of Heart Works by Intelligent Ultrasound

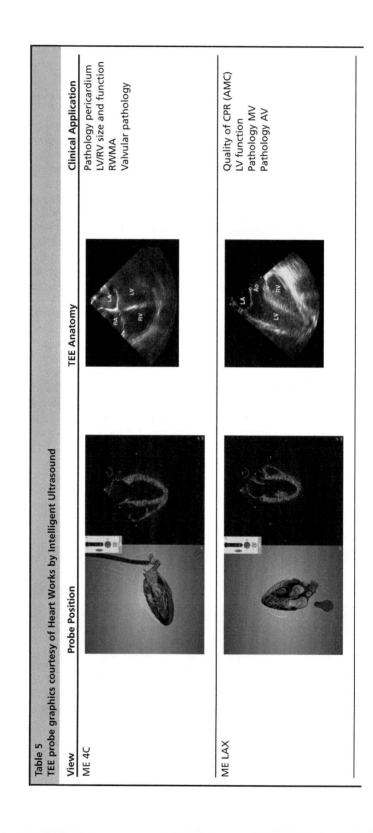

View	Probe Position	TEE Anatomy	Clinical Application
ME 4C			Pathology pericardium LV/RV size and function RWMA Valvular pathology
ME LAX			Quality of CPR (AMC) LV function Pathology MV Pathology AV

TG SAX Pap	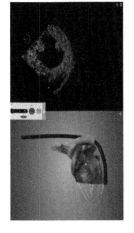	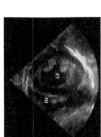	LV function RWMA Pathology pericardium
ME Bicaval	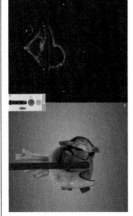	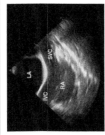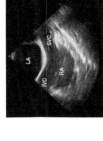	Procedure guidance Venous guidewire ECMO Volume responsiveness

Abbreviations: AMC, area of maximal compression; AV, aortic valve; CPR, cardiopulmonary resuscitation; ECMO, extracorporeal membrane oxygenation; LV, left ventricle; ME Bicaval, midesophageal bicaval; ME LAX, midesophageal long axis view; ME TG SAX Pap, midesophageal transgastric short axis papillary view; ME4C, midesophageal 4 chamber; MV, mitral valve; RV, right ventricle; RWMA, regional wall motion abnormality; TEE, transesophageal echocardiography.

3D Graphics Courtesy of Heartworks, Intelligent Ultrasound, Ltd, Abingdon, United Kingdom.

RESUSCITATIVE TRANSESOPHAGEAL ECHOCARDIOGRAPHY

Over the past 2 decades, the practice of TEE has expanded from its traditional indications (ie, patients undergoing cardiac surgery, suspected endocarditis, or cardioversion in atrial fibrillation), to assist the hemodynamic evaluation of patients with acute decompensation, shock, and cardiac arrest.[52–56] Following landmark publications demonstrating the feasibility of EP-performed TEE, a number of institutions in the United States have implemented ED-based TEE programs (**Fig. 9**). In 2017, the American College of Emergency Physicians published a Policy Statement to provide guidelines for the use of TEE in cardiac arrest.[57]

EP and intensivist-performed TEE examinations are feasible, safe, and clinically impactful in the management of critically ill patients.[56] The 4 core views in resuscitative TEE are midesophageal (ME) 4 chamber, ME long axis, transgastric short axis at the level of papillary muscles, and ME bicaval view (**Table 5**). **Fig. 10** provides an algorithm integrating the 4 core resuscitative TEE views.

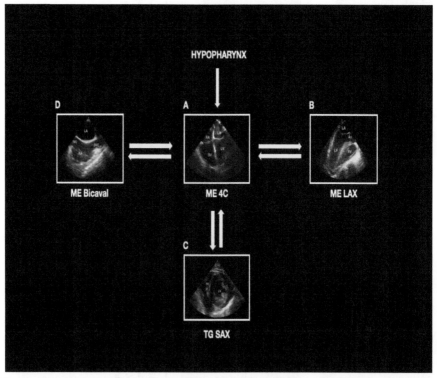

Fig. 10. Algorithm integrating 4 resuscitative TEE views. (*A*) ME4C view. ME4C represents the "home base" of resuscitative TEE and is the starting point for all examinations. This view is obtained at the mid-esophageal level (probe insertion 35–40 cm from the incisors), omniplane at 0° with sector depth at around 12–14 cm depending on the heart size. (*B*) ME LAX. From the ME 4C view, the image is centered on the LV and then the omniplane should be rotated to 130–140°. (*C*) TG SAX. From the ME 4C view, the probe is advanced out of the esophagus and into the stomach at around 40–45 cm from the incisors, with the sector depth at around 10–12 cm. As the probe exists the esophagus, gentle ante-flexion is applied to establish contact with the gastric wall. (*D*) ME Bicaval. From the ME 4C, the image is centered over the RA and then the omniplane rotated to 90°, with the sector depth at around 8–10 cm. Image courtesy of the Resuscitative TEE Project (www.resuscitativetee.com).

The primary indication for use of resuscitative TEE in the ED is during cardiac arrest.[54,58] However, TEE can be clinically influential in several other clinical scenarios:

1. Evaluation of patients in shock who have inadequate transthoracic windows.[56]
2. Assessment of fluid responsiveness in mechanically ventilated patients using SVC variation.[49]
3. The guidance of extracorporeal membrane oxygenation cannulation during initiation of extracorporeal circulation.[57]

SUMMARY

Resuscitative cardiopulmonary ultrasound is a powerful tool in the assessment of critically ill patients, and continues to rapidly grow in emergency medicine. The basic elements include the qualitative evaluation of LV and RV function, the identification of pericardial effusion, and the evaluation of preload. Advanced applications such as identification of tamponade physiology, quantitative function of the RV and LV, and hemodynamic monitoring can be incorporated with relatively simple measurements. Resuscitative cardiopulmonary ultrasound and TEE represent a dynamic and scalable field in acute care imaging. EPs can and should adapt the use of these tools to their individual needs, considering skill level, clinical environment, and wider institutional practices.

REFERENCES

1. Labovitz AJ, Noble VE, Bierig M, et al. Focused cardiac ultrasound in the emergent setting: a consensus statement of the American Society of Echocardiography and American College of Emergency Physicians. J Am Soc Echocardiogr 2010;23(12):1225–30.
2. Lang RM, Badano LP, Mor-Avi V, et al. Recommendations for cardiac chamber quantification by echocardiography in adults: An update from the American Society of Echocardiography and the European Association of Cardiovascular Imaging. Eur Heart J Cardiovasc Imaging 2015;16(3):233–71.
3. Moore CL, Rose GA, Tayal VS, et al. Determination of left ventricular function by emergency physician echocardiography of hypotensive patients. Acad Emerg Med 2002;9(3):186–93.
4. Mckaigney CJ, Krantz MJ, La Rocque CL, et al. E-point septal separation: a bedside tool for emergency physician assessment of left ventricular ejection fraction. Am J Emerg Med 2014;32(6):493–7.
5. Randazzo MR, Snoey ER, Levitt MA, et al. Accuracy of emergency physician assessment of left ventricular ejection fraction and central venous pressure using echocardiography. Acad Emerg Med 2003;10(9):973–7.
6. Shahgaldi K, Gudmundsson P, Manouras A, et al. Visually estimated ejection fraction by two dimensional and triplane echocardiography is closely correlated with quantitative ejection fraction by real-time three dimensional echocardiography. Cardiovasc Ultrasound 2009;7(1):1–7.
7. Secko MA, Lazar JM, Salciccioli LA, et al. Can junior emergency physicians use E-point septal separation to accurately estimate left ventricular function in acutely dyspneic patients? Acad Emerg Med 2011;18(11):1223–6.
8. Massie BM, Schiller NB, Ratshin RA, et al. Mitral-septal separation: new echocardiographic index of left ventricular function. Am J Cardiol 1977;39(7):1008–16.

9. Silverstein JR, Laffely NH, Rifkin RD. Quantitative estimation of left ventricular ejection fraction from mitral valve E-point to septal separation and comparison to magnetic resonance imaging. Am J Cardiol 2006;97(1):137–40.

10. Ahmadpour H, Shah AA, Allen JW, et al. Mitral E point septal separation: a reliable index of left ventricular performance in coronary artery disease. Am Heart J 1983; 106(1 PART 1):21–8.

11. Sanchez O, Trinquart L, Colombet I, et al. Prognostic value of right ventricular dysfunction in patients with haemodynamically stable pulmonary embolism: a systematic review. Eur Heart J 2008;29(12):1569–77.

12. Mekontso Dessap A, Boissier F, Charron C, et al. Acute cor pulmonale during protective ventilation for acute respiratory distress syndrome: prevalence, predictors, and clinical impact. Intensive Care Med 2016;42(5):862–70.

13. Engström AE, Vis MM, Bouma BJ, et al. Right ventricular dysfunction is an independent predictor for mortality in ST-elevation myocardial infarction patients presenting with cardiogenic shock on admission. Eur J Heart Fail 2010;12(3):276–82.

14. Weekes AJ, Johnson AK, Troha D, et al. Prognostic value of right ventricular dysfunction markers for serious adverse events in acute normotensive pulmonary embolism. J Emerg Med 2017;52(2):137–50.

15. Gaspari R, Weekes A, Adhikari S, et al. A retrospective study of pulseless electrical activity, bedside ultrasound identifies interventions during resuscitation associated with improved survival to hospital admission. A REASON Study. Resuscitation 2017;120:103–7.

16. Rutz MA, Clary JM, Kline JA, et al. Emergency physicians are able to detect right ventricular dilation with good agreement compared to cardiology. Acad Emerg Med 2017;24(7):867–74.

17. McConnell MV, Solomon SD, Rayan ME, et al. Regional right ventricular dysfunction detected by echocardiography in acute pulmonary embolism. Am J Cardiol 1996;78(4):469–73.

18. Mediratta A, Addetia K, Medvedofsky D, et al. Echocardiographic diagnosis of acute pulmonary embolism in patients with McConnell's sign. Echocardiography 2016;33(5):696–702.

19. McCutcheon JB, Schaffer P, Lyon M, et al. The McConnell sign is seen in patients with acute chest syndrome. J Ultrasound Med 2018. https://doi.org/10.1002/jum.14585.

20. Mandavia DP, Hoffner RJ, Mahaney K, et al. Bedside echocardiography by emergency physicians. Ann Emerg Med 2001;38(4 SUPPL):377–82.

21. Klein AL, Abbara S, Agler DA, et al. American Society of Echocardiography clinical recommendations for multimodality cardiovascular imaging of patients with pericardial disease: endorsed by the Society for Cardiovascular Magnetic Resonance and Society of Cardiovascular Computed Tomography. J Am Soc Echocardiogr 2013;26(9):965–1012.e15.

22. Zhang Z, Xu X, Ye S, et al. Ultrasonographic measurement of the respiratory variation in the inferior vena cava diameter is predictive of fluid responsiveness in critically ill patients: systematic review and meta-analysis. Ultrasound Med Biol 2014;40(5):845–53.

23. Long E, Oakley E, Duke T, et al, Paediatric Research in Emergency Departments International Collaborative (PREDICT). Does respiratory variation in inferior vena cava diameter predict fluid responsiveness: a systematic review and meta-analysis. Shock 2017;47(5):550–9.

24. Si X, Xu H, Liu Z, et al. Does respiratory variation in inferior vena cava diameter predict fluid responsiveness in mechanically ventilated patients? A systematic review and meta-analysis. Anesth Analg 2018;127(5):1157–64.
25. Via G, Tavazzi G, Price S. Ten situations where inferior vena cava ultrasound may fail to accurately predict fluid responsiveness: a physiologically based point of view. Intensive Care Med 2016;42(7):1164–7.
26. Corl KA, George NR, Romanoff J, et al. Inferior vena cava collapsibility detects fluid responsiveness among spontaneously breathing critically-ill patients. J Crit Care 2017;41:130–7.
27. Lee CWC, Kory PD, Arntfield RT. Development of a fluid resuscitation protocol using inferior vena cava and lung ultrasound. J Crit Care 2016;31(1):96–100.
28. Zanobetti M, Scorpiniti M, Gigli C, et al. Point-of-care ultrasonography for evaluation of acute dyspnea in the ED. Chest 2017;151(6):1295–301.
29. Buhumaid RE, St-Cyr Bourque J, Shokoohi H, et al. Integrating point-of-care ultrasound in the ED evaluation of patients presenting with chest pain and shortness of breath. Am J Emerg Med 2018. https://doi.org/10.1016/j.ajem.2018.10.059.
30. Pivetta E, Goffi A, Lupia E, et al. Lung ultrasound-implemented diagnosis of acute decompensated heart failure in the ED: A SIMEU multicenter study. Chest 2015; 148(1):202–10.
31. Wooten WM, Shaffer LET, Hamilton LA. Bedside ultrasound versus chest radiography for detection of pulmonary edema. J Ultrasound Med 2018;1–7. https://doi.org/10.1002/jum.14781.
32. Patel CJ, Bhatt HB, Parikh SN, et al. Bedside lung ultrasound in emergency protocol as a diagnostic tool in patients of acute respiratory distress presenting to emergency department. J Emerg Trauma Shock 2018;11(2):125–9.
33. Dietrich CF, Mathis G, Blaivas M, et al. Lung artefacts and their use. Med Ultrason 2016;18(4):488–99.
34. Bianco F, Bucciarelli V, Ricci F, et al. Lung ultrasonography: a practical guide for cardiologists. J Cardiovasc Med 2017;18(7):501–9.
35. Lichtenstein D, Mezière G, Biderman P, et al. The "lung point": an ultrasound sign specific to pneumothorax. Intensive Care Med 2000;26(10):1434–40.
36. Lichtenstein DA, Mezière GA, Lagoueyte JF, et al. A-lines and B-lines: lung ultrasound as a bedside tool for predicting pulmonary artery occlusion pressure in the critically ill. Chest 2009;136(4):1014–20.
37. Bataille B, Riu B, Ferre F, et al. Integrated use of bedside lung ultrasound and echocardiography in acute respiratory failure: a prospective observational study in ICU. Chest 2014;146(6):1586–93.
38. Mojoli F, Bouhemad B, Mongodi S, et al. Lung ultrasound for critically ill patients. Am J Respir Crit Care Med 2018. https://doi.org/10.1164/rccm.201802-0236CI.
39. Puchalski MD, Williams RV, Askovich B, et al. Assessment of right ventricular size and function: echo versus magnetic resonance imaging. Congenit Heart Dis 2007;2(1):27–31.
40. Huang SJ, Nalos M, Smith L, et al. The use of echocardiographic indices in defining and assessing right ventricular systolic function in critical care research. Intensive Care Med 2018;44(6):868–83.
41. Park JH, Kim JH, Lee JH, et al. Evaluation of right ventricular systolic function by the analysis of tricuspid annular motion in patients with acute pulmonary embolism. J Cardiovasc Ultrasound 2012;20(4):181–8.
42. Miller D, Farah MG, Liner A, et al. The relation between quantitative right ventricular ejection fraction and indices of tricuspid annular motion and myocardial performance. J Am Soc Echocardiogr 2004;17(5):443–7.

43. Lahham S, Fox JC, Thompson M, et al. Tricuspid annular plane of systolic excursion to prognosticate acute pulmonary symptomatic embolism (TAPSEPAPSE study). J Ultrasound Med 2018. https://doi.org/10.1002/jum.14753.

44. Dwyer KH, Rempell JS, Stone MB. Diagnosing centrally located pulmonary embolisms in the emergency department using point-of-care ultrasound. Am J Emerg Med 2018;36(7):1145–50.

45. Vakamudi S, Ho N, Cremer PC. Pericardial effusions: causes, diagnosis, and management. Prog Cardiovasc Dis 2017;59(4):380–8.

46. Appleton CP, Hatle LK, Popp RL. Cardiac tamponade and pericardial effusion: respiratory variation in transvalvular flow velocities studied by Doppler echocardiography. J Am Coll Cardiol 1988;11(5):1020–30.

47. Vincent J, Rhodes A, Perel A, et al. Clinical review: update on hemodynamic monitoring–a consensus of 16. Crit Care 2011. https://doi.org/10.1186/cc10291.

48. Porter TR, Shillcutt SK, Adams MS, et al. Guidelines for the use of echocardiography as a monitor for therapeutic intervention in adults: a report from the American Society of Echocardiography. J Am Soc Echocardiogr 2015;28(1):40–56.

49. Vieillard-Baron A, Chergui K, Rabiller A, et al. Superior vena caval collapsibility as a gauge of volume status in ventilated septic patients. Intensive Care Med 2004; 30(9):1734–9.

50. Combes A, Arnoult F, Trouillet JL. Tissue Doppler imaging estimation of pulmonary artery occlusion pressure in ICU patients. Intensive Care Med 2004;30(1): 75–81.

51. Osman D, Ridel C, Ray P, et al. Cardiac filling pressures are not appropriate to predict hemodynamic response to volume challenge. Crit Care Med 2007; 35(1):64–8.

52. Memtsoudis SG, Rosenberger P, Loffler M, et al. The usefulness of transesophageal echocardiography during intraoperative cardiac arrest in noncardiac surgery. Anesth Analg 2006;102(6):1653–7.

53. Shillcutt SK, Markin NW, Montzingo CR, et al. Use of rapid "rescue" perioperative echocardiography to improve outcomes after hemodynamic instability in noncardiac surgical patients. J Cardiothorac Vasc Anesth 2012;26(3):362–70.

54. Teran F, Dean AJ, Centeno C, et al. Evaluation of out-of-hospital cardiac arrest using transesophageal echocardiography in the emergency department. Resuscitation 2019;137:140–7.

55. Mayo PH, Narasimhan M, Koenig S. Critical care transesophageal echocardiography. Chest 2015;148(5):1323–32.

56. Arntfield R, Pace J, Hewak M, et al. Focused transesophageal echocardiography by emergency physicians is feasible and clinically influential: observational results from a novel ultrasound program. J Emerg Med 2016;50(2):286–94.

57. Fair J, Tonna J, Ockerse P, et al. Emergency physician-performed transesophageal echocardiography for extracorporeal life support vascular cannula placement. Am J Emerg Med 2016;34(8):1637–9.

58. Van Der Wouw PA, Koster RW, Delemarre BJ, et al. Diagnostic accuracy of transesophageal echocardiography during cardiopulmonary resuscitation. J Am Coll Cardiol 1997;30:780–3.

59. Dickman E, Terentiev V, Likourezos A, et al. Extension of the thoracic spine sign: a new sonographic marker of pleural effusion. J Ultrasound Med 2015;34(9): 1555–61.

Mechanical Ventilation in Hypoxemic Respiratory Failure

Shikha Kapil, MD, Jennifer G. Wilson, MD, MS*

KEYWORDS

- Hypoxemia • Respiratory failure • Mechanical ventilation • ARDS

KEY POINTS

- Acute hypoxemic respiratory failure is a common challenge faced by emergency physicians.
- Patient outcomes depend on interventions performed during the preintubation, intubation, and postintubation periods.
- There are various evidence-based methods of minimizing ventilator-induced lung injury and improving gas exchange in the acute period, including optimal utilization of mechanical ventilation.
- Therapies for worsening or refractory hypoxemia include neuromuscular blockade, prone positioning, and referral for extracorporeal membrane oxygenation consideration.

INTRODUCTION

Acute hypoxemic respiratory failure (AHRF) is a frequent and challenging condition faced by emergency physicians (EPs). The EP must simultaneously stabilize a rapidly decompensating patient, work to ascertain the cause of the hypoxemia, and prevent secondary lung injury. This concise article presents recommendations for evidence-based practice to optimally manage patients with AHRF and the acute respiratory distress syndrome (ARDS), including noninvasive support of patients with AHRF, techniques for safely intubating patients with hypoxemia, strategies for mechanical ventilation, adjunctive therapies in ARDS, and management of refractory hypoxemia.

EPIDEMIOLOGY AND CAUSES OF ACUTE HYPOXEMIC RESPIRATORY FAILURE

AHRF is responsible for 1.9 million admissions per year in the United States alone and carries a hospital mortality rate of up to 20%.[1] The most common causes include

Department of Emergency Medicine, Stanford University School of Medicine, 900 Welch Road Suite 350, Palo Alto, CA 94304, USA
* Corresponding author.
E-mail address: jennygwilson@stanford.edu

Emerg Med Clin N Am 37 (2019) 431–444
https://doi.org/10.1016/j.emc.2019.04.005
0733-8627/19/© 2019 Elsevier Inc. All rights reserved.
emed.theclinics.com

pneumonia, cardiogenic pulmonary edema, ARDS, and chronic obstructive pulmonary disease (COPD) (**Table 1**).[1] ARDS is an important syndrome of noncardiogenic edema that remains underrecognized by treating physicians; the most common risk factors for ARDS include pneumonia, nonpulmonary sepsis, and aspiration. The Berlin consensus definition of ARDS (**Table 2**) clarifies diagnostic criteria and provides the PaO_2 to fraction of inspired oxygen (FiO_2) (PaO_2/FiO_2) ratio values that are used to categorize the severity of hypoxemia.[2]

INITIAL MANAGEMENT AND NONINVASIVE SUPPORT

Initial management of the hypoxemic patient should involve immediate use of supplemental oxygen. If the patient does not require immediate endotracheal intubation (or has chosen to be on Do Not Intubate status) but fails to achieve adequate oxygenation with conventional supplemental oxygen, high-flow nasal cannula (HFNC) oxygen or noninvasive positive pressure ventilation (NIPPV) may be used (**Fig. 1**).

An HFNC provides humidified oxygen at flows up to 60 L/min. It increases Fio_2 by washing out pharyngeal deadspace, can provide low levels of positive pressure to the large airways, and offloads work-of-breathing.[3] In 1 randomized controlled trial (RCT) in subjects with AHRF without hypercapnia, subjects randomized to the HFNC group demonstrated greater ventilator-free days and an improved 90-day mortality rate compared with subjects who received NIPPV.[4] HFNC is generally well-tolerated and should be considered in any patient with AHRF not caused by cardiogenic pulmonary edema or COPD.

NIPPV, which includes both continuous positive airway pressure and bilevel positive airway pressure, is generally preferred in patients with respiratory distress due to cardiogenic pulmonary edema as opposed to immediate intubation or HFNC. In the hypertensive patient with acute cardiogenic pulmonary edema (sometimes referred to as sympathetic crashing acute pulmonary edema [SCAPE]), NIPPV and aggressive afterload reduction should be first-line treatment. This approach has been shown to decrease both the need for intubation and mortality.[5] NIPPV has also been demonstrated to be effective in reducing intubations and hospital mortality in select patients with AHRF not caused by cardiogenic pulmonary edema.[6] In a meta-analysis of 11 RCTs, subjects with AHRF (and excluding cardiogenic pulmonary edema subjects) found a significantly decreased incidence of intubation and hospital mortality (relative risk ratio 0.59 and 0.46, respectively).[7] Predictors of a favorable response to NIPPV

Table 1	
Mechanisms of hypoxemia with examples of clinical causes	
Mechanism of Hypoxemia	**Clinical Example**
Hypoventilation	Narcotic overdose, head injury, airway obstruction, neuromuscular weakness
Right-to-left shunt (anatomic or physiologic)	PFO, congenital cardiac disease, vascular malformations, atelectasis, pneumonia, pulmonary edema
Ventilation/perfusion ratio mismatch	PE, COPD
Impaired diffusion	IPF
Low inspired oxygen	Altitude

Abbreviations: IPF, Idiopathic pulmonary fibrosis; PE, pulmonary embolism; PFO, patent foramen ovale.

Table 2
Berlin definition of acute respiratory distress syndrome

Clinical Criteria	
Timing	Onset within 7 d of known clinical insult or new or worsening respiratory symptoms
Imaging	Chest radiograph or chest CT with bilateral opacities not fully explained by effusion, collapse, or nodules
Cause	Respiratory failure not entirely explained by cardiac failure or volume over
Severity	
Mild	Pao_2/Fio_2 200–300 mm Hg with PEEP $\geq$5 cm H_2O (may be delivered noninvasively)
Moderate	Pao_2/Fio_2 100–200 mm Hg with PEEP $\geq$5 cm H_2O
Severe	Pao_2/Fio_2 <100 mm Hg with PEEP $\geq$5 cm H_2O

Adapted from ARDS Definition Task Force, Ranieri VM, Rubenfeld GD, et al. Acute respiratory distress syndrome: the Berlin Definition. JAMA 2012;307(23):2526–2533; with permission.

include younger age, lower severity of illness, and signs of early clinical improvement, such as decreased heart rate.[8] It is reasonable to start with an expiratory positive airway pressure of 5 and an inspiratory positive airway pressure of 10 to 15, while titrating Fio_2 up as needed.

Not all patients benefit from NIPPV. If patients are unable to manage secretions to protect their airway, they should be intubated without a trial of NIPPV regardless of the

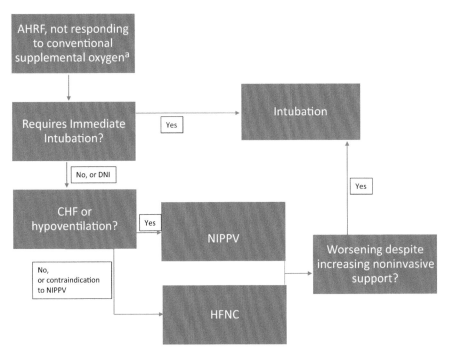

Fig. 1. Algorithm to guide decision-making in the initial management of AHRF. [a] Nasal cannula or nonrebreather mask up to 15 L supplemental oxygen. CHF, congestive heart failure; DNI, do not intubate.

cause of their hypoxemia. Similarly, if patients fail to improve on NIPPV after a time-limited trial (generally 1–2 hours) or if they worsen, timely endotracheal intubation should be considered to avoid any harm. This may be particularly true in patients who are older than 65 years of age[9] and in patients with pneumonia or ARDS, in which uncontrolled tidal volumes may result in worsened lung injury.[10] The European Respiratory Society/American Thoracic Society recommendations for application of NIPPV in acute respiratory failure are summarized in **Table 3**.[11]

INTUBATING THE HYPOXEMIC PATIENT
Rapid Sequence Intubation

Adequate preoxygenation and first-pass success are the main goals during rapid sequence intubation of the hypoxemic patient. Induction sedative should be rapidly acting (eg, etomidate or ketamine) and the paralytic should also be rapid onset (succinylcholine or high-dose rocuronium 1.2 mg/kg).[12]

Preoxygenation

Although these patients may be in respiratory distress, there is nearly always time to preoxygenate. Preoxygenation is of paramount importance for the following rationale.[13] The oxyhemoglobin dissociation curve (**Fig. 2**) demonstrates the precipitous drop in SpO_2 that occurs when Pao_2 drops below 60 mm Hg. Adequate preoxygenation extends the time before desaturation during apnea.

Adequate preoxygenation can be achieved by increasing the saturation to as close to SpO_2 of 100% as possible for at least 3 minutes if tolerated. If the patient cannot tolerate preoxygenation for 3 minutes, raising the head of the bed to 20° has been demonstrated to decrease time to adequate preoxygenation.[14] Patients should remain in head-up and/or in the sniffing position for laryngoscopy as well.[15]

In healthy patients, preoxygenation may be achieved using only a nonrebreather mask. Nasal cannula oxygen may be used underneath the nonrebreather mask to boost the flow and concentration of oxygen provided, and this can be left in place during intubation to provide apneic oxygenation (see later discussion). In critically ill and obese patients with AHRF, however, NIPPV or use of bag-valve-mask with a positive

Table 3
Summary of relevant European Respiratory Society/American Thoracic Society recommendations for application of NIV in acute respiratory failure

Cause of Hypoxemia	Recommendation	Justification
Cardiogenic pulmonary edema	BiPAP or CPAP (strong recommendation)	Significantly decreased need for intubation and decreased mortality
Immunocompromised patients with AHRF	Early NIPPV (conditional recommendation)	Significantly decreased need for intubation, decreased mortality, and decreased rates of nosocomial pneumonia
De novo respiratory failure, including pneumonia and ARDS	No recommendation	—

Abbreviations: BiPAP, bilevel positive airway pressure; CPAP, continuous positive airway pressure; NIV, non invasive ventilator.

Data from Rochwerg B, Brochard L, Elliott MW, et al. Official ERS/ATS clinical practice guidelines: noninvasive ventilation for acute respiratory failure. Eur Respir J 2017;50(2).

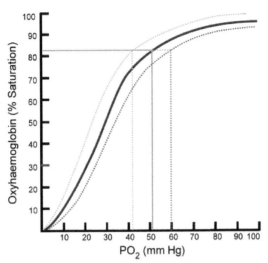

Fig. 2. The oxyhemoglobin dissociation curve, demonstrating the relationship between the Pao₂ and oxygen saturation under various conditions. (*From* Wikimedia Commons. Available at: https://commons.wikimedia.org/wiki/File:Oxyhaemoglobin_dissociation_curve.png.)

end-expiratory pressure (PEEP) valve may be required to achieve the best possible preoxygenation.[16] Not only does this strategy provide higher Fio₂ but preoxygenation with positive pressure may improve lung recruitment, thereby decreasing shunt, improving oxygenation, and prolonging safe apnea time.[12]

Finally, apneic oxygenation has also been explored as a method to prolong safe apnea time.[17,18] In 2 RCTs, nasal cannula at 5 L per minute during the apneic period prolonged safe apnea time; however, these were elective operating room cases. There is at least 1 negative trial of this technique in the critically ill, in which 15 L oxygen by nasal cannula did not increase the lowest arterial oxygen saturation during endotracheal intubation.[19] However, another recent systematic review supports its use in emergency situations.[20] On balance, available evidence suggests that apneic oxygenation may prevent critical desaturation, and is unlikely to cause harm; as such, the authors support its use.

Maximizing First-Pass Success

Although maximizing preoxygenation can extend safe apnea time in patients with AHRF, time to desaturation will still be reduced and unpredictable compared with patients with healthy lungs.[21] In addition, each repeat attempt at intubation beyond the first attempt is associated with increased risk of desaturation, as well as other adverse events, including esophageal intubation and even cardiac arrest.[22] For this reason, maximizing the likelihood of first-pass success of endotracheal intubation is especially important in patients with AHRF who may not tolerate repeat attempts. Proper positioning, use of video laryngoscopy or bougie, and requesting backup (if available) in cases in which difficult airway anatomy is anticipated can be life-saving.[23,24]

VENTILATOR MANAGEMENT
Lung Protective Ventilation

Once the hypoxemic patient is intubated, how they are ventilated can have a significant impact on their subsequent hospital course and ultimate outcome. Efforts to minimize ventilator-induced lung injury (VILI) should start in the emergency department (ED), immediately following intubation.[25]

Two decades since the publication of the landmark ARDS network trial of lower tidal volume ventilation (LTVV), targeting a tidal volume of less than or equal to 6 mL/kg predicted body weight and maintaining a plateau pressure less than 30 cm of water (H_2O) remains the best-tested method for minimizing VILI in ARDS patients, with robust evidence demonstrating that LTVV reduces mortality and increases ventilator-free days in this population.[26] All EPs should initiate lung-protective LTVV for any intubated patient who meets the criteria for ARDS. Details of the LTVV protocol used by the ARDS network are summarized in **Box 1**, though many institutions have their own lung protective ventilation protocols and order-sets in place to help clinicians adhere to this best practice in patients with ARDS. Common pitfalls when instituting lung protective ventilation in the ED include failure to use predicted body weight, failure to adjust tidal volume based on plateau pressures, and failure to adjust Fio_2 and PEEP on an ongoing basis.

What about patients who do not meet criteria for ARDS? There is increasing evidence that LTVV improves outcomes for patients without ARDS as well, suggesting that this approach should be used in all intubated patients unless there is a contraindication to its use.[27,28] Although a recent randomized trial showed no difference between LTVV and intermediate tidal volume ventilation ($\leq$10 mL/kg predicted body weight) in subjects without ARDS, it should be noted that even in the intermediate tidal volume group, tidal volume was decreased if plateau pressure exceeded 25 cm H_2O, and mean tidal volume was less than 10 mL/kg.[29] Because this trial does not rule out harm that might result from higher tidal volumes or plateau pressures, and because

---

Box 1
Sample lung protective ventilation protocol

1. Calculate PBW
   Male PBW: 50 + 2.3 (height in inches − 60)
   Female PBW: 45.5 + 2.3 (height in inches − 60)

2. Select any ventilator mode and select settings to achieve V_T of 8 mL/kg PBW

3. Reduce V_T by 1 mL/kg at intervals <2 h until V_T = 6 mL/kg PBW

4. Set initial RR to approximate baseline minute ventilation (max RR = 35)

5. Adjust V_T and RR to achieve P_{plat} and pH goals
   • If P_{plat} greater than 30 cm H_2O, reduce V_T by 1 mL/kg PBW (minimum = 4 mL/kg PBW)
   • If pH <7.30, increase RR (maximum = 35)
   • If pH <7.15, increase RR to 35, consider sodium bicarbonate administration, or increase V_T

6. Adjust Fio_2 and PEEP to achieve a Pao_2 of 55 to 80 mm Hg or SpO2 88% to 95%

   Lower PEEP or higher Fio_2 option

Fio_2	0.3	0.4	0.4	0.5	0.5	0.6	0.7	0.7	0.7	0.8	0.9	0.9	0.9	1.0
PEEP	5	5	8	8	10	10	10	12	14	14	14	16	18	18–24

   Higher PEEP/Lower Fio_2 option

Fio_2	0.3	0.3	0.3	0.3	0.3	0.4	0.4	0.5	0.5	0.5–0.8	0.8	0.9	1.0	1.0
PEEP	5	8	10	12	14	14	16	16	18	20	22	22	22	24

Abbreviations: P_{plat}, plateau pressure (airway pressure at the end of delivery of a tidal volume breath during a condition of no airflow); PBW, predicted body weight; RR, respiratory rate; V_T, tidal volume.

From the ARDSNet. Available at: http://ardsnet.org/files/ventilator_protocol_2008-07.pdf.

recognition of ARDS may be delayed, there is still a trend toward defaulting to LTVV unless contraindicated.[30]

Although there is no absolute contraindication to lower tidal volumes per se, the higher PEEP, lower oxygenation targets, and permissive hypercapnia permitted by lung protective ventilation protocols can be problematic for some patients. For example, patients with neurologic injury or significant pulmonary hypertension may require higher oxygenation targets and eucapnia, which are not the goal in standard lung protective ventilation. Other examples include patients with active airway obstruction, who may require slightly higher tidal volumes to allow for slower respiratory rates to prevent air trapping, or patients with pneumothorax who should not be placed on high PEEP. Finally, some patients tolerate LTVV poorly and develop significant ventilator dyssynchrony. In some cases the risks of the deep sedation or neuromuscular blockade (NMB) that may be required to achieve ventilator synchrony with low tidal volumes may be greater than the benefits of strict adherence to a tidal volume of less than or equal to 6 mL/kg predicted body weight.

Positive End-Expiratory Pressure and Recruitment Maneuvers

As shown by the 2 Fio_2/PEEP charts in **Box 1**, the PEEP applied during lung protective ventilation can vary. Many clinicians simply use the default FiO_2-PEEP combination that is part of their institutional LTVV protocol, or defer to institutional preferences for higher or lower PEEP. Often, the fear of barotrauma from higher PEEP supersedes concerns about underrecruitment and alveolar collapse, and the lower PEEP strategy is pursued unless a patient develops worsening hypoxemia. Indeed, understanding how to select the optimal PEEP for a patient with respiratory failure remains an open question, with conflicting data on whether a higher PEEP strategy is preferred in patients with more severe hypoxemia.[31,32] In light of this uncertainty, the authors recommend gradual adjustments in PEEP, adhering to PEEP/Fio_2 combinations that are within the range already tested by ARDS network (ie, PEEP not lower than the low PEEP/Fio_2 chart and not higher than the high PEEP/Fio_2 chart).

Based on the results of the Alveolar Recruitment for Acute Respiratory Distress Syndrome Trial (ART), which suggested possible harm associated with recruitment maneuvers, the authors recommend against the routine use of recruitment maneuvers except by experienced clinicians in specific circumstances.[26]

Alternative Modes of Ventilation

Traditionally, an assist control mode (either volume control or pressure control ventilation) is used to target low tidal volumes. Based on the results of 2 large, multicenter randomized trials published in 2013, high-frequency oscillating ventilation, in which very small tidal volumes are delivered at high frequency, is no longer a routine part of care for patients with severe ARDS or refractory hypoxemia.[33,34]

Another alternative mode of ventilation, known as airway pressure release ventilation (APRV), allows spontaneous breathing on top of high levels of PEEP with intermittent releases of applied airway pressure to allow for ventilation (**Fig. 3**). The idea behind APRV is to use higher mean airway pressure to improve alveolar recruitment and oxygenation while decreasing the atelectrauma and regional overdistension of the lung that contributes to VILI. Although there is some evidence that early use of APRV can improve outcomes in patients with ARDS,[35] the available data do not support the routine use of APRV in hypoxemic patients in the ED.

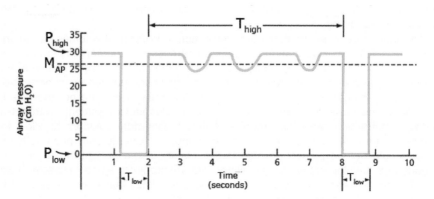

Fig. 3. Pressure versus time curve in APRV. P high, the high PEEP; P low, the low PEEP; T high, the duration of P high; T low, the duration of P low. (*From* Wikimedia Commons. Available at: https://commons.wikimedia.org/wiki/File:Airway_pressure_release_ventilation_graph.png.)

ADJUNCTIVE THERAPIES FOR THE ACUTE RESPIRATORY DISTRESS SYNDROME

ARDS is a multifactorial syndrome with heterogenous causes and phenotypes. It is likely because of this heterogeneity that any effective targeted pharmacotherapy for the syndrome is yet to be discovered. To date, no phase III drug trial has yielded any mortality benefit in ARDS, even though many potential therapies have been tested (eg, surfactant, aspirin, statins, activated protein C, and keratinocyte growth factor).[36] Management, therefore, remains focused on lung protective ventilation strategies to prevent VILI, as previously discussed, combined with adjunctive supportive therapies.

Fluid Conservative Strategy

Fluid resuscitation is strongly recommended in sepsis and is currently the first-line treatment of septic shock. In the patient with lung injury, however, aggressive fluid resuscitation must be balanced with the risk of pulmonary edema and worsening hypoxemia. Before the 2006 Fluids and Catheter Treatment trial (FACTT), which compared a liberal versus a conservative fluid administration strategy in ARDS, there was no definitive evidence regarding appropriate fluid administration in such patients.[37] Though no mortality benefit was shown, subjects assigned to the fluid conservative arm had significantly more ventilator-free days without increased need for dialysis. As such, after initial resuscitation, fluid administration should be minimized in patients with ARDS, unless the patient remains in shock that is likely to be volume responsive.

Glucocorticoids

As previously discussed, ARDS is a heterogenous syndrome; retrospective analyses of large ARDS trials have revealed 2 distinct subphenotypes, 1 of which is marked by greater inflammation and worse outcomes.[38] This may explain why evidence supporting the use of glucocorticoids in unselected patients with ARDS is equivalent at best. It also raises the question, however, if appropriately selected ARDS patients may in fact benefit from steroid administration. Indeed, current Society of Critical Care Medicine and European Society of Intensive Care Unit (ICU) Medicine guidelines recommend the use of methylprednisolone (1 mg/kg/d) early in the course of moderate to severe ARDS, though is only a conditional recommendation supported by moderate quality evidence.[39] The authors look forward to further studies examining the use of steroids in more carefully selected ARDS subjects.

MANAGEMENT OF SEVERE OR REFRACTORY HYPOXEMIA

Even after successful intubation and initiation of appropriate lung protective ventilation, many patients develop worsening hypoxemia despite increasing levels of Fio_2 and PEEP. In this case, the authors suggest clinicians troubleshoot for easily reversible causes before escalating to more intensive interventions.

Troubleshooting

Any new or worsening hypoxemia in the mechanically ventilated patient requires immediate assessment. The EP should examine the patient, noting changes in vital signs, chest expansion, and lung sounds. One commonly used checklist to thoroughly evaluate postintubation hypoxemia is the DOPES mnemonic (**Fig. 4**). The ventilator should be checked for the appropriateness of the settings (ie, adequate PEEP) or problems with patient–ventilator interaction (eg, breath stacking or ventilator dyssynchrony). In most cases, repeat lung ultrasound and chest radiograph should be obtained as soon as possible to evaluate for pneumothorax; endotracheal tube malpositioning; worsening edema, consolidation, or effusion; or lobar collapse. During this evaluation, the patient may require bag ventilation at an Fio_2 of 1 to maintain adequate arterial oxygen saturation.

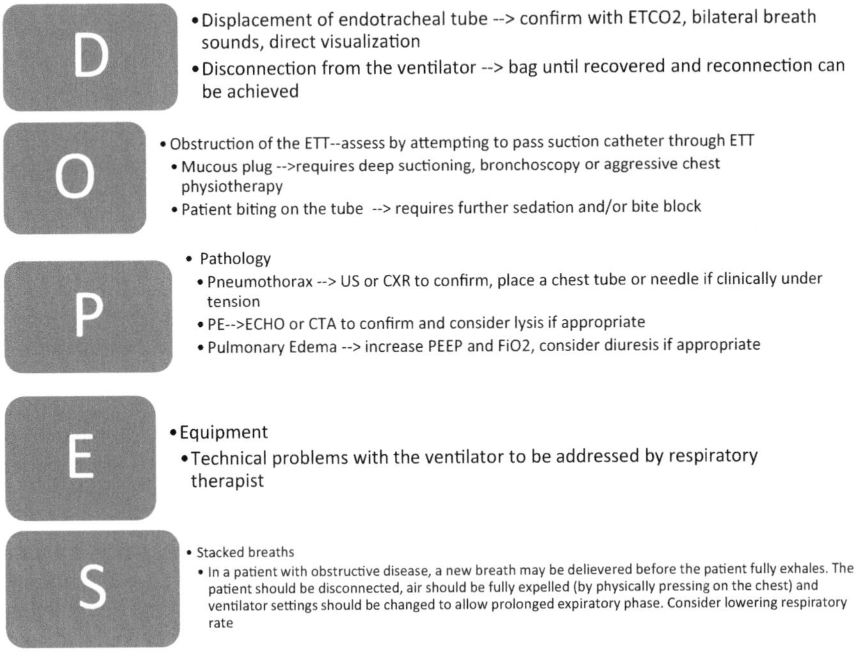

D
- Displacement of endotracheal tube --> confirm with ETCO2, bilateral breath sounds, direct visualization
- Disconnection from the ventilator --> bag until recovered and reconnection can be achieved

O
- Obstruction of the ETT--assess by attempting to pass suction catheter through ETT
- Mucous plug -->requires deep suctioning, bronchoscopy or aggressive chest physiotherapy
- Patient biting on the tube --> requires further sedation and/or bite block

P
- Pathology
  - Pneumothorax --> US or CXR to confirm, place a chest tube or needle if clinically under tension
  - PE-->ECHO or CTA to confirm and consider lysis if appropriate
  - Pulmonary Edema --> increase PEEP and FiO2, consider diuresis if appropriate

E
- Equipment
- Technical problems with the ventilator to be addressed by respiratory therapist

S
- Stacked breaths
  - In a patient with obstructive disease, a new breath may be delievered before the patient fully exhales. The patient should be disconnected, air should be fully expelled (by physically pressing on the chest) and ventilator settings should be changed to allow prolonged expiratory phase. Consider lowering respiratory rate

Fig. 4. Algorithm for assessing postintubation hypoxemia. CTA, computed tomography with angiography; CXR, chest radiograph; Echo, echocardiogram; ETCO2, end-tidal carbon dioxide; ETT, endotracheal tube; PE, pulmonary embolism; US, ultrasound.

If hypoxemia persists after any easily reversible causes have been addressed, there are several additional tools that may be available to the EP to support the patient and improve gas exchange.

Paralytics

NMB is an important tool in the management of patients with worsening hypoxemia or significant ventilator dyssynchrony that is not responsive to deeper sedation. Currently, the best available data suggest that the early use of NMB in patients with moderate-to-severe ARDS is associated with both a mortality benefit and increased ventilator-free days without increasing rates of ICU-acquired muscle weakness.[40] Prolonged infusions such as cisatracurium are most often used, starting at a dose of 1 to 2 mcg/kg/min and titrating to train-of-4. It is important to note this was a single-center study that applies only to patients in the first 48 hours of ARDS. Funded by the National Institutes of Health, the Prevention and Early Treatment of Acute Lung Injury (PETAL) trials network is currently analyzing data from a multicenter RCT to clarify the use of continuous NMB in moderate-to-severe ARDS. In the interim, the authors suggest that, provided the patient is adequately sedated, initiating NMB in the ED should be considered for any patient with a Pao_2/Fio_2 ratio less than 150, especially if there is any component of ventilator dyssynchrony.

Prone Positioning

Based on the results of a multicenter European RCT of prone positioning showing a significant reduction in mortality in patients with ARDS and a sustained Pao_2/Fio_2 ratio less than 150, many ICUs will place patients with severe ARDS in the prone position.[41] Prone positioning is believed to improve outcomes through promoting more homogenous alveolar recruitment, improving ventilation to perfusion ratio matching, and decreasing stress and strain on the lungs. However, due to the associated logistical challenges, lack of experienced providers, and shorter lengths-of-stay, prone positioning is likely outside the scope of routine ED care.

Inhaled Vasodilators

Though no mortality benefit has been demonstrated with the use of inhaled vasodilators (eg, epoprostenol or nitric oxide), they do improve the Pao_2.[42] Although these therapies can be a used as a bridge to more definitive care, they are often not readily available, and the EP and respiratory therapists must be familiar with their use. In addition, these medications can increase preload to the left heart and should be used with caution in patients with severe left-sided heart failure. The authors, therefore, recommend against their routine use by EPs, except in consultation with an intensivist.

Extracorporeal Membrane Oxygenation

As a final resort for truly refractory hypoxemia, the EP should consult for initiation of venovenous extracorporeal membrane oxygenation (ECMO) in appropriately selected patients. ECMO offers complete pulmonary support and is used to oxygenate blood while the lungs are essentially nonfunctional.

The Murray lung score (**Table 4**) may be useful in deciding when to initiate the process of transferring or consulting for ECMO.[43] A Murray lung score of 3 or greater in selected ARDS patients (ie, patients without contraindications to anticoagulation, other likely terminal conditions, or poor neurologic prognosis) has been used as a trigger for consultation to an ECMO service.[44]

To date, the 2 most well-designed studies of ECMO for ARDS are the CESAR trial and the extracorporeal membrane oxygenation for severe Acute respiratory distress

Table 4 The Murray lung injury score	
Murray Acute Lung Injury Score	
Chest Radiograph Score	
No alveolar consolidation	0
Alveolar consolidation confined to 1 quadrant	1
Alveolar consolidation confined to 2 quadrants	2
Alveolar consolidation confined to 3 quadrants	3
Alveolar consolidation confined to all 4 quadrants	4
Hypoxemia Score	
$Pao_2/Fio_2 \geq 300$ mm Hg	0
Pao_2/Fio_2 225–299 mm Hg	1
Pao_2/Fio_2 175–224 mm Hg	2
Pao_2/Fio_2 100–174 mm Hg	3
$Pao_2/Fio_2 <100$ mm Hg	4
PEEP Score	
PEEP ≤ 5	0
PEEP 6–8	1
PEEP 9–11	2
PEEP 12–14	3
PEEP ≥ 15	4
Respiratory Compliance (Tv/[PIP-PEEP])	
≥ 80	0
60–79	1
40–59	2
20–39	3
≤ 19	4

Abbreviations: PIP, positive inspiratory pressure; Tv, tidal volume.
   A score of 3 or greater, or a pH lower than 7.20, should prompt consideration of consultation to an ECMO service in cases of potentially reversible respiratory failure.
   Reprinted with permission of the American Thoracic Society. Copyright © 2019 American Thoracic Society. Murray JF, Matthay MA, Luce JM, and Flick MR. An expanded definition of the adult respiratory distress syndrome. Am Rev Respir Dis. 1988;138:720-3. The American Journal of Respiratory and Critical Care Medicine is an official journal of the American Thoracic Society.

syndrome (EOLIA) trial. The conventional ventilatory support vs extracorporeal membrane oxygenation for severe adult respiratory failure (CESAR) trial demonstrated a significant survival benefit of ECMO in ARDS; however, it remained unclear whether the benefit was derived from ECMO itself, or due to simultaneous interventions and expert management at the ECMO-referral center.[38] In contrast, The EOLIA trial was stopped for futility after 5 years of data collection.[45] Although there was an 11% reduction in all-cause mortality in the ECMO arm ($P = .07$) at the time the trial was stopped, this difference was not projected to meet predetermined goals for statistical significance. Additionally, nearly one-third of the control group required crossover to the ECMO arm of the study, further suggesting the utility of veno-venous ECMO despite the nominally negative result. These considerations contribute to ongoing debate within the critical care community and do not definitively rule out the benefit of ECMO in severe ARDS.

   Based on existing data, EPs should still consider consultation for ECMO as a salvage for appropriate patients with severe ARDS and a Murray lung score of 3 or greater, who have not improved despite initiation of appropriate lung protective ventilation and supportive therapies. It may be that only a transfer to an ECMO-capable center can benefit such patients. It is the authors' experience that early initiation of these conversations helps facilitate efficient transitions of care in these vulnerable AHRF patients.

SUMMARY

AHRF is a common challenge faced by EPs. Although noninvasive support may be sufficient in many cases, a significant portion of patients progress to require endotracheal intubation. During intubation, maximizing preoxygenation (to the extent possible) and first-pass intubation success are of vital importance. Once intubated, meticulous attention to ventilator management can help reduce VILI and improve outcomes. LTVV targeting a tidal volume of less than or equal to 6 mL/kg predicted body weight and maintaining a plateau pressure less than 30 cm H_2O remains the cornerstone of supportive care for patients with ARDS, and lower tidal volumes and plateau pressures may even benefit intubated patients who do not meet criteria for ARDS. For patients who develop worsening or refractory hypoxemia, NMB and referral for ECMO consideration may be necessary. Understanding this step-wise approach to managing the patient with AHRF is important even in early stages of illness and is key to improving downstream outcomes for AHRF patients requiring mechanical ventilation in the ED.

REFERENCES

1. Stefan MS, Shieh MS, Pekow PS, et al. Epidemiology and outcomes of acute respiratory failure in the United States, 2001 to 2009: a national survey. J Hosp Med 2013;8(2):76–82.
2. Ranieri VM, Rubenfeld GD, Thompson BT, et al. Acute respiratory distress syndrome: the Berlin definition. JAMA 2012;307(23):2526–33.
3. Zhao H, Wang H, Sun F, et al. High-flow nasal cannula oxygen therapy is superior to conventional oxygen therapy but not to noninvasive mechanical ventilation on intubation rate: a systematic review and meta-analysis. Crit Care 2017;21:184.
4. Frat JP, Thille AW, Mercat A, et al. High-flow oxygen through nasal cannula in acute hypoxemic respiratory failure. N Engl J Med 2015;372(23):2185–96.
5. Mebazaa A, Gheorghiade M, Piña IL, et al. Practical recommendations for prehospital and early in-hospital management of patients presenting with acute heart failure syndromes. Crit Care Med 2008;36(1 Suppl):S129–39.
6. International Consensus Conferences in Intensive care medicine: noninvasive positive pressure ventilation in acute respiratory failure. Am J Respir Crit Care Med 2001;163(1):283–91.
7. Xu XP, Zhang XC, Hu SL, et al. Noninvasive ventilation in acute hypoxemic non-hypercapnic respiratory failure: a systematic review and meta-analysis. Crit Care Med 2017;45(7):e727–33.
8. Antonelli M, Conti G, Moro ML, et al. Predictors of failure of noninvasive positive pressure ventilation in patients with acute hypoxemic respiratory failure: a multicenter study. Intensive Care Med 2001;27(11):1718–28.
9. Valley TS, Walkey AJ, Lindenauer PK, et al. Association between noninvasive ventilation and mortality among older patients with pneumonia. Crit Care Med 2017;45(3):e246–54.
10. Carteaux G, Millan-Guilarte T, De Prost N, et al. Failure of noninvasive ventilation for de novo acute hypoxemic respiratory failure: role of tidal volume. Crit Care Med 2016;44(2):282–90.

11. Rochwerg B, Brochard L, Elliott MW, et al. Official ERS/ATS clinical practice guidelines: noninvasive ventilation for acute respiratory failure. Eur Respir J 2017;50(2).

12. Ahmed A, Azim A. Difficult tracheal intubation in critically ill. J Intensive Care 2018;6:49.

13. Weingart SD, Levitan RM. Preoxygenation and prevention of desaturation during emergency airway management. Ann Emerg Med 2012;59(3):165–75.e1.

14. Lane S, Saunders D, Schofield A, et al. A prospective, randomised controlled trial comparing the efficacy of pre-oxygenation in the 20 degrees head-up vs supine position. Anaesthesia 2005;60(11):1064–7.

15. Altermatt FR, Munoz HR, Delfino AE, et al. Pre-oxygenation in the obese patient: effects of position on tolerance to apnoea. Br J Anaesth 2005;95(5):706–9.

16. El-Khatib MF, Kanazi G, Baraka AS. Noninvasive bilevel positive airway pressure for preoxygenation of the critically ill morbidly obese patient. Can J Anaesth 2007; 54(9):744–7.

17. Ramachandran SK, Cosnowski A, Shanks A, et al. Apneic oxygenation during prolonged laryngoscopy in obese patients: a randomized, controlled trial of nasal oxygen administration. J Clin Anesth 2010;22(3):164–8.

18. Taha SK, Siddik-Sayyid SM, El-Khatib MF, et al. Nasopharyngeal oxygen insufflation following pre-oxygenation using the four deep breath technique. Anaesthesia 2006;61(5):427–30.

19. Semler MW, Janz DR, Lentz RJ, et al. Randomized trial of apneic oxygenation during endotracheal intubation of the critically ill. Am J Respir Crit Care Med 2016;193(3):273–80.

20. Oliveira J E Silva L, Cabrera D, Barrionuevo P, et al. Effectiveness of Apneic oxygenation during intubation: a systematic review and meta-analysis. Ann Emerg Med 2017;70(4):483–94.

21. Farmery AD, Roe PG. A model to describe the rate of oxyhaemoglobin desaturation during apnoea. Br J Anaesth 1996;76(2):284–91.

22. Sakles JC, Chiu S, Mosier J, et al. The importance of first pass success when performing orotracheal intubation in the emergency department. Acad Emerg Med 2013;20:71–8.

23. Lewis SR, Butler AR, Parker J, et al. Videolaryngoscopy versus direct laryngoscopy for adult patients requiring tracheal intubation. Cochrane Database Syst Rev 2016;(11):CD011136.

24. Driver B, Dodd K, Klein LR, et al. The Bougie and first-pass success in the emergency department. Ann Emerg Med 2017;70(4):473–8.

25. Fuller BM, Mohr NM, Miller CN, et al. Mechanical ventilation and ARDS in the ED: a multicenter, observational, prospective, cross-sectional study. Chest 2015; 148(2):365–74.

26. Acute Respiratory Distress Syndrome Network, Brower RG, Matthay MA, Morris A, et al. Ventilation with lower tidal volumes as compared with traditional tidal volumes for acute lung injury and the acute respiratory distress syndrome. N Engl J Med 2000;342(18):1301–8.

27. Serpa Neto A, Cardoso SO, Manetta JA, et al. Association between use of lung-protective ventilation with lower tidal volumes and clinical outcomes among patients without acute respiratory distress syn- drome: a meta-analysis. JAMA 2012;308(16):1651–9.

28. Futier E, Constantin JM, Paugam-Burtz C, et al. A trial of intraopera- tive low-tidal-volume ventilation in abdominal surgery. N Engl J Med 2013;369(5):428–37.

29. Writing Group for the PReVENT Investigators, Simonis FD, Serpa Neto A, Binnekade JM, et al. Effect of a low vs intermediate tidal volume strategy on ventilator-free days in intensive care unit patients without ARDS: a randomized clinical trial. JAMA 2018;320(18):1872–80.

30. Sjoding MW, Gong MN, Haas CF, et al. Evaluating delivery of low tidal volume ventilation in six ICUs using electronic health record data. Crit Care Med 2019; 47(1):56–61.

31. Briel M, Meade M, Mercat A, et al. Higher vs lower positive end- expiratory pressure in patients with acute lung injury and acute respiratory distress syndrome: systematic review and meta-analysis. JAMA 2010;303(9):865–73.

32. Writing Group for the Alveolar Recruitment for Acute Respiratory Distress Syndrome Trial (ART) Investigators, Cavalcanti AB, Suzumura ÉA, Laranjeira LN, et al. Effect of lung recruitment and titrated positive end-expiratory pressure (PEEP) vs low PEEP on mortality in patients with acute respiratory distress syndrome: a randomized clinical trial. JAMA 2017;318:1335–45.

33. Young D, Lamb SE, Shah S, et al. High-frequency oscillation for acute respiratory distress syndrome. N Engl J Med 2013;368(9):806–13.

34. Ferguson ND, Cook DJ, Guyatt GH, et al. High-frequency oscillation in early acute respiratory distress syndrome. N Engl J Med 2013;368(9):795–805.

35. Zhou Y, Jin X, Lv Y, et al. Early application of airway pressure release ventilation may reduce the duration of mechanical ventilation in acute respiratory distress syndrome. Intensive Care Med 2017;43:1648–59.

36. Wilson JG, Matthay MA. Mechanical ventilation in acute hypoxemic respiratory failure: a review of new strategies for the practicing hospitalist. J Hosp Med 2014;9(7):469–75.

37. National Heart, Lung, and Blood Institute Acute Respiratory Distress Syndrome (ARDS) Clinical Trials Network, Wiedemann HP, Wheeler AP, Bernard GR, et al. Comparison of two fluid-management strategies in acute lung injury. N Engl J Med 2006;354(24):2564–75.

38. Calfee CS, Delucchi K, Parsons PE, et al. Subphenotypes in acute respiratory distress syndrome: latent class analysis of data from two randomised controlled trials. Lancet Respir Med 2014;2(8):611–20.

39. Annane D, Pastores SM, Rochwerg B, et al. Guidelines for the diagnosis and management of critical illness-related corticosteroid insufficiency (CIRCI) in critically ill patients (part i): society of critical care medicine (SCCM) and European Society of Intensive Care Medicine (ESICM) 2017. Crit Care Med 2017;45(12):2078–88.

40. Papazian L, Forel JM, Gacouin A, et al. Neuromuscular blockers in early acute respiratory distress syndrome. N Engl J Med 2010;363(12):1107–16.

41. Guerin C, Reignier J, Richard JC, et al. Prone positioning in severe acute respiratory distress syndrome. N Engl J Med 2013;368(23):2159–68.

42. Cherian SV, Kumar A, Akasapu K, et al. Salvage therapies for refractory hypoxemia in ARDS. Respir Med 2018;141:150–8.

43. Murray JF, Matthay MA, Luce JM, et al. An expanded definition of the adult respiratory distress syndrome. Am Rev Respir Dis 1988;138:720–3.

44. Peek GJ, Mugford M, Tiruvoipati R, et al. Efficacy and economic assessment of conventional ventilatory support versus extracorporeal membrane oxygenation for severe adult respiratory failure (CESAR): a multicentre randomised controlled trial. Lancet 2009;374(9698):1351–63.

45. Combes A, Hajage D, Capellier G, et al. Extracorporeal membrane oxygenation for severe acute respiratory distress syndrome. N Engl J Med 2018;378(21): 1965–75.

Mechanical Ventilation Strategies for the Patient with Severe Obstructive Lung Disease

Jarrod M. Mosier, MD[a,b,*], Cameron D. Hypes, MD, MPH[a,b]

KEYWORDS

- Ventilatory failure • Emergency department • Auto-PEEP • Air trapping
- Mechanical ventilation • Dynamic hyperinflation • Bronchospasm

KEY POINTS

- Noninvasive methods of respiratory support to improve work of breathing should be attempted to avoid the untoward difficulties of invasive mechanical ventilation.
- Patients with severe obstructive lung disease are often dyssynchronous with the ventilator and require deep sedation and often neuromuscular blockade to prevent ventilator-associated injuries.
- Adequate exhalation time should be monitored by assessing the expiratory flow waveform on the ventilator.
- Air trapping and auto-positive end-expiratory pressure should be evaluated and managed to prevent decompensation from high intrathoracic pressure and ventilator-induced lung injury.
- Allow permissive hypercapnia as long as the patient has hemodynamic stability and lacks contraindications such as pregnancy or elevated intracranial pressure.

INTRODUCTION

Most critically ill patients who are admitted to the intensive care unit (ICU) come through the emergency department (ED), and many of them spend a significant time in the ED.[1] Mechanical ventilation is one of the most common therapies required in those patients while in the ED, thus it is important for emergency physicians to skillfully

[a] Department of Emergency Medicine, University of Arizona College of Medicine, 1501 North Campbell Avenue, PO Box 245057, Tucson, AZ 85724-5057, USA; [b] Department of Medicine, Division of Pulmonary, Allergy, Critical Care and Sleep, University of Arizona College of Medicine, Tucson, AZ, USA
* Corresponding author. Department of Emergency Medicine, University of Arizona College of Medicine, University of Arizona, 1501 North Campbell Avenue, PO Box 245057, Tucson, AZ 85724-5057, USA.
E-mail address: JMosier@aemrc.arizona.edu

Emerg Med Clin N Am 37 (2019) 445–458
https://doi.org/10.1016/j.emc.2019.04.003
0733-8627/19/© 2019 Elsevier Inc. All rights reserved.

manage challenging patients on mechanical ventilation. Currently, patients in the ED often do not receive optimal lung protective ventilatory strategies. Of all intubated patients in the ED, lung protective ventilation was shown to be used in only half of all patients, and 15% developed acute respiratory distress syndrome (ARDS) with a mean onset of 2 days after hospital admission.[2] Wilcox reported that in addition to injurious tidal volumes, most patients are ventilated with low positive end-expiratory pressure and high fraction of inspired oxygen,[3] which are significant risk factors for ventilator-induced lung injury and the development or worsening of ARDS. Worse, few ventilator changes are ever made until the patient gets out of the ED. Thus, the quality and safety of mechanical ventilation represents a large target for improvement for our specialty regardless of cause.

Common goals of mechanical ventilation include optimizing patient-ventilator synchrony, reducing iatrogenic injury, and supporting gas exchange in a way that accounts underlying pathophysiology. The authors use the workflow in **Fig. 1** and summarize the salient points further.

Patient-ventilator synchrony: ventilators work by opening a valve to allow the flow of gas into the circuit to either a pressure or a volume target. Once that target is reached, the inspiratory valve is closed and an expiratory valve is opened to allow the efflux of respiratory gases. The valves can be opened by the ventilator itself if the patient is not breathing, or they can be opened by patient effort crossing a flow or pressure trigger threshold. Optimal outcomes come from when the patient and the ventilator are synchronous, not just in terms of patient comfort but in avoiding lung injury from volutrauma or barotrauma. Often in the setting of acute critical illness this requires deep sedation and sometimes continuous neuromuscular blockade. The first priority when establishing patient-ventilator synchrony is adequate sedation. The details of analgosedation strategy for mechanically ventilated patients are discussed further in Christopher Noel and Haney Mallemat's article, "Sedation and Analgesia for Mechanically Ventilated Patients in the Emergency Department," in this issue, but are briefly summarized here, as it is critical for managing the ventilator in these challenging patients.

Principally, postintubation sedation is based around the concept of analgosedation—address *analgesia* first.[4] A narcotic is started for analgesia, and at higher doses narcotics such as fentanyl have sedative properties as well. Of the commonly available narcotic infusions, fentanyl is the optimal for analgosedation, as it has a rapid onset, is easily titratable, has a sedative effect, and is hemodynamically neutral. The typical starting dose is 150 to 250 mcg/h, with 50 to 100 mcg boluses at the time of initiation and then intermittently as necessary. Many patients in the ED who require intubation are in the early resuscitation phase and require painful procedures, transport, etc., and thus a deeper sedation level is usually required. Ideally, one would start with intermittent sedative boluses; however, given the logistical constraints of the ED and early resuscitation period, a continuous sedative infusion is often required. Propofol is an excellent choice as a continuous sedative for the same reasons as fentanyl. Dexmedetomidine is also a good choice but will not achieve the same depth of sedation as propofol. Midazolam is another option, although benzodiazepine infusions for sedation have been associated with a higher incidence of delirium in these patients, and it is better used in bolus dosing regimens rather than as a continuous infusion if possible.[4] All drugs should be titrated to a specified goal level of sedation, as oversedation, while clinically less dramatic than undersedation, is also harmful (**Box 1**). A sedation scoring regimen such as the Richmond Agitation-Sedation Scale[5] (see Table 1 in Ref 5) should be implemented in both the ED and ICU to facilitate precise and appropriate sedation for a given clinical scenario.

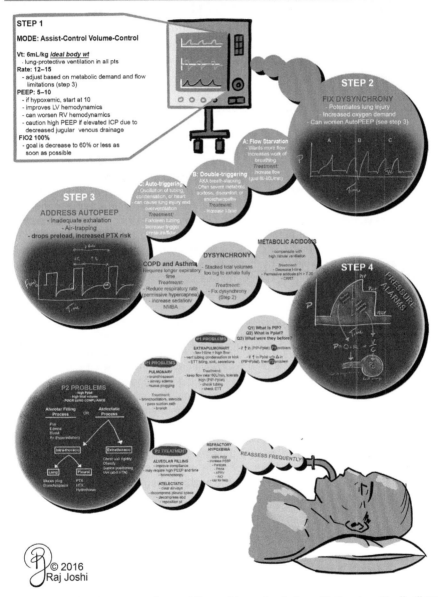

Fig. 1. Infographic illustrating the workflow with mechanical ventilation in critically ill ED patients. Credit: Raj Joshi, MD for developing the infographic for the authors' emergency medicine residents.

Box 1
Pearls for routine postintubation care in the emergency department

1. Continuous fentanyl infusion—start 150 mcg/h, bolus 100mcg IV, and titrate infusion rate up as needed.

2. Continuous sedative infusion—start propofol at 20 to 60mcg/kg/h.

3. RASS goal −3 until painful procedures, neuromuscular blockade, and transport are complete, then goal 0.

4. Elevate head of the bed to 30°.

5. Gastric decompression.

Reduce iatrogenic injury: iatrogenic injury related to mechanical ventilation involves infectious (ventilator-associated pneumonia) and mechanical causes (ventilator-induced lung injury). There are many ventilator-associated pneumonia bundles in existence; however, some simple and effective methods of reducing ventilator-associated pneumonia are to elevate the head of the bed to 30 degrees and place an oro- or nasogastric tube to prevent aspiration of gastric contents.[6] Mechanical complications include barotrauma and volutrauma, among others, collectively termed "ventilator-induced lung injury" and are a result of injurious volumes and transalveolar pressures. These are avoided by carefully choosing ventilator settings, achieving patient-ventilatory synchrony and then reassessing frequently as these are dynamic variables.

Support gas exchange while respecting the underlying pathophysiology: this article focuses on patients with obstructive lung disease, mainly chronic obstructive pulmonary disease (COPD) and asthma. Patients with dynamic hyperinflation in COPD have an outflow obstruction, meaning that inspiratory flow is preserved but on exhalation the air is trapped by airway collapse. Similarly in asthma there is a fixed obstruction from bronchospasm and airway edema that disproportionately reduces expiratory flow. As additional gas is retained with each breath, the only way to continue ventilation is to breathe at an increasingly higher residual intrathoracic volume, reducing inspiratory muscle efficiency and tidal volumes, resulting in fatigue, increased dead space fraction, and ventilatory failure. The primary goals of mechanical ventilation in obstructive lung pathophysiologies are to reduce the work of breathing, maintain an acceptable blood pH, and limit auto-positive end-expiratory pressure (auto-PEEP) while targeted therapies work to reduce the outflow obstruction. Mechanical ventilation is the bridge that provides the time for other therapies to exert their effect.

NONINVASIVE STRATEGIES FOR OBSTRUCTIVE LUNG DISEASE

One attractive method of avoiding patient-ventilator dyssynchrony is to avoid intubation altogether. There are 2 commonly used methods of noninvasive respiratory support: noninvasive positive pressure ventilation (often known as continuous positive airway pressure [CPAP]/bilevel positive airway pressure [BiPAP]) and high-flow nasal insufflation. Noninvasive positive pressure ventilation has been shown to reduce intubation rate and improve work of breathing in patients with COPD exacerbations.[7–9] Thus, it has become a standard therapy in patients presenting to the ED with respiratory failure secondary to COPD but preserved mentation. Work of breathing is improved with the application of pressure support (inspiratory positive airway pressure [IPAP]) and externally applied PEEP (expiratory positive airway pressure [EPAP]) to offset auto-PEEP (also known as intrinsic PEEP, caused by dynamic hyperinflation). High-flow nasal insufflation has been shown to be useful in this patient population as well but robust data are lacking.[10,11] In patients with asthma, the literature is unclear regarding the optimal use of noninvasive ventilation or high-flow nasal insufflation. Regardless, if a patient with asthma exacerbation is developing respiratory failure secondary to high work of breathing, it is reasonable to think either therapy may reduce the risk of intubation. The pressure differential between the IPAP and the EPAP drives ventilation with a larger pressure difference, resulting in larger tidal volumes and increased ventilation. Tidal volumes and minute ventilation should be monitored closely before and after any noninvasive positive pressure ventilation (NIPPV) setting changes so that any effect can be detected in real-time. In patients with respiratory failure secondary to an obstructive upper airway lesion, noninvasive strategies should not be attempted and patients are generally easy to manage on the ventilator once the tracheal tube bypasses the obstruction (**Table 1**).

INVASIVE STRATEGIES FOR OBSTRUCTIVE LUNG DISEASE

Ventilator mode selection: in patients who require invasive mechanical ventilation with an endotracheal tube, the first task is to choose a mode of ventilation that targets either a pressure or a volume when the inspiratory valve is opened. There are advantages and disadvantages to both modes, and when one mode is not working oftentimes the answer to improve patient ventilator synchrony is to change to the other mode. In pressure-targeted modes, once the inspiratory valve is open the ventilator allows an inspiratory flow of gases (composition based on the set Fio_2) until the target pressure is reached (pressure is set, volume is dependent). When the exhalation valve is opened, dead space and alveolar gas effluxes from the lungs until the desired PEEP

Table 1
Pearls for managing noninvasive respiratory support

Noninvasive Positive Pressure Ventilation	High-Flow Nasal Insufflation
Start: 1. COPD: EPAP 5–8, IPAP 5–10, Fio_2 80%–100% 2. Asthma: EPAP 0–5, IPAP 5–10 Fio_2 100%	Start: 1. Flow: 50% of maximum 2. Fio_2: 100%
Adjust: 1. Titrate up IPAP (asthma and COPD) and EPAP (COPD) as tolerated to reduce work of breathing—monitor changes in tidal volume and minute ventilation 2. To increase ventilation, increase the gradient between IPAP:EPAP 3. Wean Fio_2 as tolerated to keep O2 sat >88%	Adjust: 1. Increase flow to reduce work of breathing and increase CO2 clearance 2. Wean Fio_2 as tolerated to keep O2 sat >88%
Wean: 1. Reduce IPAP:EPAP gradient as work of breathing improves	Wean: 1. Reduce flow as work of breathing improves

is reached at which point the valve closes. In patients with poor lung compliance or high airways resistance, these pressures are reached quite rapidly resulting in low tidal volumes. When the inspiratory valve is opened in volume-targeted modes, inspiratory gases flow until a set tidal volume is reached and then the efflux of gases occurs until the desired PEEP is reached. In this mode, patients with poor lung compliance can have high peak and plateau pressures as a result. During the early phase of resuscitation, patients typically require deep sedation and sometimes continuous neuromuscular blockade to allow for sufficient expiratory time to achieve adequate exhalation. In this early phase the authors recommend becoming very familiar with one mode of mechanical ventilation, the most common being a volume-targeted mode.

Respiratory rate, inspiratory:expiratory time selection: the most important principle during the mechanical ventilation of the patient with obstructive lung disease is to allow adequate exhalation, preventing dynamic hyperinflation. This is best and most easily achieved by simply starting with a low respiratory rate such as 6 to 10, as fewer inspirations per minute means the patient must spend a greater proportion of the respiratory cycle in passive exhalation. The consequence of a low respiratory rate, of course, is hypoventilation, which can also lead to respiratory acidosis. Generally, hypercapnia is well tolerated and permissive hypercapnia should be allowed with a pH goal greater than 7.20 as long as the patient remains hemodynamically stable or is not in a high-risk group such as those who are pregnant, have intracranial hypertension, or pulmonary arterial hypertension.[12] Counterintuitively, providing adequate exhalation will facilitate improved ventilation by reducing dead space fraction and limiting breath stacking, hyperinflation, and auto-PEEP. Although lowering the respiratory rate is the most important and first intervention aimed at extending expiratory time, it can also be increased by decreasing the time needed for inhalation. This is accomplished by increasing the inspiratory flow rate, allowing the ventilator to more quickly deliver the set tidal volume. This method of increasing the expiratory time is limited because the increased rate of flow will cause higher inspiratory pressures triggering the ventilator's peak pressure alarm system. Raising the peak pressure alarm trigger can be helpful, but risks patient harm when done incorrectly and should probably be reserved to those with extensive experience or training in mechanical ventilation as well as to use after more basic interventions such as reducing the respiratory rate, paralysis, and permissive hypercapnia have failed.

Tidal volume selection: a higher tidal volume can be used to preserve minute ventilation despite a low respiratory rate. Although lung protective tidal volumes of 6 to 8 mL per kilogram ideal body weight is a standard tidal volume goal to prevent ventilator-induced lung injury, this rule occasionally must be violated to maintain an adequate blood pH. There are some recent data that suggest that this strategy is safe in patients without ARDS, although other data are conflicting.[13–16] Tidal volume and exhalation time go hand-in-hand, in that any additional volume inhaled must be exhaled and increasing tidal volume may result in air trapping for any given expiratory time. Any increase in tidal volume should be followed by a reevaluation of air trapping. In patients with COPD, who have parenchymal destruction leading to more compliant lungs, increased tidal volume is well tolerated. However, in asthmatics with fixed obstruction secondary to bronchospasm and a regional distribution of gas flow secondary to mucous plugs, an increased tidal volume may result in pneumothoraces and barotrauma. If an increased tidal volume is to be given while maintaining a constant or increased expiratory time, then the rate of inspiratory flow must be increased. High inspiratory flows make peak-pressure alarms more likely.

Waveforms and airway pressures: the second principle in the mechanical ventilation in patients with obstructive lung disease is to monitor flow waveforms and airway pressures to assess air trapping and auto-PEEP. The single most important ventilator waveform to monitor is the flow waveform (**Fig. 2**). This waveform gives a global assessment of the expiratory egress of respiratory gases. When the expiratory limb of the flow waveform returns to baseline before the next breath, the patient has adequately exhaled the tidal volume. If the next breath begins before the waveform reaching the baseline, there is residual pulmonary gas that is not exhaled, which leads to dynamic hyperinflation. Thus, one way to initiate and monitor mechanical ventilation in patients with obstructive lung disease is to start with a low respiratory rate (eg, 6 breaths per minute) to allow for the expiratory limb of the flow waveform to return to baseline and slowly increase the respiratory rate until breath stacking occurs and then reduce the respiratory rate by one. Doing so requires a patient breathing passively at the ventilator set rate and not triggering breaths, typically achieved through deep sedation and paralysis. As bronchospasm and obstruction resolve, the respiratory rate can be increased as long as air trapping does not occur. When auto-PEEP is suspected the flow waveforms should be examined, as air trapping it is the most likely culprit.

As previously recommended using volume-targeted modes in this early phase of resuscitation, the authors focus on airway pressures related to that mode.

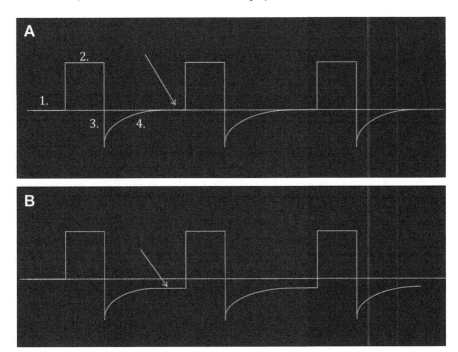

Fig. 2. Flow waveform and air trapping. This figure shows the typical flow waveform seen on commonly used ventilators in the ED and ICU. The waveform shows time on the X-axis and flow on the Y-axis. (A) At steady state, there is no flow either to or from the lungs (1). With inspiration, there is a sharp increase in flow that either plateaus in a constant flow mode (as shown here) or tapers off in the decelerating flow mode (2). With exhalation, flow reverses direction (3) and slowly progresses toward the baseline as the small airways empty (4). The flow waveform should return to baseline before the next inhalation (*arrow*). In (B), breaths are not fully exhaled prior the initiation of the next inspiratory cycle (*arrow*), leading to retention of that volume of gas in the lungs with the next inspiratory volume added to it, which is air trapping and hyperinflation.

Pressure-targeted modes can be successfully used but require significantly greater vigilance. In a volume-targeted mode, the ventilator delivers a set tidal volume with airway pressures being dependent on the resistance and compliance of the pulmonary system. The pressure measured at the airway opening can be divided into the pressure to overcome resistance in the airways and the pressure to overcome the elasticity of the lung and chest wall (**Fig. 3**). With few exceptions, the peak pressure represents the total pressure required to overcome both resistive (eg, bronchospasm, airway edema) and elastic forces (eg, stiff lungs or chest wall), whereas the plateau pressure represents only the contribution of elastic forces, as it is measured in the absence of gas flow. Patients with obstructive lung disease often have high peak pressures due to the resistance from bronchospasm and airflow obstruction. The peak inspiratory pressure is evaluated continuously without any maneuvers on the ventilator, as it is the pressure read at the airway opening at the end of inspiration (typically <30cmH$_2$O, with high pressure alarms set by institutional protocol, typically at 40–60cmH$_2$O). When high peak pressure is encountered, plateau pressure must be measured to see if it exceeds a goal pressure of less than 30cmH$_2$O. The plateau pressure is determined by performing an inspiratory hold on the ventilator that closes the inspiratory valve at end-inspiration and allows the pressure to equilibrate with the alveoli in the absence of gas flow. Patients who have dynamic hyperinflation and significant auto-PEEP will have both high peak and plateau pressures and are at risk of pneumothorax, which is why mechanical ventilation in asthmatics can be dangerous. Although peak pressure greater than 50 and plateau pressure greater than 30 have been associated with barotrauma, it is unlikely that these represent threshold values and risk likely increases with increasing pressure.[17,18] Elevated peak pressure should only confer risk of barotrauma when it is symptomatic of elevated plateau pressure. When the plateau pressure is elevated, one must evaluate factors reducing respiratory system compliance, often auto-PEEP and air trapping in the context of obstructive lung disease (**Table 2**).

Auto-PEEP is measured by performing an expiratory hold on the ventilator, which closes the expiratory valve and allows pressure to equilibrate with the alveoli at rest. The total pressure measured will be higher than the set PEEP (**Fig. 4**) in the presence of auto-PEEP. Auto-PEEP may be grossly underestimated due to regional obstruction, which is most pronounced in patients with the fixed bronchospasm

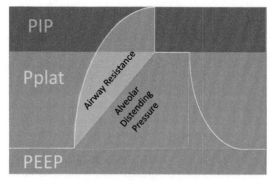

Fig. 3. Airway pressures. This pressure waveform on the ventilator shows time on the X-axis and pressure on the Y-axis. The ventilator must overcome 2 pressures to deliver a breath, the airway resistive pressure, and the alveolar distending pressure. The starting and ending pressure for each breath will be from the set PEEP.

Table 2
Causes of high peak pressure

High Peak Pressure, Normal or Lower Plateau Pressure	High Peak Pressure and High Plateau Pressure
Mechanism: Increased respiratory system *resistance* to flow	Mechanism: Decreased respiratory system *compliance* (increased stiffness)
Causes: 1. Bronchospasm 2. Mucous plugging 3. Obstructed (secretions) or kinked tracheal tube or ventilator tubing 4. Endobronchial tumors 5. Extrinsic compression 6. Foreign body aspiration	Causes: 1. Lung overdistension—dynamic hyperinflation—"breath stacking," auto-PEEP, right mainstem intubation 2. Decreased lung compliance—ARDS, edema, fibrosis, collapse, consolidation 3. Pleural factors—effusion, tension pneumothorax 4. External factors—obesity, ascites, burn eschar, supine positioning, abdominal hypertension

and mucous plugs with normal to decreased lung compliance as seen in asthma as opposed to dynamic airway collapse and increased lung compliance as seen in patients with emphysema and COPD. If a lung unit has an auto-PEEP that exceeds the pressure required to obstruct the efflux of gas, the pressure will not be reflected at the airway opening, underestimating the total PEEP. In cases of obstructive lung disease with significant auto-PEEP, externally applied PEEP may reduce work of breathing by lowering the threshold pressure needed to trigger the ventilator but it is a double-edged sword. Externally applied PEEP greater than this threshold will

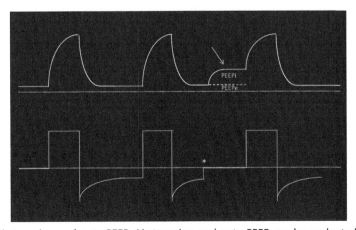

Fig. 4. Air trapping and auto-PEEP. Air trapping and auto-PEEP can be evaluated with an expiratory hold maneuver. If the expiratory limb of the flow waveform (*bottom green*) does not return to baseline before the subsequent breath, that volume of gas is "trapped" in the lung while the next volume-targeted breath is delivered as seen here. Holding the expiratory valve closed with an expiratory hold maneuver on the ventilator (*asterisk*) will allow the pressures to equilibrate between the alveoli and the airway opening. This will demonstrate a total PEEP (*arrow*), with the components being extrinsically set PEEP and the difference between the total PEEP and set PEEP being the intrinsic, or auto-PEEP.

worsen dynamic hyperinflation and increase the risk of pneumothorax. This is the risk of PEEP both invasively and noninvasively in patients with respiratory failure secondary to obstructive lung disease. The analogy of a "respiratory waterfall" has been proposed to conceptualize this effect of applied PEEP. In this case, the water flowing over the waterfall represents the auto-PEEP or gas flowing out of the alveolus down its pressure gradient during expiration and the pool of water below the waterfall represents the applied PEEP. As long as the upstream pressure (auto-PEEP) is higher than the downstream pressure (applied PEEP) there will be no effect of increasing applied PEEP on hyperinflation just as there is no effect of raising the height of the pool of water below the waterfall until its height reaches that of the water above. However, by raising the lower pool, the potential (pressure) difference between the pools is reduced. This reduces the negative pressure that must be generated by muscular effort to accomplish ventilator triggering, reducing work of breathing, and the risk of ineffective triggering.[19,20]

VENTILATOR ALARMS

Peak pressure alarms are frequently encountered in patients undergoing mechanical ventilation for obstructive lung disease. These alarms occur when the ventilator senses the peak pressure during a breath going over a pre-set maximum. At most institutions these maximums are set by protocol and typically not directly ordered by the physician unless some deviation from the protocol is requested. In the setting of a high peak pressure with a normal plateau pressure, one might reasonably assume that the alarm is of little consequence, as they are a consequence of airways resistance and not transmitted to the lung parenchyma. However, this is not the case and "alarm" is a bit of a misnomer, as when the pressure threshold is reached for the alarm, the ventilator acts as a pop-off valve and stops delivering the breath, which results in tidal volumes less than the set volume even in volume control modes, sometimes severely decreasing minute ventilation. Peak pressure alarms in an unstable patient should result in disconnection of the ventilator and hand ventilation of the patient. Troubleshooting stable patients is done on the ventilator by first observing the actual delivered tidal volume and then measuring the plateau pressure to develop a differential. Causes of both high peak and plateau pressures are factors that reduce the compliance of the respiratory system, whereas factors that cause increased resistance to airflow elevate only the peak pressure (see **Table 2**). If peak pressure alarming persists despite considering this differential and treating the modifiable causes, most importantly auto-PEEP, then the peak pressure alarm setting may be increased, accepting that this may be associated with an increased risk of barotrauma, particularly in cases where respiratory system compliance is reduced. Increasing the peak pressure alarm can be helpful but risks patient harm when done incorrectly, namely when decreased compliance is the cause of the elevated peak pressure (plateau pressure is elevated).

All patients on mechanical ventilation should be monitored with continuous waveform capnography. However, patients with obstructive lung disease commonly have high dead space fractions and the end-tidal CO2 will typically underestimate the Pa_{CO_2} (**Fig. 5**).

CASES

Case #1: a 56-year-old woman presents to the ED by emergency medical services (EMS) with respiratory distress. The patient has a history of severe COPD and has had a change in her sputum and increased cough for the last 5 days. She has been out of her nebulized bronchodilators for the last 3 days and has been increasing her

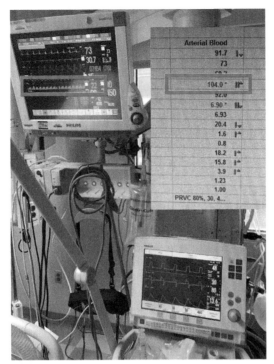

Fig. 5. Capnography in dead space. This figure shows the pitfall of capnography in patients with dead space. Because of the ineffective ventilation, the CO2 measured at the airway opening by the ETCO2 sensor will underestimate the partial pressure of arterial, or venous, CO2. The degree of underestimation will be determined by the dead space fraction.

home oxygen from her baseline 2 L/min to 6 L/min. Chest radiograph shows hyperexpanded lung fields, flattened diaphragms, and interstitial infiltrate in the right upper lobe. A venous blood gas is obtained, which shows a pH of 7.25 with a Pco_2 of 88. On examination, the patient has tripod posture and is tachypneic with pursed lipped breathing.

How to manage this patient: there may be a role for high-flow nasal insufflation in these patients, but the data are lacking as of the time of this writing. The authors' strategy is to start with BiPAP in these patients with impending respiratory arrest, as the respiratory muscles need immediate assistance. We start with 5 of PEEP and 5 of IPAP to allow the patient to get used to the mask. Most BiPAP failure early on is due to mask intolerance; so starting low and quickly titrating up can be useful to avoid early failure. When patients cannot tolerate the mask despite starting low, there are 3 options. The first option is to change to a high-flow nasal insufflation. When doing this, the authors start at 100% Fio_2 and roughly 50% of the maximum flow of the HFNC system and increase the flow greater than 5 to 10 minutes to the maximum tolerated flow while adjusting the Fio_2 to maintain an oxygen saturation between 88% and 93%. The second option is to give medication to allow mask tolerance. We prefer dexmedetomidine or ketamine over benzodiazepines. The third option is to intubate and mechanically ventilate. Each maneuver has its benefits and risks that each need to be weighed. The authors' strategy is to start with NIPPV and titrate up to higher pressures while checking a blood gas to get a baseline Pa/vCO2 and placing an inline waveform capnograph. To increase ventilation, one must increase the gradient between IPAP and EPAP. The EPAP is useful to offset auto-PEEP, and the mask seal is typically maintained up to about 20cmH2O. If patients cannot tolerate the mask, a trial of an HFNC is reasonable. If the patient does fail and require intubation, high-dose fentanyl and propofol will be started for synchrony. Start initially with assist-control/volume-control mode with 100% Fio_2 (weaned quickly by pulse oximetry), PEEP 5, tidal volume of 6 to 8 mL/kg predicted body weight, and rate of 6 to 8. The flow waveform is monitored to ensure no air trapping and the respiratory rate progressively increased if none. Serial blood gases are followed.

Case #2: a 26-year-old woman with a history of asthma presents to the ED by EMS in respiratory failure. The patient takes chronic steroids and a long-acting beta agonist for moderate persistent asthma and has never required intubation in the past. The patient is difficult to mask ventilate and is obtunded requiring invasive mechanical ventilation. The patient is intubated on arrival for impending cardiopulmonary arrest.

How to manage this patient: the first priority is patient ventilator synchrony. High-dose fentanyl and propofol infusions should be started immediately. The authors prefer to start neuromuscular blockade from the beginning in patients with respiratory failure from pure asthma. Cisatracurium is the neuromuscular blocker of choice if a continuous infusion is to be used as its elimination is not changed by renal or hepatic dysfunction. The patient is placed on assist-control/volume control mode on the ventilator. An initial tidal volume of 6 mL/kg predicted body weight is selected, PEEP of 5, Fio_2 of 100% (weaned down rapidly by pulse oximetry), and a rate of 6 to 8. Inspiratory flows are increased as tolerated to allow for a longer expiration time, typically targeting 50 L/min or more. The flow waveform is observed and returns to baseline before the next breath, so the rate is increased by one until breath stacking occurs and then backed off by one. End-tidal CO2 is connected and a blood gas is evaluated, aiming for a pH greater than 7.2 but allowing permissive hypercapnia. Continuous bronchodilators, magnesium, and steroids are started. Intravenous fluids are administered to replace insensible loss and volume depletion from the high work of breathing.

SUMMARY RECOMMENDATIONS

1. Noninvasive methods of respiratory support to improve work of breathing should be attempted to avoid the untoward difficulties of invasive mechanical ventilation. The current literature supports noninvasive ventilation as the first-line therapy, although we recommend high-flow nasal insufflation in patients who cannot tolerate the tight fitting facemask.
2. For patients who require invasive mechanical ventilation, the first action is to optimize patient-ventilator synchrony using continuous high-dose fentanyl and a sedative agent—the authors prefer propofol. Elevate the head of the bed to 30° and place an orogastric feeding tube. Many patients also require an initial period of neuromuscular blockade for patient-ventilator synchrony and optimal exhalation time.
3. Exhalation time should be maximized using a low respiratory rate and the expiratory flow waveform observed to ensure complete exhalation in the absence of air trapping. Initial tidal volume should be set at 6 to 8 mL/kg ideal body weight, but it is not clear that lung protective tidal volumes must be strictly adhered to in the absence of ARDS and presence of a compelling reason to adjust them otherwise.
4. Perform inspiratory and expiratory hold maneuvers to evaluate plateau pressure and auto-PEEP. Apply external PEEP to reduce work of breathing and prevent cyclic opening and closing of compliant alveolar units and reevaluate auto-PEEP.

Table 3
What do I do if....?

I cannot achieve adequate patient-ventilator synchrony:	1. Ensure adequate analgosedation 2. Evaluate ventilator waveforms 3. Administer a neuromuscular blocking agent 4. Consider a pressure-targeted mode
I cannot achieve a respiratory rate that eliminates breath stacking:	1. Reduce tidal volume 2. Deepen sedation 3. Consider NMBA 4. Rescue maneuvers—extracorporeal CO2 removal with venovenous ECMO or induced hypothermia 5. Increase inspiratory flow rate/increase peak pressure alarm setting
I cannot maintain an adequate pH despite ventilator settings required to eliminate breath stacking and auto-PEEP:	1. If hemodynamically stable, may consider allowing a lower pH if closely monitored. 2. Rescue maneuvers—infusion of a buffer (sodium bicarbonate), extracorporeal CO2 removal with venovenous ECMO, or induced hypothermia
My patient is tolerating noninvasive support, but the venous blood gas is not improving:	1. Increase IPAP:EPAP gradient if on BiPAP 2. Increase flow if on HFNC 3. Invasive mechanical ventilation (exception: asthmatics)
My patient becomes suddenly hypotensive:	1. Disconnect ventilator and decompress the chest. 2. Evaluate for pneumothorax.
The peak pressure continues to alarm:	1. Evaluate plateau pressure 2. Low plateau pressure—bronchodilators, pulmonary toilette, eliminate endotracheal tube biting, or obstruction 3. High plateau pressure—evaluate and treat causes of decreased respiratory compliance, particularly dynamic hyperinflation in the context of obstructive lung disease. 4. Reduce inspiratory flow if patient factors allow, consider expert consultation, consider increasing peak pressure alarm setting as a last resort.

Abbreviation: ECMO, extracorporeal membrane oxygenation.

5. Waveform capnography should be started and calibrated to a peripheral blood gas. In the absence of oxygenation abnormalities, a venous blood gas is sufficient. This will allow an evaluation of dead space.
6. Allow permissive hypercapnia as long as the patient has hemodynamic stability and lacks contraindications such as pregnancy or elevated intracranial pressure. Tidal volume may be increased to improve minute ventilation, which is below the threshold for permissive hypercapnia. If tidal volume is increased, expiratory flow waveform and alveolar pressures should be reevaluated.
7. See **Table 3** for recommendations in patients with refractory disease.

REFERENCES

1. Rose L, Scales DC, Atzema C, et al. Emergency department length of stay for critical care admissions. a population-based study. Ann Am Thorac Soc 2016; 13(8):1324–32.

2. Fuller BM, Mohr NM, Miller CN, et al. Mechanical ventilation and ARDS in the ED: a multicenter, observational, prospective, cross-sectional study. Chest 2015; 148(2):365–74.
3. Wilcox SR, Richards JB, Fisher DF, et al. Initial mechanical ventilator settings and lung protective ventilation in the ED. Am J Emerg Med 2016;34(8):1446–51.
4. Devlin JW, Skrobik Y, Gelinas C, et al. Clinical practice guidelines for the prevention and management of pain, agitation/sedation, delirium, immobility, and sleep disruption in adult patients in the ICU. Crit Care Med 2018;46(9):e825–73.
5. Sessler CN, Gosnell MS, Grap MJ, et al. The Richmond Agitation-Sedation Scale: validity and reliability in adult intensive care unit patients. Am J Respir Crit Care Med 2002;166(10):1338–44.
6. Klompas M, Branson R, Eichenwald EC, et al. Strategies to prevent ventilator-associated pneumonia in acute care hospitals: 2014 update. Infect Control Hosp Epidemiol 2014;35(8):915–36.
7. Keenan SP, Kernerman PD, Cook DJ, et al. Effect of noninvasive positive pressure ventilation on mortality in patients admitted with acute respiratory failure: a meta-analysis. Crit Care Med 1997;25(10):1685–92.
8. Schnell D, Timsit JF, Darmon M, et al. Noninvasive mechanical ventilation in acute respiratory failure: trends in use and outcomes. Intensive Care Med 2014;40(4):582–91.
9. Kramer N, Meyer TJ, Meharg J, et al. Randomized, prospective trial of noninvasive positive pressure ventilation in acute respiratory failure. Am J Respir Crit Care Med 1995;151(6):1799–806.
10. Doshi P, Whittle JS, Bublewicz M, et al. High-velocity nasal insufflation in the treatment of respiratory failure: a randomized clinical trial. Ann Emerg Med 2018; 72(1):73–83 e75.
11. Braunlich J, Kohler M, Wirtz H. Nasal highflow improves ventilation in patients with COPD. Int J Chron Obstruct Pulmon Dis 2016;11:1077–85.
12. Hickling KG, Henderson SJ, Jackson R. Low mortality associated with low volume pressure limited ventilation with permissive hypercapnia in severe adult respiratory distress syndrome. Intensive Care Med 1990;16(6):372–7.
13. Futier E, Constantin JM, Paugam-Burtz C, et al. A trial of intraoperative low-tidal-volume ventilation in abdominal surgery. N Engl J Med 2013;369(5):428–37.
14. Serpa Neto A, Simonis FD, Barbas CS, et al. Association between tidal volume size, duration of ventilation, and sedation needs in patients without acute respiratory distress syndrome: an individual patient data meta-analysis. Intensive Care Med 2014;40(7):950–7.
15. Wanderer JP, Blum JM, Ehrenfeld JM. Intraoperative low-tidal-volume ventilation. N Engl J Med 2013;369(19):1861.
16. Writing Group for the PReVENT Investigators, Simonis FD, Serpa Neto A, Binnekade JM, et al. Effect of a low vs intermediate tidal volume strategy on ventilator-free days in intensive care unit patients without ARDS: a randomized clinical trial. JAMA 2018;320(18):1872–80.
17. Petersen GW, Baier H. Incidence of pulmonary barotrauma in a medical ICU. Crit Care Med 1983;11(2):67–9.
18. Ioannidis G, Lazaridis G, Baka S, et al. Barotrauma and pneumothorax. J Thorac Dis 2015;7(Suppl 1):S38–43.
19. Leatherman JW, Ravenscraft SA. Low measured auto-positive end-expiratory pressure during mechanical ventilation of patients with severe asthma: hidden auto-positive end-expiratory pressure. Crit Care Med 1996;24(3):541–6.
20. Mughal MM, Culver DA, Minai OA, et al. Auto-positive end-expiratory pressure: mechanisms and treatment. Cleve Clin J Med 2005;72(9):801–9.

Emergency Department Management of Acute Kidney Injury, Electrolyte Abnormalities, and Renal Replacement Therapy in the Critically Ill

Ivan Co, MD[a,b,*], Kyle Gunnerson, MD, FCCM[c,d,e]

KEYWORDS

- Acute kidney injury • Acute renal failure • Electrolyte derangement • Acidosis

KEY POINTS

- Acute kidney injury is a common diagnosis with multiple sequelae and consequences.
- Treatment and management rely on astute diagnosis of the cause for acute kidney injury.
- Renal replacement therapy or hemodialysis is the treatment modality when conservative management fails.

INTRODUCTION AND DEFINITION

Acute kidney injury (AKI), formerly called acute renal failure, is a common diagnosis in the emergency department (ED) and in the critically ill.[1] Numerous studies have found

Disclosures: None.
[a] Department of Emergency Medicine, University of Michigan Health System, 1500 East Medical Center Drive SPC 5301, Ann Arbor, MI 48109, USA; [b] Department of Internal Medicine, Division of Pulmonary Critical Care, University of Michigan Health System, 1500 East Medical Center Drive SPC 5301, Ann Arbor, MI 48109, USA; [c] Department of Emergency Medicine, Division of Emergency Critical Care, Massey Family Foundation Emergency Critical Center (EC3), University of Michigan Health System, 1500 East Medical Center Drive, Ann Arbor, MI 48109-5303, USA; [d] Department of Anesthesiology, Division of Emergency Critical Care, Massey Family Foundation Emergency Critical Center (EC3), University of Michigan Health System, 1500 East Medical Center Drive, Ann Arbor, MI 48109-5303, USA; [e] Department of Internal Medicine, Division of Emergency Critical Care, Massey Family Foundation Emergency Critical Center (EC3), University of Michigan Health System, 1500 East Medical Center Drive, Ann Arbor, MI 48109-5303, USA
* Corresponding author. Department of Internal Medicine, Division of Pulmonary Critical Care, University of Michigan Health System, 1500 East Medical Center Drive SPC 5301, Ann Arbor, MI 48109.
E-mail address: coivan@med.umich.edu

Emerg Med Clin N Am 37 (2019) 459–471
https://doi.org/10.1016/j.emc.2019.04.006
0733-8627/19/© 2019 Elsevier Inc. All rights reserved.
emed.theclinics.com

significant morbidity and mortality regardless of patient characteristics, comorbidities, and clinical context.[2–5] Mortality has been estimated to occur in 15% to 80% of critically ill patients. Therapeutic interventions often target correcting electrolyte abnormalities, preventing secondary injury with hemodynamic support, and initiation of emergent hemodialysis in patients with advanced metabolic derangements. Patient outcome varies depending on the provider's ability to identify the patient's AKI early and provide appropriate treatment interventions.

The definition of AKI has undergone multiple revisions over the past few decades. The RIFLE (risk, injury, failure, loss, end-stage renal disease) criteria were initially proposed in 2004, and later modified in 2007 to include absolute serum creatinine (SCr) level increase. In addition, in 2012, both definitions were combined into what is currently used: the KDIGO (Kidney Disease; Improving Global Outcomes) definition (**Box 1**).

EVALUATION AND GENERAL MANAGEMENT OF PATIENTS WITH ACUTE KIDNEY INJURY

Critically ill patients in the ED may have several contributing causes for their acute injuries. A careful review of their history, examination, and known comorbidities may provide early clues toward identifying the cause of their reduced renal function. AKI cause can be subdivided into 3 broad categories: prerenal, intrinsic, and postrenal causes.

AKI rarely causes any symptoms. Most clinical symptoms are a result of the primary underlying disease leading to the development of AKI rather than the kidney injury itself. Outside of clinical history, examination, and comorbidities, laboratory testing may help delineate the 3 categories of AKI: urine osmolarity, urine electrolytes, renal ultrasonography, urinalysis with microscopy. Urine electrolyte levels can be obtained to calculate the fractional excretion of sodium (FENa) or urea (FEUrea) if the patient is taking diuretic medications. A FENa less than 1% or FEUrea less than 35% suggests a prerenal cause of AKI, whereas a FENa greater than 2% or FEUrea greater than 35% is more consistent with an intrinsic disease process. Cutoff values may be less helpful in patients with chronic kidney disease or mild cases of AKI. Urinalysis with microscopy is another diagnostic test that can help differentiate the AKI cause by the presence or absence of casts. Keep in mind that no single value is absolute in diagnosing AKI.

Prerenal Acute Kidney Injury

Prerenal AKI is often a manifestation of decreased renal perfusion caused by intravascular volume depletion or a decreased renal perfusion pressure leading to a reduced glomerular filtration rate (GFR). Approximately 70% of patients presenting with AKI have a prerenal cause.[6] Sepsis and septic shock continue to be the most important

---

Box 1
Kidney Disease; Improving Global Outcomes definitions of acute kidney injury

AKI can be diagnosed if the patient has any of the following:
1. Increase in SCr level by at least 0.3 mg/dL within 48 hours
2. Increase in SCr level to greater than 1.5× baseline occurring within 7 days
3. Urine output less than 0.5 mL/kg/h for 6 hours

Data from Kidney Disease: Improving Global Outcomes (KDIGO) Acute Kidney Injury Work Group. KDIGO clinical practice guideline for acute kidney injury. Kidney Int Suppl 2012;2:1–138.

Table 1 Causes of prerenal acute kidney injury	
Causes of Poor Renal Perfusion Leading to Prerenal Acute Kidney Injury	**Potential Causes**
Volume depletion	Diuretics Diarrhea Blood loss anemia Osmotic diuresis Diuretic overuse Burns Vomiting

Decreased arterial
  pressure
	Medication: NSAIDs, cyclosporine, tacrolimus,
	  angiotensin receptor blocker
	Cardiorenal syndrome
	Hepatorenal syndrome
	Intra-abdominal hypertension
	Systemic vasodilation: sepsis

Abbreviation: NSAIDs, nonsteroidal antiinflammatory drugs.
Data from Rahman M, Shad F, Smith M. Acute kidney injury: a guide to diagnosis and management. Am Fam Physician 2012;86(7):631–639.

causes of AKI in critically ill patients and account for more than 50% of patients with AKI admitted to the intensive care unit.[7]

Several pathophysiologic derangements that can cause a prerenal AKI are not a result of volume depletion. AKI as a result of decreased arterial pressure secondary to intravascular fluid overload can be found in patients with congestive heart failure resulting in cardiorenal syndrome. This kind of prerenal AKI can be treated with diuretic therapy. Patients with hepatorenal syndrome can manifest as having prerenal disease; however, intervention with volume expansion or diuretics may be necessary depending on their clinical state and laboratory findings. Common causes of prerenal AKI are noted in **Table 1**.

Intrinsic (Renal) Acute Kidney Injury

Intrinsic renal injury develops when the primary cause of AKI is parenchymal injury, often caused by medications, toxins, or ischemia. Components of the kidney that are affected include the tubules, glomerulus, vascular, and the interstitium. Common causes of intrinsic AKI are listed in **Table 2**.

Acute tubular necrosis (ATN) is the most common intrinsic cause of AKI, often the result of prolonged hypotension resulting in ischemic renal tubular injury. There is no specific intervention to reverse ATN once it develops. Prevention of additional secondary insults is important for renal recovery. Acute interstitial nephritis is the second most common cause of intrinsic AKI, often a consequence of certain medications or infections. Prolonged prerenal disease, if not promptly identified and intervened on, will eventually progress to intrinsic disease.

Postrenal Acute Kidney Injury

Postrenal AKI is a result of renal congestion caused by a blockage of urinary flow. Common causes include prostatic hypertrophy, renal calculi, and an external mass compressing the ureter or the urethra. Postrenal AKI is almost always associated with some form of hydronephrosis. Despite being the rarest of the 3 causes of AKI,

Table 2 Common causes of intrinsic acute kidney injury	
Common Types of Intrinsic AKI	**Potential Causes**
Tubular	Ischemia
	Nephrotoxins: endogenous toxins such as calcium, uric acid, hemolysis, rhabdomyolysis, contrast media, chemotoxic agents
Interstitial	Medications: aminoglycosides, cephalosporin, penicillin
	Infection: *Streptococcus*, Epstein-Barr virus
	Systemic disease: lupus, sarcoidosis
Glomerular	Postinfection
	Glomerulonephritis
Vascular	Renal thrombosis
	Malignant hypertension

Data from Rahman M, Shad F, Smith M. Acute kidney injury: a guide to diagnosis and management. Am Fam Physician. 2012;86(7):631–639.

diagnosis can often be made with a thorough clinical examination and diagnostic ultrasonography to identify the location of the anatomic obstruction.

ACID-BASE DERANGEMENT IN THE CRITICALLY ILL

Before treatment initiation, a solid understanding of the patient's acid-base derangement is paramount. Patients with AKI may present with a metabolic acidosis, often classified as either an anion-gap or non-anion gap metabolic acidosis.[8]

Acid-base homeostasis is normally achieved by the kidney's ability to excrete acid load, through the Na^+/H^+ transporter, which excretes approximately 1 mEq of H^+ ions per kilogram per day in the urine.[9] Metabolic acidosis occurs once the mechanism to excrete H^+ is overwhelmed by excessive acid production, inability to reabsorb a bicarbonate buffer, or decreased H^+ excretion.[9]

AKI associated non–anion-gap metabolic acidosis (NAGMA) occurs purely from a loss of bicarbonate without concomitant increase in exogenous acid production. This condition occurs most commonly in patients with severe hypovolemia secondary to diarrhea where the large bowel has impaired ability to reabsorb bicarbonate. Worsening chronic renal dysfunction can also cause NAGMA, as well as renal tubular acidosis (RTA). Patients with an acute RTA have impaired bicarbonate reabsorption secondary to ion transporter dysfunction.

Anion-gap metabolic acidosis (AGMA) often occurs because of an increased acid production that the kidneys are unable to excrete because of an acute decrease in GFR. Bicarbonate in the body is used to buffer the excess ion to no avail, resulting in a worsening metabolic acidosis.[9] Most common causes of AGMA in the critically ill include lactic acidosis and ketoacidosis. Other causes of AGMA are listed in **Table 3**.

The most common AGMA encountered in critically ill patients is lactic acidosis. Lactate production often occurs as a result of poor tissue perfusion and inadequate oxygen delivery. Malperfused tissues transition from aerobic to anaerobic glycolysis metabolism to supplement inefficient ATP production to match the patient's metabolic demand.[10] Lactate generation results in a metabolic acidosis that can cause myocardial depression, catecholamine resistance, and progressive vasodilatory shock. Vasodilatory shock occurs when vascular wall smooth muscle is unable to constrict despite a maximum level of plasma catecholamines (released in response to hypoperfusion)

Table 3 Common causes of anion-gap metabolic acidosis	
AGMA Mnemonic	**Causes**
M	Methanol
U	Uremia
D	Diabetic, alcohol, starvation ketoacidosis
P	Paracetamol/acetaminophen
I	Isoniazid, iron ingestion, inborn error of metabolism
L	Lactic acidosis
E	Ethanol, ethylene glycol
S	Salicylates

and inappropriate activation of other vasodilatory mechanisms.[11] Transient correction of the acidic environment with sodium bicarbonate or dialysis can help mitigate the patient's vasodilatory shock, but effective treatment should be focused on reversing the inciting event.[11]

MEDICAL MANAGEMENT OF ACUTE KIDNEY INJURY

Therapy targeted to improve a patient's AKI should focus on supportive interventions that include optimizing hemodynamics, intravascular fluid status, correcting electrolyte abnormalities, improving severe pH derangements, and minimizing interventions that could further reduce the patient's GFR. In addition to supportive measures, identifying potential nephrotoxic agents and appropriate pharmacologic dosing adjustments to the patient's GFR are of utmost importance.[12]

Fluid Resuscitation

In patients with a prerenal AKI caused by severe hypovolemia, intravenous crystalloid resuscitation is often the initial and primary therapy. Fluid resuscitation improves cardiac output and ultimately improves renal perfusion and GFR. There is increasing evidence to suggest that resuscitation using high-chloride-load fluids may be harmful, causing a worsening NAGMA, renal acidosis, and renal function.[13–15] In patients with prerenal, hypovolemic AKI, lactated Ringer or a balanced crystalloid solution is currently the resuscitative fluid of choice.[16]

Hemodynamic Optimization with Vasopressor Therapy

In patients who continue to have hemodynamic instability with a low mean arterial pressure (MAP) despite fluid resuscitation (or diuresis), vasopressor administration may be necessary to achieve adequate renal perfusion.[17] Vasopressor administration should be initiated to target an initial MAP of greater than or equal to 65 mm Hg, potentially titrating up to a higher MAP target in patients with a history of hypertension and clinical improvement with higher blood pressure target.[10]

No specific vasopressor has been proved to be more effective for the treatment and/or prevention of AKI in patients with shock. Vasopressor choice should be catered toward the patient's primary clinical pathophysiology. Norepinephrine (NE) has been found to improve creatinine clearance in patients with distributive shock.[18] In a comparative study comparing NE with dopamine, there was no significant difference between renal function or mortality outcome.[19] Dopamine was found to have an increased incidence of tachydysrhythmias and adverse events.[19] Administration of, renal-dose dopamine to achieve renal vasodilation has not been found to reduce the incidence of AKI, need for renal replacement therapy, or patient mortality.[20] In fact, dopamine may worsen both renal perfusion and GFR.[21–23] As a result, KDIGO has provided a 1A recommendation against using low-dose dopamine in patients with AKI.[16]

Management of Electrolyte Derangements

Hyperkalemia is the most common life-threatening electrolyte derangement as a sequela of AKI. Breakdown in potassium homeostasis, whether a result of reduced renal excretion (secondary to decreased GFR), excessive intake, worsening acidosis, or leakage of potassium into the extracellular compartment can rapidly increase serum potassium levels.[24]

Hyperkalemia is diagnosed by any serum potassium level greater than 5.5 mEq/L. There are no specific physical examination findings or clinical symptoms that correlate with the degree of hyperkalemia. Cardiac rhythm disturbances, most commonly nonspecific repolarization abnormalities, peaked T waves, widening of the QRS complex, and ST depression, are common sequelae of hyperkalemia.[24] The degree of cardiac rhythm disturbances does not correlate with the degree of hyperkalemia (**Fig. 1**).

Hyperkalemia therapy should not be solely guided by the potassium level but by additional clinical symptoms such as cardiac arrhythmias, nausea, vomiting, degree of metabolic acidosis, and the ability for respiratory compensation.[25] Medical therapy for hyperkalemia involves transient cardiac membrane stabilization and intracellular shift of potassium until the kidney is able to provide adequate elimination.[26] Treatment options include:

- Calcium gluconate: stabilizes cardiac membrane potential in hyperkalemia-induced conduction abnormalities.
- Intravenous insulin with dextrose: insulin stimulates the Na^+/K^+ ATPase pump to shift excess K^+ to the intracellular compartment, whereas dextrose prevents hypoglycemia.

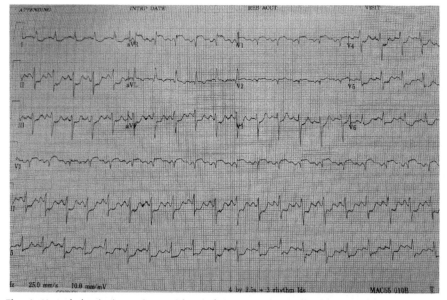

Fig. 1. Hyperkalemia in patient with K of 6.5 mEq/L manifesting as ST depression and peaked T waves.

- Beta-adrenergic agonists: stimulate K^+ shift from extracellular to intracellular space via Na^+/K^+ ATPase pump.

Increased potassium excretion can be considered in outpatients with hyperkalemia; however, caution should be exercised in critically ill patients because sequelae from therapy may result in significant clinical complications. These include:

- Loop diuretics: inhibit Na/K/Cl channel, allowing more K to be excreted from the kidneys. Patients with hypovolemic, prerenal AKI may develop hemodynamic compromise and reduced GFR.
- Ion-exchange resins: prevent enteral reabsorption of potassium by binding potassium into the resin. In patient with shock and decreased gut perfusion, ion-exchange resin administration may precipitate gut ischemia and necrosis.[27]

Increasing potassium excretion is often challenging in critically ill patients with concomitant renal impairment, and emergent renal replacement therapy may be required.

Calcium derangement is common, often a result of the increased serum phosphorus levels that can occur with a decreased GFR. Therapeutic intervention in patients with hypocalcemia usually involves correction of hyperphosphatemia with oral phosphate binders. In patients with symptomatic hypocalcemia, the lowest possible dose of intravenous calcium should be administered to relieve symptoms to avoid excessive supplementation, which can lead to calcium phosphate crystal formation.

Tumor lysis syndrome (TLS) is an oncologic emergency that often presents with significant hypocalcemia, hyperphosphatemia, hyperkalemia, and hyperuricemia. Patients with recent initiation of chemotherapy to treat hematologic malignancies are particularly at risk for TLS, because of a massive lysis of tumor cells resulting in a large release of potassium and phosphorus into the circulatory system. Hyperphosphatemia often precipitates with extracellular calcium to form calcium phosphate crystals that can impair end-organ blood flow.[28] Patients with TLS should be initially treated with intravenous crystalloids to further prevent calcium phosphate crystal formation. Early hemodialysis should be considered in oliguric patients with severe hyperphosphatemia and symptomatic hypocalcemia.

Sodium Bicarbonate Therapy

Administration of sodium bicarbonate in patients with AKI has been controversial, particularly in those patients with concomitant AGMA.[29–31] Treatment goals for patients with AGMA should be focused on treating the underlying cause. Administration of sodium bicarbonate alone improves acidemia and serum pH without reversing the cause of acid production.

Sodium bicarbonate therapy may be warranted in patients with severe metabolic acidosis as a temporizing measure while the clinician attempts to reverse the underlying cause. In patients with a pH less than 7.1, bicarbonate therapy may help temporize profound hemodynamic instability and improve vasopressor sensitivity.[32]

The recently published BICAR-ICU (Sodium Bicarbonate Therapy for Patients with Severe Metabolic Acidaemia in the Intensive Care Unit) trial, randomized 389 critically ill patients with mean serum bicarbonate level less than 13 mmol/L and acidemia (mean pH of 7.15) to receive bicarbonate versus placebo to maintain serum pH greater than 7.3. The study found no difference between 28-day mortality or organ failure at 7 days between treatment and control groups. However, patients with severe AKI who received bicarbonate therapy did show a trend toward decreased need for renal replacement therapy.[33]

Clinicians should be aware of some clinically significant side effects of sodium bicarbonate therapy. Sodium bicarbonate ultimately gets metabolized to CO_2, causing a transient increase in arterial P_{CO_2}, which may be detrimental for patients with an already extreme minute ventilation.[34]

Diuretic Therapy

Loop and thiazide diuretic therapy should be administered only to patients who have renal injury as a result of fluid overload causing renal congestion and reduced GFR. Diuretic therapy may stimulate urine output and shift fluid overloaded patients' volume status in a favorable direction, but diuretics do not seem to reduce mortality or future need for renal replacement therapy.[35] Diuretics should be avoided in patients with a hypovolemic, prerenal AKI because this may further reduce renal perfusion.[16] Despite the renoprotective properties of loop diuretics, KDIGO does not recommend the use of loop diuretics to prevent the worsening of renal function.[16,36]

In patients with intrinsic or prerenal AKI from cardiorenal syndrome, complicated by volume overload and hypoxic respiratory failure, the use of diuretics has been shown to help facilitate fluid removal and improve oxygenation and the tolerance of lung protective ventilation. Despite the increase in urine output with the assistance of diuretics in these patients, there were no clinical outcome benefits noted in terms of expedited recovery from AKI or shorter duration of renal replacement therapy (RRT).[37]

RENAL REPLACEMENT THERAPY

A small subgroup of patients who present with a severe AKI fail medical management and require emergent hemodialysis to correct their acid-base disturbances or electrolyte abnormalities (hyperkalemia). The timing for initiation of RRT is highly debated. KDIGO recommends initiating RRT for life-threatening changes in fluid balance, electrolytes, and acid-base levels but provides no specific objective criteria.[16] Life-threatening indications for emergent hemodialysis are listed in **Table 4**.

Initiation of Renal Replacement Therapy

Initiation of RRT in critically ill patients often requires nephrology consultation as well as temporary vascular access. Current guideline recommendations suggest the use of a 10-French or 12-French, double-lumen, central venous dialysis catheter to facilitate emergent RRT. Emergently placed temporary hemodialysis catheters can be placed with ultrasonography guidance, in a nontunneled fashion, preferentially in the right

Table 4 Mnemonic for emergent hemodialysis indications	
A	Acidemia: severe metabolic acidosis despite adequate medical optimization (pH<7.1)
E	Electrolytes: particularly hyperkalemia refractory to medical therapy
I	Ingestion: poisoning by drugs that are able to be eliminated with RRT
O	Overload: volume overload resulting in hypoxic respiratory failure necessitating mechanical ventilation
U	Uremia: complications secondary to increased BUN (bleeding, pericarditis, encephalopathy)

Abbreviation: BUN, blood urea nitrogen level.
Data from Nee P, Bailey D, Todd V, et al. Critical care in the emergency department: acute kidney injury. Emerg Med J 2016;33:361–365.

internal jugular vein (**Fig. 2**). If the right internal jugular vein is unable to be accessed, femoral vein access is preferred to left internal jugular vein cannulation. Subclavian vein access should be avoided, because temporary hemodialysis catheters are associated with higher rates of central vein stenosis, which may prevent the use of the ipsilateral arm as a site for long-term hemodialysis access (arteriovenous graft or fistula) in the future.[38]

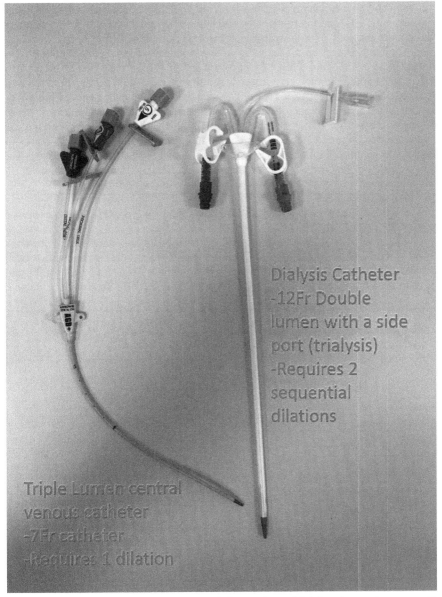

Fig. 2. Difference between temporary hemodialysis catheter (*right*) and central venous catheter (*left*).

In order to optimize catheter blood flow, the temporary hemodialysis catheter's distal tip must be located within a large central vessel. Catheter length is an important consideration, and in general should be 12 to 15 cm for right internal jugular, 15 to 20 cm for left internal jugular, and 19 to 24 cm for femoral vein access. Optimal catheter placement is important for establishing an effective venovenous hemodialysis circuit to provide adequate extracorporeal blood flow for fluid and/or solute removal.[39]

Mode of Renal Replacement Therapy

Once appropriate vascular access has been obtained and confirmed in the right location, delivering RRT via intermittent or continuous hemodialysis should be decided. This delivery requires an understanding of the indication for initiation of hemodialysis, hemodynamics, as well as the logistics needed to initiate either mode (**Table 5**).

Intermittent hemodialysis (iHD) can provide external blood filtration at blood flow rates of 300 to 500 mL/min, and is often the preferred mode for RRT for rapid removal of toxins (poisoning), electrolytes (hyperkalemia), and intravascular fluid volume. A single hemodialysis session can often be completed in 2 to 4 hours. Hemodynamic stability is generally required before initiation of iHD. Critically ill patients with hypotension or vasopressor dependence are often unable to increase cardiac output to compensate for the volume of blood that is being filtered by the extracorporeal circuit. iHD also has a higher resource demand, because these machines often require an additional technician if hemodialysis is being performed at the bedside.[40,41]

Continuous RRT (CRRT) is run at a much slower blood flow rate (usually 20–40 mL/kg/h) to achieve the same effects of iHD, but over a 24-hour period. It is the preferred mode of RRT in patients who have unstable hemodynamics or require vasoactive support. Fluid balance is able to be controlled by intensivists and individualized to each patient's needs. The negatives of CRRT are its inability to rapidly clear toxins secondary to its low blood flow rate, the need for anticoagulation to prevent circuit clot formation, and prolonged limitations to patient mobility. There is also an increased nursing

Table 5
Comparison between the 2 common hemodialysis modalities in critically ill patients

	Intermittent (iHD)	Continuous (CRRT)
Indication	Ambulatory, hemodynamically stable, electrolyte and poison clearance	Critically ill, nonambulatory
Solute Transport	Diffusion	Convection
Blood Flow (mL/min)	300–400	150–200
Dialysate (L/min)	30	1
Efficiency	High	Low
Hemodynamic Stability	Poor	Good
Duration	Average 3 h	Continuous 24 h until discontinued
Anticoagulation	Not required secondary to high blood flow rate	Required (within CRRT filter)
Logistics	Need tap water supply, technically difficult to initiate	High workload, immobility, costly

Abbreviations: CRRT, continuous RRT; iHD; intermittent hemodialysis.
Data from Alvarez G, Chrusch C, Hulme T, et al. Renal replacement therapy: a practical update. Can J Anesth 2019;66:593–604.

resource burden, which includes frequently changing the CRRT machine's dialysate bath and laboratory draws.[40]

SUMMARY

Effective treatment of critically ill patients with AKI requires astute clinicians who can rapidly obtain a detailed history, perform a thorough physical examination, and identify high-risk elements contributing to the patient's decreased renal function. Most patients improve with conservative therapy, including normalizing fluid status, hemodynamic support, removal of offending agents, and addressing the patient's underlying disorder. The utility of sodium bicarbonate administration remains unclear. Sodium bicarbonate therapy may be useful in patients with a severe metabolic acidosis (arterial pH <7.1) as a temporizing intervention until the underlying disorder can be treated and reversed.

Despite aggressive medical intervention, a subgroup of patients with AKI require initiation of emergent RRT. Important considerations include RRT mode, appropriate temporary dialysis catheter equipment, and insertion site. Timely interventions that address these needs in critically ill patients with AKI are imperative to ensure the best long-term chances of recovery.

REFERENCES

1. Challiner R, Ritchie J, Fullwood C, et al. Incidence and consequence of Acute Kidney Injury in unselected emergency admissions to a large acute UK hospital trust. BMC Nephrol 2014;15:84.
2. Pickering JW, James MT, Palmer SC. Acute kidney injury and prognosis after cardiopulmonary bypass: a meta-analysis of cohort studies. Am J Kidney Dis 2015; 65:283–93.
3. Bagshaw SM, George C, Gibney RTN, et al. A multi-center evaluation of early acute kidney injury in critically ill trauma patients. Ren Fail 2008;30:581–9.
4. Bellomo R, Ronco C, Kellum JA, et al. Acute renal failure- definition, outcome measures, animal model, fluid therapy, and information technology needs: the Second International Consensus Conference of the Acute Dialysis Quality Initiative (ADQI) Group. Crit Care 2004;8(4):R204–12.
5. Mehta RL, Kellum JA, Shah SV, et al, Acute Kidney Injury Network. Acute Kidney Injury Network: report of an initiative to improve outcomes in acute kidney injury. Crit Care 2007;11(2):R31.
6. Kaufman J, Dhakal M, Patel B, et al. Community-acquired acute renal failure. Am J Kidney Dis 1991;17(2):191–8.
7. Uchino S, Kellum JA, Bellomo R, et al, Beginning and Ending Supportive Therapy for the Kidney (BEST Kidney) Investigators. Acute renal failure in the critically ill; a multinational, multicenter study. JAMA 2005;294(7):813–8.
8. Hertzberg D, Ryden L, Pickering J, et al. Acute kidney injury- an overview of diagnostic methods and clinical management. Clin Kidney J 2017;10(3):323–31.
9. Moe OW, Rector FC, Alpern RJ. Renal regulation of acid-base metabolism. In: Narins RG, editor. Maxwell and Kleeman's clinical disorders of fluid and electrolyte metabolism. 5th edition. New York: McGraw-Hill, Inc.; 1994. p. 203.
10. Cecconi M, Backer DD, Antonelli M, et al. Consensus on circulatory shock and hemodynamic monitoring. Task Force of the European Society of Intensive Care Medicine. Intensive Care Med 2014;40:1795–815.
11. Landry D, Oliver J. The pathogenesis of vasodilatory shock. N Engl J Med 2001; 345(8):588–95.

12. Harty J. Prevention and management of acute kidney injury. Ulster Med J 2014; 83:149–57.

13. Yunos NM, Bellomo R, Hegarty C, et al. Association between a chloride-liberal vs chloride-restrictive intravenous fluid administration strategy and kidney injury in critically ill adults. JAMA 2012;308:1566–72.

14. Young P, Bailey M, Beasley R, et al. Effect of a buffered crystalloid solution vs saline on acute kidney injury among patients in the intensive care unit: the SPLIT randomized clinical trial. JAMA 2015;314:1701–10.

15. Self W, Semler M, Wanderer J, et al. Balanced crystalloid versus saline in noncritically ill adults. N Engl J Med 2018;378:819–28.

16. KDIGO clinical practice guideline for Acute Kidney Injury. International Society of Nephrology 2012;2:1.

17. Bellomo R, Kellum JA, Wisniewski SR, et al. Effects of norepinephrine on the renal vasculature in normal and endotoxemic dogs. Am J Respir Crit Care Med 1999; 159:1186–92.

18. Redl-Wenzl EM, Armbruster C, Edelmann G, et al. The effects of norepinephrine on hemodynamics and renal function in severe septic shock states. Intensive Care Med 1993;19:151–4.

19. De Backer D, Biston P, Devriendt J, et al. Comparison of dopamine and norepinephrine in the treatment of shock. N Engl J Med 2010;362:779–89.

20. Bellomo R, Chapman M, Finfer S, et al. Low-dose dopamine in patients with early renal dysfunction: a placebo-controlled randomised trial. Australian and New Zealand Intensive Care Society (ANZICS) Clinical Trials Group. Lancet 2000; 356:2139–43.

21. Murray PT. Use of dopaminergic agents for renoprotection in the ICU. Yearbook of intensive care and emergency medicine. Berlin: Springer-Verlag; 2003. p. 637–48.

22. Lauschke A, Teichgraber UK, Frei U, et al. 'Low-dose' dopamine worsens renal perfusion in patients with acute renal failure. Kidney Int 2006;69:1669–74.

23. Kellum JA, M Decker J. Use of dopamine in acute renal failure: a meta-analysis. Crit Care Med 2001;29:1526–31.

24. Lehnhardt A, Kemper M. Pathogenesis, diagnosis, and management of hyperkalemia. Pediatr Nephrol 2011;26:377–84.

25. Montague BT, Ouellette JR, Buller GK. Retrospective review of the frequency of ECG changes in hyperkalemia. Clin J Am Soc Nephrol 2008;3:324–30.

26. Aslam S, Friedman EA, Ifudu O. Electrocardiography is unreliable in detecting potentially lethal hyperkalaemia in haemodialysis patients. Nephrol Dial Transplant 2002;17:1639–42.

27. Watson M, Baker T, Nguyen A, et al. Association of prescription of oral sodium polystyrene sulfonate with sorbitol in an inpatient setting with colonic necrosis: a retrospective cohort study. Am J Kidney Dis 2012;60(3):409–16.

28. Criscuolo M, Fianchi L, Dragonetti G, et al. Tumor lysis syndrome: review of pathogenesis, risk factors and management of a medical emergency. Expert Rev Hematol 2016;9(2):197–208.

29. Kraut JA, Kurtz I. Use of base in the treatment of severe academic state. Am J Kidney Dis 2001;38(4):703.

30. Forsythe SM, Schmidt GA. Sodium Bicarbonate for the treatment of lactic acidosis. Chest 2000;117(1):260.

31. Stacpoole PW. Lactic acidosis: the case against bicarbonate therapy. Ann Intern Med 1986;105(2):276.

32. Kraut JA, Madias NE. Treatment of acute metabolic acidosis: a pathophysiologic approach. Nat Rev Nephrol 2012;8(10):58–601.
33. Jaber S, Paugam C, Futier E, et al. Sodium bicarbonate therapy for patients with severe metabolic acidaemia in the intensive care unit (BICAR-ICU): a multicenter, open-label, randomized controlled, phase-3 trial. Lancet 2018;392:31–40.
34. Androgue HJ, Rashad MN, Gorin AB, et al. Assessing acid-base status in circulatory failure. Difference between arterial and central venous blood. N Engl J Med 1989;320(20):1312.
35. Bagshaw SM, Delaney A, Haase M, et al. Loop diuretics in the management of acute renal failure: a systematic review and meta-analysis. Crit Care Resusc 2007;9(1):60–8.
36. Cantarovich F, Rangoonwala B, Lorenz H, et al. High-dose furosemide for established ARF: a prospective, randomized, double-blind, placebo controlled, multicenter trial. Am J Kidney Dis 2004;44:402–9.
37. Van der Voort PH, Boerma EC, Koopmans M, et al. Furosemide does not improve renal recovery after hemofiltration for acute renal failure in critically ill patients: a double blind randomized controlled trial. Crit Care Med 2009;37:533–8.
38. Macrae JM, Ahmed A, Johnson N, et al. Central vein stenosis: a common problem in patients on hemodialysis. ASAIO J 2005;51(1):77–81.
39. Oliver MJ. Acute dialysis catheters. Semin Dial 2001;14:432–5.
40. Rabindranath K, Adams J, Macleod AM, et al. Intermittent versus continuous renal replacement therapy for acute renal failure in adults. Cochrane Database Syst Rev 2007;(3):CD003773.
41. Bagshaw SM, Mortis G, Godinez-Luna T, et al. Renal recovery after severe acute renal failure. Int J Artif Organs 2006;29:1023–30.

Advances in Emergent Airway Management in Pediatrics

Kelsey A. Miller, MD, Joshua Nagler, MD, MHPEd*

KEYWORDS

- Pediatric airway • Endotracheal intubation • Bag-mask ventilation
- Videolaryngoscopy • Difficult airway

KEY POINTS

- Predictable anatomic and physiologic differences in children are addressed to facilitate success with endotracheal intubation.
- Maximizing preoxygenation and using apneic oxygenation may help address the rapid desaturation that commonly occurs during intubation of children.
- Noninvasive ventilation including high-flow nasal cannula, CPAP, and BPAP is used effectively as an alternative to endotracheal intubation in many pediatric patients with respiratory compromise.
- Videolaryngoscopy is being increasingly used in pediatric airway management with demonstrated improvement in glottic visualization, and the potential for higher intubation success. Video recordings can also be used for education and quality improvement afterward.
- Limited clinical exposure to advanced airway management is supplemented by simulation, operating room experiences, or use of recorded videos to help maintain comfort and procedural competence.

 Video content accompanies this article at http://www.emed.theclinics.com.

INTRODUCTION

Airway management is the cornerstone to resuscitation efforts for many critically ill pediatric patients presenting for emergency care. The cause of arrest in children is more commonly from a respiratory than a cardiac process, and therefore, early and effective

---

Disclosure Statement: The authors have no financial disclosures of conflicts of interest to report.
Division of Emergency Medicine, Boston Children's Hospital, 300 Longwood Avenue, Boston, MA 02115, USA
* Corresponding author.
E-mail address: Joshua.Nagler@childrens.harvard.edu

Emerg Med Clin N Am 37 (2019) 473–491
https://doi.org/10.1016/j.emc.2019.03.006
0733-8627/19/© 2019 Elsevier Inc. All rights reserved.

airway management is life-saving.[1] However, critical illness and injury is much less common in pediatric patients than in adults.[2–5] Therefore, clinical opportunities for emergency medicine providers to manage pediatric airways may be limited. In addition, lack of familiarity with anatomic and physiologic differences in children can further complicate performance of this critical procedure. This article reviews current understanding and recent advances in pediatric airway management. We provide background information, review relevant anatomic and physiologic differences in children, and offer strategies to optimize procedural success. In addition, we include tips for effective bag-mask ventilation, laryngoscopy (direct and video), and intubation; modifications to rapid sequence intubation (RSI); and approaches to predict and manage anatomically and physiologically difficult pediatric airways.

EPIDEMIOLOGY OF PEDIATRIC EMERGENT AIRWAY MANAGEMENT

Only a small proportion of pediatric patients ultimately require advanced airway management. Data suggest that the need for endotracheal intubation in children presenting to the emergency department (ED) ranges from 0.6 to 3.3 cases per thousand visits.[6,7] Characteristics of children requiring intubation vary by center, with median reported ages varying from 2 to 7 years, although a disproportionate number are 1 year of age or younger.[8–12] Broadly, there are approximately equal number of intubations for trauma and medical indications in children, though proportions vary widely by institution, given differences in patient populations, trauma center designations, and regionalization of pediatric care.[8,12]

ANATOMIC AND PHYSIOLOGIC DIFFERENCES BETWEEN PEDIATRIC AND ADULT AIRWAYS

There are several predictable anatomic and physiologic differences in children that affect airway management (**Table 1**). Infants have a large occiput causing natural flexion of the airway in neutral position. The larynx in children is anatomically high in the neck. Although commonly referred to as anterior, it is this superior position that can create the acute angle needed to see the glottis, making visualization challenging. The epiglottis in children is commonly large and often floppy and can obstruct visualization. The shape of the airway in children has been described historically to be funnel shaped; widest in the supraglottic region and the narrowest portion at the cricoid cartilage. This understanding

Table 1 Anatomic and physiologic differences in children and strategies to address them	
Anatomic/Physiologic Difference	**Strategy to Address**
Large occiput	Position patient appropriately (align external auditory meatus with sternal notch)
Superior airway	Look "up" during laryngoscopy
Large epiglottis	Lift with straight blade Engage the hypoepiglottic ligament
Airway shape (elliptical, not funneled)	Consider cuffed endotracheal tubes
Smaller lung volume	Use the "pop-off" valve during mask ventilation to avoid inadvertent barotrauma
Rapid desaturation	Preoxygenation Apneic oxygenation

contributed to the recommendation for using uncuffed endotracheal tubes in children. However more recently, a series of studies using bronchoscopy, MRI, and airway computed tomography have demonstrated proportional cross-sectional area of the subglottis in children, similar to adults, although more elliptical in shape.[13–17] Finally, children have smaller lungs, and therefore proportionally smaller tidal volumes than adults.

There are numerous physiologic differences between children and adults; however, the one most relevant to airway management is the more rapid rate of desaturation. Children have a smaller functional residual capacity.[18,19] Therefore, even with appropriate preoxygenation, the stores of oxygenated airspace from which to draw is smaller. In addition, children have a higher metabolic rate and therefore consume oxygen at a rate that may be twice that of adults, on a per kilogram basis. These factors combine to create a shorter safe apnea time.

ROLE FOR NONINVASIVE VENTILATION

In considering urgent and emergent airway management in pediatric patients, providers should tailor airway interventions to the clinical need. Noninvasive ventilation (NIV) can provide increased support in children with hypoxic and hypercarbic respiratory failure, and obviate endotracheal intubation in many of these patients. A brief review of high-flow nasal cannula (HFNC) and continuous positive airway pressure (CPAP) and bilevel positive airway support (BPAP) is included here. For more details on these topics, readers are referred to a separate recent review of this material.[20]

High-Flow Nasal Cannula

Traditional low-flow nasal cannula cannot match inspiratory flow rates in infants and children outside the neonatal period without causing nasal mucosal injury. HFNC devices deliver heated, humidified air that match or exceed patients' inspiratory flow rates. This limits entrainment of room air and assists respiratory effort through several different mechanisms (**Box 1**). The flow should be adjusted based on patient age.

HFNC devices have demonstrable clinical benefits in various pediatric populations, including those with bronchiolitis and respiratory distress from other causes.[21] Adequate respiratory support with HFNC devices can obviate sedation and the risk of endotracheal intubation, mechanical ventilation, and ventilator-associated pneumonia. In addition, even in the setting of low oxygen requirements, HFNC devices may be preferred over facemasks, which are less well tolerated in pediatric patients and make speaking and feeding more difficult. HFNC has an excellent safety profile in pediatrics, with complications rarely reported.

Noninvasive Ventilation

NIV encompasses mechanical respiratory support without endotracheal intubation through either CPAP or BPAP. Both modalities are delivered through a range of

---

Box 1
Mechanisms of action for high-flow nasal cannula

Washout of nasopharyngeal dead space

Minimizing nasopharyngeal airway resistance

Improved conductance and lung compliance

Reduction in metabolic expenditure for gas conditioning

Positive distending pressure

interfaces, included nasal cannula, nasal mask, full-face mask, or helmet. Identifying an appropriate interface is often the greatest challenge in pediatrics. Interfaces should be chosen balancing the desire to maximize comfort and compliance while ensuring minimal leak. In addition to positive pressure, NIV can also deliver supplemental oxygen and is compatible with inhaled therapies, such as albuterol and racemic epinephrine.

Similar to HFNC, NIV is used for acute hypoxic and/or hypercarbic respiratory failure. Published experience supports the use of NIV for acute respiratory failure caused by bronchiolitis, status asthmaticus, pneumonia, pulmonary edema, cystic fibrosis, acute chest syndrome, and dynamic upper airway obstruction.[22] CPAP may be appropriate when hypoxemia is the primary indication. Because it delivers higher mean airway pressures while offloading inspiratory effort, BPAP is used for more severe hypoxemia and to address hypercapnia. As in adults, NIV should not be used in patients requiring immediate endotracheal intubation, such as those in cardiopulmonary arrest, those with impaired mental status or requiring airway protection, and those with high aspiration risk. Relative contraindications include facial injury, upper gastrointestinal bleeding, untreated pneumothorax, and significant or escalating vasopressor support.[23,24]

NIV provides benefit through three primary mechanisms: (1) decreasing work of breathing, (2) maintaining patency of the respiratory tract to reduce obstructive apnea and facilitate expiratory flow, and (3) recruiting alveoli to increase functional residual capacity and decrease ventilation-perfusion mismatching. Most children, with appropriate coaching and provider patience during initiation, tolerate NIV, although some require minimal anxiolysis or sedation.

Multiple parameters are titrated with NIV, including CPAP (typically 5–10 cm H_2O), expiratory positive airway pressure (EPAP) and inspiratory positive airway pressure (IPAP) (typically 5–10 cm H_2O and 8–22 cm H_2O, respectively), fraction of inspired oxygen, and back-up ventilation rate if patient is experiencing intermittent apnea or hypopnea.[23,25]

To ensure an adequate response to NIV, patients should be closely monitored with noninvasive measurement of respiratory rate, heart rate, oxygen requirement, and pulse oximetry and monitoring for hypercarbia through blood gas analysis, or end-tidal CO_2 devices.[26–28] Complications include barotrauma, aspiration, and hemodynamic instability caused by decreased venous return. Minor complications frequently associated with ill-fitting interfaces may include skin breakdown, eye irritation, and nasal mucosal trauma.

STRATEGIES FOR SUCCESSFUL ADVANCED AIRWAY MANAGEMENT

Children may require endotracheal intubation because of failure to oxygenate or ventilate, failure to maintain or protect their airway, or because of their anticipated clinical course. Several strategies may be effective in addressing the predictable anatomic and physiologic differences in pediatric airways described previously (see **Table 1**). In addition, modifications to RSI and use of optimal equipment are helpful.

Strategies to Address Anatomic Differences in the Pediatric Airway

Given the large occiput in young infants, using a shoulder roll can help align the airway. Toddlers and school age children are often well anatomically aligned with supine without support, and older children and adolescents frequently benefit from elevation of the head, similar to adults. A consistent approach that can obviate the need to remember position by age group is to align the external auditory meatus with the sternal notch. Data support that this strategy improves glottic visualization during laryngoscopy.[29]

Given the superior location of the larynx in pediatric patients, one should anticipate the glottic opening will be located at the top of the visual field during direct laryngoscopy. The wider viewing angles available through videolaryngoscopes may also facilitate visualization of the glottic structures.

The large, floppy epiglottis is addressed using two techniques. Common teaching is to use a straight blade to lift the epiglottis directly. However, curved blades can also be used in pediatric airway management, with the blade placed along the base of the tongue to indirectly lift the epiglottis. Depressing or engaging the hyoepiglottic ligament within the vallecula is particularly helpful in elevating the epiglottis (**Fig. 1**, Video 1).[30]

Recent recognition that the airway in children is not funnel shaped, combined with changes in the size and design of endotracheal tubes has contributed to the increased use of cuffed tubes in pediatric patients. Cuffed endotracheal tubes reduce the need for tube exchange without increasing risk of tracheal injury using postextubation stridor as a proxy.[31] Current pediatric advanced life support (PALS) guidelines suggest that cuffed and uncuffed endotracheal tubes are acceptable, and that cuffed tubes may be preferred in cases of poor lung compliance or high airway resistance, and that cuffed tubes may decrease the risk of aspiration.[32,33] Therefore, most indications for pediatric intubations in emergency medicine are included in these "cuffed preferred" conditions. Given these advantages (**Box 2**), it is the authors' practice to use cuffed endotracheal tubes in essentially all pediatric intubations in the ED, with careful attention paid to correct positioning of the endotracheal tube and avoidance of overinflation of the cuff.

Bag-mask ventilation may be performed to provide transient respiratory support, or in the context of endotracheal intubation. Delivering effective but safe breaths is key. Motor memory for providers caring primarily for adult patients might result in excessive breath volumes when squeezing a bag. Therefore, many pediatric bags are equipped with "pop-off" valves, designed to limit maximal pressure to a preset limit (often 35–40 cm H_2O). This valve can be opened (creating a maximal allowable pressure) or closed (no limit to the pressure that is delivered) (**Fig. 2**). Most providers use this safety device in the open position to avoid inadvertent overventilation or barotrauma; however, it is important to recognize that in some patients closure of the valve may be necessary to achieve effective ventilation.[34]

Strategies to Address Physiologic Differences in Children

Strategies to avoid desaturation during intubation of pediatric patients include maximizing preoxygenation, using apneic oxygenation, and limiting duration of attempts.

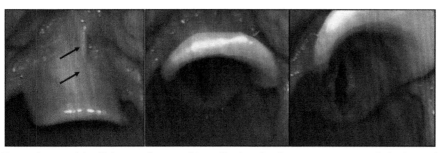

Fig. 1. Sequential still images from a video clip showing how engagement of the hyoepiglottic ligament (*arrows*) within the vallecula can elevate the epiglottis and improve glottic visualization.

> **Box 2**
> **Advantages of using cuffed endotracheal tubes in children**
> - Fit well into elliptical-shaped pediatric airway
> - Favored in patients with poor lung compliance or airway obstruction
> - May help prevent aspiration
> - Reduce need for tube exchange in critically ill patients
> - No increased risk of tracheal injury with proper cuff inflation pressure

Preoxygenation in children in the ED is traditionally performed using a nonbreather mask often with additional nasal cannula oxygen delivery. Although self-inflating bags are commonly used in adults, spontaneously breathing infants and young children may not have the inspiratory force to open the one-way valve in these devices. Therefore, the bag must be squeezed, ideally synchronized to the patient's breaths, to facilitate oxygen delivery. Alternatively, flow-inflating bags do not have a one-way valve and are used without delivery of assisted breaths. Flush rate oxygen delivery has been shown to be effective in improving preoxygenation in adults[35,36]; however, it is not clear if such high rates are similarly beneficial in pediatric patients who have fractionally lower minute ventilation.

Apneic oxygenation is well suited for airway management of children and many centers are now using it routinely,[37] although data regarding use in pediatric patients in the ED are limited.[38] Importantly, flow rates to provide optimal physiologic benefit without increased risk (eg, distending the esophagus or filling the gastrum with air) are not known. Multiple recommendations have been proposed as safe and likely beneficial (**Table 2**). Even with adequate preapneic and apneic oxygenation, many pediatric patients require mask ventilation between attempts if intubation is not achieved quickly. If the nasal cannula used for apneic oxygenation impedes adequate mask seal, it should be immediately removed.

Finally, limiting lengths of laryngoscopic attempts may be valuable. Although common practice is to continue attempts until oxygen saturation falls lower than some predetermined level (often 90%–92%), others have suggested that limiting attempts by length of time (eg, 30–45 seconds) may reduce the frequency of hypoxia without affecting success rates.[39]

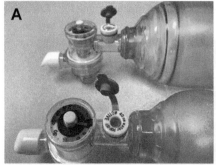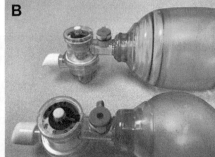

Fig. 2. The "pop-off" valve on neonatal and pediatric self-inflating bags is designed to prevent inadvertent barotrauma. (*A*) When open, the maximal deliverable pressure is limited by the preset value on the valve (40 cm H_2O on these bags). (*B*) The pop-off valve is closed to delivery higher pressures if lung compliance or airway resistance is high.

Table 2
Proposed recommendations for nasal cannula flow rates during apneic oxygenation in children

	Adjusted per Year of Age[69]	Stepwise Approach[70]	Infant/Child Versus Adolescent[71]
General recommendations	1–2 L/min per year of age (max 15 L/min)	<3 y old: 2 L/min 3–8 y old: 4 L/min >8 y old: 6 L/min	Infants/children: 5 L/min Adolescents: 15 L/min
Applying Each Recommendation Across Sample Ages			
1 y old	1–2 L/min	2 L/min	5 L/min
5 y old	5–10 L/min	4 L/min	5 L/min
16 y old	15 L/min	6 L/min	15 L/min

Data from Refs.[69–71]

Modifications Used in Rapid Sequence Intubation for Children

RSI is the mainstay of pediatric emergent airway management. Modifications in approach may be beneficial when caring for pediatric patients.

Modified rapid sequence intubation

"True" or "pure" RSI avoids positive pressure breaths after medication delivery to minimize insufflation of air into the stomach, which might increase the risk of aspiration. Given that children are apt to desaturate during intubation, positive pressure ventilation is commonly used to restore oxygenation at some point during the procedure. This delivery of slow, gentle positive pressure breaths after medication administration is referred to as "modified" or "controlled" RSI. This approach has been demonstrated to be safe in the operating room setting, and is common in pediatric emergent intubations.[40]

Use of Neuromuscular Blocking Agents

There is a temptation to intubate pediatric patients without using neuromuscular blocking agents. This likely stems from the recognition of the ability to overpower infants and children without neuromuscular blocking agents, and reluctance to relinquish spontaneous respirations based on concern for inability to successfully secure the airway in this less familiar patient population. However, data suggest that intubation success rates are higher when RSI is performed.[12,41] Ensuring effective bag-mask ventilation before medication delivery can help predict the ability to mask ventilate if intubation is not successful and alleviate some concerns. If there is difficulty with preintubation bag-mask ventilation, or if there are other predictors of airway difficulty including significant airway obstruction, the decision to administer neuromuscular blocking agents should be carefully considered.

Atropine

The use of atropine as a premedication for pediatric patients is controversial. Bradycardia is common during pediatric intubation; however, this most commonly results from associated hypoxemia. Atropine is not predicted to prevent hypoxia-induced bradycardia. The premise for atropine use as a premedication is to attenuate the high vagal tone common in young infants, which is triggered by the placement of the laryngoscope in the hypopharynx. PALS guidelines have acknowledged that data regarding the efficacy of atropine are conflicting, although citing one study suggesting improved clinical outcome.[33] The recommendations are not to use atropine routinely, but as a premedication in circumstances where there may be a higher risk of bradycardia. Our practice, therefore, is to use atropine in our youngest patients (<1 year of age) in whom vagal-mediated bradycardia is most likely to occur.

Use of Videolaryngoscopy in Pediatrics

Use of videolaryngoscopy (VL) for endotracheal intubation is increasing in pediatrics.[8,11] Although originally considered rescue devices, videolaryngoscopes are now used as first-line devices by many providers. Several of the currently available videolaryngoscopes may be used in children, including some with a full complement of pediatric blade sizes ranging from neonatal through adolescent/adult. Much of the currently available data in children have shown that VL improves glottic visualization, although with mixed data on first-pass success, and with some studies showing longer time to intubation.[42] The failure of improved view to consistently translate into improved success may be explained by: (1) longer time to intubation with VL is not well tolerated given rapid desaturation in children, (2) bulkier blades and handles are more cumbersome in the smaller pediatric oropharynx and hypopharynx, (3) indirect tube passage in the superiorly positioned airway is challenging, and (4) the infrequency in performing this procedure in any given pediatric age group with these devices may affect procedural competence.

Data from select age groups and devices have shown improvement in pediatric intubation performance with using VL.[8,11] In addition to this potential procedural benefit, VL offers additional advantages not necessary captured when using first-pass success as a metric. The shared view of the airway anatomy and procedural progress allows other clinicians to offer real-time guidance to the primary laryngoscopist. VL also has an important role as a teaching tool, with demonstrated improvement in subsequent intubation performance and confidence. In addition, many VL devices allow attempts to be recorded and incorporated into subsequent teaching.[43,44] Such recordings can also be reviewed for quality assurance purposes to assess performance metrics, such as number of attempts, time to intubation, and complications.

Although there are several VL devices for use with children, three of the most commonly used with blade sizes that encompass all pediatric ages are reviewed here (**Table 3**). Given nuances with the use of each videolaryngoscope, it is recommended that providers choose one or two devices to gain comfort with use in children, rather than attempt to master all available options.

IDENTIFICATION AND MANAGEMENT OF DIFFICULT PEDIATRIC AIRWAYS
Definition

The American Society of Anesthesia defines a difficult airway as the clinical situation in which there is difficulty with facemask ventilation of the upper airway, difficulty with tracheal intubation, or both.[45] Difficulty can arise from any combination of patient factors, the clinical setting, and skills of the practitioner attempting to secure the airway. Such difficulties have been shown to be common in pediatric patients, specifically those 1 year of age and younger, and are devestating.[46–48] Difficult mask ventilation may occur in up to 6% of children.[49] Difficult intubation is less common, occurring in 0.5% to 1% of pediatric patients, but 5% in infants less than 1 year of age.[47,48,50]

Predicting Difficult Airways in Pediatric Patients

Providers must keep in mind several unique considerations when confronted with difficult pediatric airways. Traditional tools used to assess the adult airway, including the

Three commonly used pediatric video laryngoscopes

Device	Images Demonstrating Use	Advantages and Technique Tips	Troubleshooting Difficulties
C-MAC	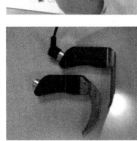	Can be used as a direct or video laryngoscope. Helpful for shared viewing with DL or if the camera lens becomes obscured. Familiar technique for those comfortable with DL. The indirect video view is often better than the simultaneous DL view. A pediatric D-blade with increased angulation is available for use with superior airways or c-spine immobilization. New Mac 0 blade is narrower than Miller and works well in small infants.	Given DL capabilities, troubleshoot difficulties with this device using similar approaches to a traditional laryngoscope. Larger handle size may partially obstruct smaller mouths making blade manipulation potentially challenging. The pediatric D-blade may be too large for use with young infants. Tube delivery is often more challenging than obtaining a glottic view when using the D-blade. A shallow insertion to create a "birds-eye" view of the glottis facilitates tube insertion.
Glidescope	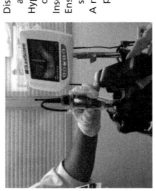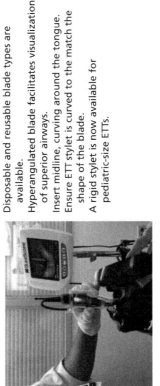	Disposable and reusable blade types are available. Hyperangulated blade facilitates visualization of superior airways. Insert midline, curving around the tongue. Ensure ETT stylet is curved to the match the shape of the blade. A rigid stylet is now available for pediatric-size ETTs.	Look directly in the mouth when inserting the scope or the ETT to avoid inadvertent trauma to the lip, dentition, or palate. Tube delivery is often more challenging than obtaining a glottic view. A shallow insertion to create a "birds-eye" view of the glottis facilitates tube insertion. Consider a smaller than expected blade size to facilitate broader view. If the angulation of the stylet causes the ETT to be directed into the anterior tracheal wall, pull the stylet out of the ETT 1–2 cm and then advance the ETT.

(continued on next page)

Table 3
(continued)

Device	Images Demonstrating Use	Advantages and Technique Tips	Troubleshooting Difficulties
Airtraq		Disposable, single-use versions available, with optional attachable Wi-Fi camera hood. Look through eyepiece/screen early in the insertion to allow progressive visualization of anatomy. Designed to be midline insertion. Ensure proper lubrication of nonstyletted tube to ease delivery through the channel and facilitate disengaging from the device.	When advancing the tube, if the tip dives below the glottic opening, lift the device upward toward the ceiling rather than rock it backward to avoid dental/lip trauma. Disengaging the ETT from the device can result in accidental extubation. Care must be taken to stabilize the ETT during device removal.

Abbreviation: DL, direct laryngoscopy; ETT, endotracheal tube.

Mallampati test and the hyomental and thyromental distances, are poorly characterized for pediatric patients.[51]

Several anatomic features have been identified that can make airway management difficult in children. These may predispose to potential challenges with bag-mask ventilation and/or intubation in pediatric patients.[46,52] These characteristics, their associated conditions, and potential strategies to address them are reviewed in **Table 4**.

Table 4
Anatomic features associated with difficult airways in children

Anatomic Feature	Associated Conditions	Impact on Airway Management	Possible Strategies
Impingement on airway lumen	Thermal injury Angioedema Vascular malformations External compression (abscesses or tumors)	Difficulty with BMV Difficulty visualizing the glottis Difficulty with tube passage	Close pop-off valve for higher BMV pressure Early intervention in rapidly progressive conditions Smaller tube size (cuffed)
Cervical spine abnormalities (instability or limited mobility)	Cervical spine immobilization Trisomy 21 Rheumatologic disease Prior spinal fusion	Inability to align oropharyngeal, laryngeal, and tracheal axes May limit visualization of the laryngeal structures	Open collar, perform in-line stabilization Videolaryngoscopy (hyperangulated blade)
Macroglossia	Trauma to the tongue Allergic reaction Trisomy 21 Mucopolysaccharidoses	Anatomic airway obstruction Difficulty with BMV Difficulty visualizing glottis	Jaw thrust Oral or nasal airway use Supraglottic airway may bypass obstruction Early intervention if progressive
Micrognathia (mandibular hypoplasia)	Can be normal anatomic variant Pierre Robin sequence Treacher Collins syndrome	Anatomic airway obstruction Difficulty with BMV Difficulty visualizing the glottis	Jaw thrust Oral or nasal airway use Supraglottic airway may bypass obstruction Videolaryngoscopy (hyperangulated blade)
Cleft palate	May be additional airway abnormalities Associated with congenital heart disease	Increased risk of airway obstruction Difficulty with laryngoscope blade movement Heart disease may affect RSI	Nasal airway use Rotational placement of supraglottic airways Hemodynamically stable medications

Abbreviation: BMV, bag-mask ventilation.
[a] Careful consideration should be given before administering neuromuscular blocking agents in any pediatric patient with a potentially difficult airway.

Approaches to the Difficult Airway

For anticipated difficult intubations in pediatrics, it is essential to plan ahead; have all equipment available; and to recruit appropriate assistance, such as an anesthesiologist and/or otolaryngologist, or other providers with significant pediatric airway experience. Optimization of intubating conditions by ensuring adequate preoxygenation and apneic oxygenation is also critical. Depending on the reasons for anticipated difficulty, certain strategies may be more or less appropriate in children.

Videolaryngoscopy

VL may help with visualization in many congenital and acquired conditions, and may limit cervical spine movement. However, tube passage under indirect visualization may still be challenging.[53]

Tracheal tube introducer

The bougie is commonly used in adults to help facilitate intubation if either visualization or tube passage is difficult, and therefore would likely be equally efficacious in managing adolescent airways. Although pediatric bougies exist, experience with use during intubation of children is limited to small case series in select populations of children. It is unclear if the tactile stimulation (ie, "clicks") received when the angled tip strikes the tracheal rings is as pronounced in infants and young children, or if the risk of injury to glottic structures or the tracheobronchial tree is higher when using this technique in less mature airways.

Sedation-only induction

When intubation of a child predicted to have a difficult airway is unavoidable, providers should aim to move the patient to an operating room setting whenever possible. This allows for additional personal, equipment, and the availability of inhaled anesthetics. When more emergent intervention is required, sedation-only induction should be considered to preserve spontaneous respiration. This is achieved with careful titration of propofol or ketamine without the use of neuromuscular blockade.

Rescue devices

Of greatest concern is the "can't intubate can't ventilate" or "can't intubate can't oxygenate" scenario, in which a child cannot be effectively ventilated or oxygenated by facemask and tracheal intubation is unsuccessful. Providers should ensure that all appropriate steps have been taken to maximize potential success with bag-mask ventilation including head extension, jaw thrust, two-operator mask ventilation, suctioning, and trial of an oral and/or nasal airway.[54] If despite such optimization maneuvers the patient cannot be ventilated, the American Society of Anesthesia protocols call for rescue devices to sustain effective assisted ventilation until the airway is secured.[55] They are advantageous in patients with craniofacial abnormalities, either congenital or traumatic, in whom it is difficult or impossible to achieve an adequate seal for bag-mask ventilation with a facemask.[56]

The most common rescue device is the laryngeal mask airway.[54,57,58] A range of sizes and manufacturers (LMA, Air-Q, I-gel) of laryngeal airways exist, permitting their use in newborns through adults. The packaging and/or device provides information on patient size and required air volume for cuff inflation, obviating memorization of these details. Laryngeal airways are easy to place and use, with low complication rates among pediatric patients.[59] Second-generation devices have now been developed across pediatric sizes. These permit higher seal pressures and gastric decompression through esophageal lumens, which may be particularly valuable in children with gastric distention secondary to preceding bag-mask ventilation.

Table 5
Management of physiologically difficult airways

Physiologic Condition	Impact on Airway Management	Potential Strategies
Asthma	Positive pressure ventilation can worsen hyperinflation Changing from negative to positive intrathoracic pressure reduces venous return and preload Manipulation of the airway can worsen bronchospasm Prolonged expiratory time	Fluid resuscitation before induction to ensure sufficient preload Ketamine offers bronchodilatory effects Set ventilator for low respiratory rate and prolonged expiratory time (lower I:E ratio)
Heart disease (congenital or acquired)	Risk of decompensated systolic heart failure Risk of dysrhythmia Risk of arrest	Intubate where ECMO is available when possible Place defibrillator pads and backboard before induction Ketamine and/or fentanyl may minimize myocardial depression Vasopressors (epinephrine and dopamine) should be readily available
DKA/metabolic acidosis	Hypovolemia compromises preload Acidosis impairs cardiac contractility Induced apnea prevents physiologic respiratory compensation	Avoid intubation whenever possible Fluid resuscitation before induction Avoid prolonged apnea (consider, sedation-only intubation, mask ventilate until immediately before laryngoscopy, avoid prolonged attempts) Postintubation hyperventilation to match physiologic compensation
Sepsis/septic shock	Often hemodynamically unstable May have critical metabolic acidosis that is worsened by induced apnea during induction Risk of arrest	Fluid resuscitation before induction Consider use of vasopressors before induction Ketamine is most commonly preferred agent Use of etomidate is controversial
Trauma	Cervical spine immobilization impairs anatomic alignment Induced apnea results in cerebral vasodilation, which may increase ICP Noxious stimulus from intubation may increase ICP Hypoperfusion to injured brain may have negative effects on outcome	Cervical spine immobilization is addressed in **Table 4** Maximize preoxygenation and apneic oxygenation Avoid prolonged laryngoscopic attempts Aim to avoid hypotension or hypertension Lidocaine as premedication is not supported by data Etomidate is favored induction agent Ketamine use is supported even with head injury, although alternatives should be considered in hypertensive patients

Abbreviations: DKA, diabetic ketoacidosis; ECMO, extracorporeal membrane oxygenation; ICP, intracranial pressure.

In cases where a patient cannot be successfully intubated and the use of a rescue device to maintain oxygenation and ventilation has failed, providers must resort to invasive techniques including needle or surgical cricothyroidotomy.

Physiologically Difficult Intubations

In addition, obtaining an adequate view of the glottic opening and successfully passing an endotracheal tube, intubation frequently involves sedation, neuromuscular blockade, and mechanical ventilation. These interventions can result in physiologically challenging intubations, even in the absence of an anatomically difficult airway. Many patients intubated in the pediatric ED setting are critically ill from processes that pose unique difficulties in managing the physiologic changes during the peri-intubation period. Select conditions and associated strategies are reviewed in **Table 5**.

CHALLENGES AND STRATEGIES FOR MAINTAINING AIRWAY MANAGEMENT SKILLS

Pediatric airway management is a critical but infrequently performed procedure in the ED setting. Even in high-volume pediatric EDs, more than 60% of faculty do not perform a single successful intubation in a year.[60] Among providers working in general EDs, 25% do not feel comfortable performing endotracheal intubation and other potentially life-saving procedures.[61] As such, maintaining procedural competence is an important consideration for ED providers who care for children.

Reliance on clinical opportunities for airway management in children is likely to be insufficient to achieve and maintain competency in endotracheal intubation, and to a lesser extent bag-mask ventilation.[62] To address this issue, alternative approaches may include low- and high-fidelity simulation, animal or cadaver laboratory experience, operating room rotations, or advanced trauma life support/PALS trainings.[62] Simulation has been shown to improve procedural proficiency, but requires high-fidelity simulators and instructors with significant airway management experience to be most effective.[63,64] Operating room rotations are the preferred learning modality for endotracheal intubation among pediatric ED physicians.[65]

Finally, the videolaryngoscope has become an important tool in procedural instruction around intubation. The shared view allows for real-time instruction and guidance that has been shown to improve intubation performance.[66–68] Additionally, video clips obtained during intubations can be used remotely from procedural attempts to foster familiarity with native airway anatomy and laryngoscopic technique, and ultimately improve intubation performance.[44]

SUMMARY

Managing the airway in critically ill children in the ED is challenging for many emergency providers. Lack of familiarity with anatomic and physiologic differences in pediatric patients, coupled with relative infrequency of clinical exposure are contributing factors. Modification of approach, such as use of alternative personnel, equipment including videolaryngoscopes, or pharmacologic regimens based on predictable differences, is helpful. Finally, it is incumbent on emergency providers to identify opportunities to maintain procedural skills outside the ED when clinical exposure is limited.

SUPPLEMENTARY DATA

Supplementary data related to this article can be found online at https://doi.org/10.1016/j.emc.2019.03.006.

REFERENCES

1. Atkins DL, Berger S, Duff JP, et al. Part 11: pediatric basic life support and cardiopulmonary resuscitation quality: 2015 American Heart Association guidelines update for cardiopulmonary resuscitation and emergency cardiovascular care. Circulation 2015;132(18):S519–25.

2. Green SM. Emergency department patient acuity varies by age. Ann Emerg Med 2012;60(2):147–51.

3. Chen EH, Cho CS, Shofer FS, et al. Resident exposure to critical patients in a pediatric emergency department. Pediatr Emerg Care 2007;23(11):774–8.

4. Chen EH, Shofer FS, Baren JM. Emergency medicine resident rotation in pediatric emergency medicine: what kind of experience are we providing? Acad Emerg Med 2004;11(7):771–3. Available at: http://www.ncbi.nlm.nih.gov/pubmed/15231469. Accessed April 4, 2017.

5. Green SM, Ruben J. Emergency department children are not as sick as adults: implications for critical care skills retention in an exclusively pediatric emergency medicine practice. J Emerg Med 2009;37(4):359–68.

6. Nguyen LD, Craig S. Paediatric critical procedures in the emergency department: incidence, trends and the physician experience. Emerg Med Australas 2016;28(1):78–83.

7. Losek JD, Olson LR, Dobson JV, et al. Tracheal intubation practice and maintaining skill competency: survey of pediatric emergency department medical directors. Pediatr Emerg Care 2008;24(5):294–9.

8. Pallin DJ, Dwyer RC, Walls RM, et al. Techniques and trends, success rates, and adverse events in emergency department pediatric intubations: a report from the national emergency airway registry. Ann Emerg Med 2016;67(5):610–5.e1.

9. Pek JH, Ong GY. Emergency intubations in a high-volume pediatric emergency department. Pediatr Emerg Care 2018. https://doi.org/10.1097/PEC.0000000000001355.

10. Kerrey BT, Rinderknecht AS, Geis GL, et al. Rapid sequence intubation for pediatric emergency patients: higher frequency of failed attempts and adverse effects found by video review. Ann Emerg Med 2012;60(3):251–9.

11. Eisenberg MA, Green-Hopkins I, Werner H, et al. Comparison between direct and video-assisted laryngoscopy for intubations in a pediatric emergency department. Acad Emerg Med 2016;23(8). https://doi.org/10.1111/acem.13015.

12. Sagarin MJ, Chiang V, Sakles JC, et al. Rapid sequence intubation for pediatric emergency airway management. Pediatr Emerg Care 2002;18(6):417–23. Available at: http://www.ncbi.nlm.nih.gov/pubmed/12488834. Accessed August 5, 2015.

13. Litman RS, Weissend EE, Shibata D, et al. Developmental changes of laryngeal dimensions in unparalyzed, sedated children. Anesthesiology 2003;98(1):41–5. Available at: http://www.ncbi.nlm.nih.gov/pubmed/12502977. Accessed December 16, 2018.

14. Dalal PG, Murray D, Messner AH, et al. Pediatric laryngeal dimensions: an age-based analysis. Anesth Analg 2009;108(5):1475–9.

15. Wani TM, Rafiq M, Talpur S, et al. Pediatric upper airway dimensions using three-dimensional computed tomography imaging. Paediatr Anaesth 2017;27(6):604–8.

16. Wani TM, Rafiq M, Akhter N, et al. Upper airway in infants-a computed tomography-based analysis. Paediatr Anaesth 2017;27(5):501–5.

17. Wani TM, Bissonnette B, Rafiq Malik M, et al. Age-based analysis of pediatric upper airway dimensions using computed tomography imaging. Pediatr Pulmonol 2016;51(3):267–71.
18. Gerhardt T, Reifenberg L, Hehre D, et al. Functional residual capacity in normal neonates and children up to 5 years of age determined by a N2 washout method. Pediatr Res 1986;20(7):668–71.
19. Stocks J, Quanjer PH. Reference values for residual volume, functional residual capacity and total lung capacity. ATS workshop on lung volume measurements. Official Statement of The European Respiratory Society. Eur Respir J 1995;8(3): 492–506. Available at: http://www.ncbi.nlm.nih.gov/pubmed/7789503. Accessed December 16, 2018.
20. Viscusi CD, Pacheco GS. Pediatric emergency noninvasive ventilation. Emerg Med Clin North Am 2018;36(2):387–400.
21. Lee M, Nagler J. High-flow nasal cannula therapy beyond the perinatal period. Curr Opin Pediatr 2017;29(3):291–6.
22. Najaf-Zadeh A, Leclerc F. Noninvasive positive pressure ventilation for acute respiratory failure in children: a concise review. Ann Intensive Care 2011; 1(1):15.
23. Akingbola OA, Hopkins RL. Pediatric noninvasive positive pressure ventilation. Pediatr Crit Care Med 2001;2(2):164–9. Available at: http://www.ncbi.nlm.nih. gov/pubmed/12797876.
24. Calderini E, Chidini G, Pelosi P. What are the current indications for noninvasive ventilation in children? Curr Opin Anaesthesiol 2010;23(3):368–74.
25. Abadesso C, Nunes P, Silvestre C, et al. Non-invasive ventilation in acute respiratory failure in children. Pediatr Rep 2012;4(2):e16.
26. Dohna-Schwake C, Stehling F, Tschiedel E, et al. Non-invasive ventilation on a pediatric intensive care unit: feasibility, efficacy, and predictors of success. Pediatr Pulmonol 2011;46(11):1114–20.
27. Mayordomo-Colunga J, Medina A, Rey C, et al. Non-invasive ventilation in pediatric status asthmaticus: a prospective observational study. Pediatr Pulmonol 2011;46(10):949–55.
28. Fortenberry JD, Del Toro J, Jefferson LS, et al. Management of pediatric acute hypoxemic respiratory insufficiency with bilevel positive pressure (BiPAP) nasal mask ventilation. Chest 1995;108(4):1059–64.
29. Kim EH, Lee JH, Song IK, et al. Effect of head position on laryngeal visualisation with the McGrath MAC videolaryngoscope in paediatric patients. Eur J Anaesthesiol 2016;33(7):528–34.
30. Murphy MF, Hung OR, Law JA. Tracheal intubation: tricks of the trade. Emerg Med Clin North Am 2008;26(4):1001–14.
31. Weiss M, Dullenkopf A, Fischer JE, et al. Prospective randomized controlled multi-centre trial of cuffed or uncuffed endotracheal tubes in small children. Br J Anaesth 2009;103(6):867–73.
32. Kleinman ME, Chameides L, Schexnayder SM, et al. Part 14: Pediatric advanced life support: 2010 American Heart Association guidelines for cardiopulmonary resuscitation and emergency cardiovascular care. Circulation 2010;122(SUPPL. 3). https://doi.org/10.1161/CIRCULATIONAHA.110.971101.
33. De Caen AR, Berg MD, Chameides L, et al. Part 12: Pediatric advanced life support: 2015 American Heart Association guidelines update for cardiopulmonary resuscitation and emergency cardiovascular care. Circulation 2015;132(18): S526–42.

34. O'Neill J, Scott C, Kissoon N, et al. Pediatric self-inflating resuscitators: the dangers of improper setup. J Emerg Med 2011;41(6):607–12.
35. Driver BE, Klein LR, Carlson K, et al. Preoxygenation with flush rate oxygen: comparing the nonrebreather mask with the bag-valve mask. Ann Emerg Med 2018;71(3):381–6.
36. Driver BE, Prekker ME, Kornas RL, et al. Flush rate oxygen for emergency airway preoxygenation. Ann Emerg Med 2017;69(1):1–6.
37. Oliveira J E Silva L, Cabrera D, Barrionuevo P, et al. Effectiveness of apneic oxygenation during intubation: a systematic review and meta-analysis. Ann Emerg Med 2017;70(4):483–94.e11.
38. Vukovic AA, Hanson HR, Murphy SL, et al. Apneic oxygenation reduces hypoxemia during endotracheal intubation in the pediatric emergency department. Am J Emerg Med 2018;37(1):27–32.
39. Rinderknecht AS, Mittiga MR, Meinzen-Derr J, et al. Factors associated with oxyhemoglobin desaturation during rapid sequence intubation in a pediatric emergency department: findings from multivariable analyses of video review data. Acad Emerg Med 2015;22(4):431–40.
40. Neuhaus D, Schmitz A, Gerber A, et al. Controlled rapid sequence induction and intubation: an analysis of 1001 children. Paediatr Anaesth 2013;23(8):734–40.
41. Zeiler FA, Teitelbaum J, West M, et al. The ketamine effect on ICP in traumatic brain injury. Neurocrit Care 2014;21(1):163–73.
42. Sun Y, Lu Y, Huang Y, et al. Pediatric video laryngoscope versus direct laryngoscope: a meta-analysis of randomized controlled trials. Paediatr Anaesth 2014; 24(10):1056–65.
43. Nagler J, Nagler A, Bachur RG. Development and assessment of an advanced pediatric airway management curriculum with integrated intubation videos. Pediatr Emerg Care 2017;33(4). https://doi.org/10.1097/PEC.0000000000000777.
44. Miller KA, Monuteaux MC, Aftab S, et al. A randomized controlled trial of a video-enhanced advanced airway curriculum for pediatric residents. Acad Med 2018;1. https://doi.org/10.1097/ACM.0000000000002392.
45. Apfelbaum JL, Hagberg CA, Caplan RA, et al. Practice guidelines for management of the difficult airway. Anesthesiology 2013;118(2):251–70. https://doi.org/10.1097/ALN.0b013e31827773b2.
46. Belanger J, Kossick M. Methods of identifying and managing the difficult airway in the pediatric population. AANA J 2015;83(1):35–41.
47. Heinrich S, Birkholz T, Ihmsen H, et al. Incidence and predictors of difficult laryngoscopy in 11,219 pediatric anesthesia procedures. Paediatr Anaesth 2012; 22(8):729–36.
48. Fiadjoe JE, Nishisaki A, Jagannathan N, et al. Airway management complications in children with difficult tracheal intubation from the Pediatric Difficult Intubation (PeDI) registry: a prospective cohort analysis. Lancet Respir Med 2016;4(1): 37–48.
49. Valois-Gõmez T, Oofuvong M, Auer G, et al. Incidence of difficult bag-mask ventilation in children: a prospective observational study. Paediatr Anaesth 2013; 23(10):920–6.
50. Graciano AL, Tamburro R, Thompson AE, et al. Incidence and associated factors of difficult tracheal intubations in pediatric ICUs: a report from National Emergency Airway Registry for Children: NEAR4KIDS. Intensive Care Med 2014; 40(11):1659–69.
51. Mansano AM, Módolo NSP, Silva LM, et al. Bedside tests to predict laryngoscopic difficulty in pediatric patients. Int J Pediatr Otorhinolaryngol 2016;83:63–8.

52. Russo SG, Becke K. Expected difficult airway in children. Curr Opin Anaesthesiol 2015;28(3):321–6.
53. Holm-Knudsen R. The difficult pediatric airway: a review of new devices for indirect laryngoscopy in children younger than two years of age. Paediatr Anaesth 2011;21(2):98–103.
54. Walker RWM, Ellwood J. The management of difficult intubation in children. Paediatr Anaesth 2009;19(Suppl 1):77–87.
55. Bhaskar CS, Vidhale NN, Berad BN. Synthesis of some ??-picolinyl-I,2,4,5-dithiadiazine and their antimicrobial activity. Asian J Chem 2002;14(1):162–8.
56. Fiadjoe J, Stricker P. Pediatric difficult airway management: current devices and techniques. Anesthesiol Clin 2009;27(2):185–95.
57. Jagannathan N, Ramsey MA, White MC, et al. An update on newer pediatric supraglottic airways with recommendations for clinical use. Paediatr Anaesth 2015;25(4):334–45.
58. Ostermayer DG, Gausche-Hill M. Supraglottic airways: the history and current state of prehospital airway adjuncts. Prehosp Emerg Care 2014;18(1):106–15.
59. Kleine-Brueggeney M, Gottfried A, Nabecker S, et al. Pediatric supraglottic airway devices in clinical practice: a prospective observational study. BMC Anesthesiol 2017;17(1):119.
60. Mittiga MR, Geis GL, Kerrey BT, et al. The spectrum and frequency of critical procedures performed in a pediatric emergency department: implications of a provider-level view matthew. Ann Emerg Med 2013;61(3). https://doi.org/10.1016/j.annemergmed.2012.06.021.
61. Simon HK, Sullivan F. Confidence in performance of pediatric emergency medicine procedures by community emergency practitioners. Pediatr Emerg Care 1996;12(5):336–9. Available at: http://www.ncbi.nlm.nih.gov/pubmed/8897539. Accessed April 4, 2017.
62. Mittiga MR, Fitzgerald MR, Kerrey BT. A survey assessment of perceived importance and methods of maintenance of critical procedural skills in pediatric emergency medicine. Pediatr Emerg Care 2016. [Epub ahead of print].
63. Mills DM, Williams DC, Dobson JV. Simulation training as a mechanism for procedural and resuscitation education for pediatric residents: a systematic review. Hosp Pediatr 2013;3(2):167–76. Available at: http://www.ncbi.nlm.nih.gov/pubmed/24340419. Accessed October 26, 2016.
64. Yang D, Wei Y-K, Xue F-S, et al. Simulation-based airway management training: application and looking forward. J Anesth 2016;30(2):284–9.
65. Craig SS, Auerbach M, Cheek JA, et al. Preferred learning modalities and practice for critical skills: a global survey of paediatric emergency medicine clinicians. Emerg Med J 2018. https://doi.org/10.1136/emermed-2017-207384.
66. Ayoub CM, Kanazi GE, Al Alami A, et al. Tracheal intubation following training with the GlideScope compared to direct laryngoscopy. Anaesthesia 2010;65(7):674–8.
67. Moussa A, Luangxay Y, Tremblay S, et al. Videolaryngoscope for teaching neonatal endotracheal intubation: a randomized controlled trial. Pediatrics 2016;137(3):e20152156.
68. Howard-Quijano KJ, Huang YM, Matevosian R, et al. Video-assisted instruction improves the success rate for tracheal intubation by novices. Br J Anaesth 2008;101(4):568–72.
69. The Airway Card™ v 4.5. Available at: theairwaysite.com. Accessed January 15, 2019.

70. Mittiga MR, Rinderknecht AS, Kerrey BT. A modern and practical review of rapid-sequence intubation in pediatric emergencies. Clin Pediatr Emerg Med 2015; 16(3):172–85.
71. Nagler J, Mick NW. Airway management for the pediatric patient. In: Walls RM, Hockberger RS, Marianne G-H, editors. Rosen's emergency medicine: concepts and clinical practice. 9th edition. Philadelphia: Elsevier Inc; 2018. p. 1997.

Nonischemic Causes of Cardiogenic Shock

Susan R. Wilcox, MD

KEYWORDS

- Cardiogenic shock • Volume overload • Vasopressors • Inotropes
- Mechanical circulatory support

KEY POINTS

- Most cardiogenic shock is caused by myocardial infarction, but nonischemic etiologies are important to identify.
- Once cardiogenic shock is recognized, clinicians must assess and optimize preload, contractility, and afterload.
- Understanding indications and options for mechanical circulatory support is important for timely consultation or transfer as indicated.

INTRODUCTION

Acute heart failure is a syndrome with a wide spectrum of presentations, from mild volume overload to florid cardiogenic shock (CS). The term "cardiogenic shock" simply indicates inadequate cardiac output to meet the metabolic demands of the body, but this final common pathway can arise from disorders of any cardiac structure.[1] Without timely intervention, this primarily cardiac disorder produces organ congestion and hypoperfusion, and leads to multiorgan system failure and ultimately death.[2,3]

Distributive shock is by far the most common cause of shock presenting to the emergency department (ED) (**Fig. 1**).[4] Although CS accounts for only approximately 5% of acute heart failure presentations,[2,5] mortality remains approximately 40% to 60%.[2,6–8] The hallmark feature of CS is decreased cardiac output, but other structural and clinical conditions can present with a similar hemodynamic profile. Some patients have high or low preload, and high or low systemic vascular resistance.[4] Patients with heart failure[9–11] and shock[1] alike are categorized by volume status and perfusion (**Fig. 2**).

CS may be challenging to recognize on initial presentation, often confused for more mild heart failure or other etiologies of shock. Definitions for CS commonly used in the

Disclosure Statement: The author has no financial disclosures to report.
Division of Critical Care, Department of Emergency Medicine, Massachusetts General Hospital, Zero Emerson Place, Suite 3B, Boston, MA 02114, USA
E-mail address: Swilcox1@partners.org

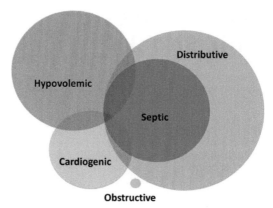

Fig. 1. Schematic illustrating relative incidence of types of shock in emergency medicine.

literature involve cardiac indices and pulmonary capillary wedge pressures, which are not available on presentation to the ED.[12] Most studies on CS are derived from the cardiology and critical care literature,[13,14] with few studies of this population in emergency medicine.

CAUSE OF CARDIOGENIC SHOCK

The most common cause of CS is acute coronary syndrome, accounting for about 70% to 80% of CS cases.[2,6,13] Although not the focus of this review, emergency medicine clinicians should be aware that most CS is caused by acute coronary syndrome and evaluate for ischemia accordingly.[2] **Table 1** outlines etiologies of CS.

Other causes of CS predominantly include the decompensation of chronic heart failure[6,15] and right ventricular (RV) failure in about 5% of cases.[16] RV failure may be a

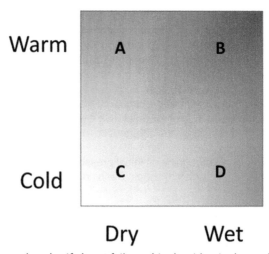

Fig. 2. Commonly used to classify heart failure, this algorithm is also useful for considering the cause of patients in shock. "A" profiles indicate a distributive picture, whereas "B" is consistent with distributive with chronic heart failure or a mixed picture. "C" is consistent with hypovolemic or euvolemic cardiogenic causes, and "D" is most consistent with classic cardiogenic shock.[1]

Table 1
Causes of cardiogenic shock

Etiology	Clinical Considerations

Postischemic
  Papillary muscle
    rupture/acute mitral
    regurgitation
  VSD
  Free wall rupture
	Consider in any patient presenting in shock within 2 wk of an MI
	Higher mortality than other CS
	Needs prompt recognition, cardiac surgery consultation

Ischemic cardiomyopathy	History of prior ischemic events, common cause of cardiomyopathy Acute decompensation of chronic condition

Stress cardiomyopathy
  (takotsubos
  cardiomyopathy)
	LV dysfunction related to stress within 1–5 d
	1%–2% of patients with suspected acute coronary syndrome, most
	  common in postmenopausal women
	ECG: STE or STD, TWI, QTc prolongation
	Echo: LV WMA beyond single coronary artery distribution; assess
	  for LVOTO
	Mild elevation of troponin, very elevated BNP
	Treatment depends on presence of LVOTO; with LVOTO, avoid
	  inotropes to prevent further obstruction; phenylephrine or
	  vasopressin for hypotension
	Without LVOTO, standard supportive care appropriate

Hypertrophic
  cardiomyopathy
	Suspect with history of syncope or family history sudden cardiac
	  death
	ECG: LVH, may have a deep, narrow Q wave inferiorly or laterally
	Echo: asymmetric ventricular hypertrophy, especially in the
	  parasternal long view, may have LVOTO
	Hypovolemia is deleterious, especially in patients with LVOTO
	Consider phenylephrine or vasopressin to reduce gradient across
	  LVOTO
	Avoid decreasing preload or afterload or increasing contractility

Other nonischemic
  cardiomyopathies
  Viral
  Autoimmune
  Nutritional deficiencies
  Endocrinologic
  Alcohol
  Genetic conditions
  Medication-related,
    including
    chemotherapy
  Restrictive
  Infiltrative
  Peripartum
  Idiopathic
	Wide array of causes
	If new presentation, will require inpatient work-up for cause and
	  management of CS
	Additional specific therapies vary with the cause, such as treating
	  thyrotoxicosis or thiamine deficiency

Myocarditis	Long differential diagnosis, associated with viral and bacterial
	  infections, reactions to medications, and underlying
	  autoimmune diseases
	ECG: variable, conduction delays, nonspecific T-wave and ST
	  changes, STE, arrhythmias
	Echo: evaluate chamber sizes, wall thickness, function
	Some etiologies require immunosuppression; treatment otherwise
	  supportive

(continued on next page)

Table 1 (continued)	
Etiology	Clinical Considerations
Valvular disease	May have acute decompensation of chronic condition
Aortic insufficiency	AS is preload dependent; hypotension can lead to decreased
AS	coronary perfusion
MR	Aortic insufficiency is a contraindication to most MCS
Mitral stenosis	Can be primary pathology or secondary to LV (MR) or RV (TR)
TR	enlargement
Arrhythmias	May be primary or secondary cause of CS
Tachydysrhythmias	Can exacerbate existing cardiomyopathy, triggering CS
Bradydysrhythmias	Low threshold to cardiovert tachydysrhythmias
	Note that sinus tachycardia may be a compensatory mechanism for low stroke volume and as such, should not be slowed
	Avoid BB and CCB in CS
	Atropine, chronotropes, transcutaneous pacing, and transvenous pacing should be used as required for bradydysrhythmias
	In cases of CS from BB or CCB overdose, treat with HIE, intravenous calcium, or intralipid while providing supportive care

Abbreviations: AS, aortic stenosis; BB, beta-blocker; BNP, B-type natriuretic peptide; CCB, calcium channel blocker; ECG, electrocardiogram; Echo, echocardiography; HIE, hyperinsulinemia euglycemia; LV, left ventricle; LVH, left ventricular hypertrophy; LVOTO, left ventricular outflow tract obstruction; MCS, mechanical circulatory support; MI, myocardial infarction; MR, mitral regurgitation; RV, right ventricle; TR, tricuspid regurgitation; VSD, ventricular septal defect WMA, wall motion abnormalities.

result of infarction,[16] long-standing pulmonary hypertension,[17] or pulmonary embolism (although pulmonary embolism is typically considered an obstructive cause of shock). RV dysfunction can also develop as a result of acute respiratory distress syndrome or other causes of severe hypoxemia (**Fig. 3**).

Although a rare cause of CS, patients with left ventricular (LV) outflow tract obstruction, such as hypertrophic cardiomyopathy, deserve special mention.[18] Because of the configuration of the myocardium, patients with hypertrophic cardiomyopathy have a small LV cavity and the outflow tract to the aorta can be compressed during systole. Management with diuretics or inotropic therapy could precipitate or worsen CS.

Takotsubo cardiomyopathy, or stress-induced cardiomyopathy, can present after any potential stressor.[19] Although patients usually have only mild hemodynamic consequences, it can present with CS and may require temporary mechanical support.[1,20] Myocarditis can present with a range of phenotypes, from a mild illness to fulminant shock.[21,22]

Dysrhythmias can present as a primary cause of shock or secondary to a primary cardiac or metabolic insult. Cardiovascular medications, such as β-blockers, calcium channel blockers, and occasionally digoxin, can inhibit a compensatory increase in cardiac output during periods of increased physiologic demand and can also lead to a primary dysrhythmia in the setting of overdose.[23]

ASSESSMENT OF CARDIOGENIC SHOCK
History and Physical Examination

Patients presenting with CS may present with vague symptoms, such as dyspnea,[24] orthopnea, abdominal pain, or loss of appetite. A review of the patient's past medical

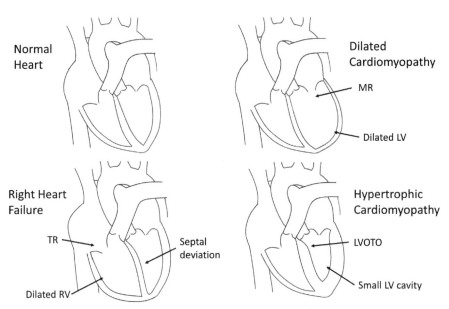

Fig. 3. Representation of various cardiomyopathies. Dilated cardiomyopathies result in poor systolic function and the development of mitral regurgitation. In right heart failure, the RV becomes dilated and/or hypertrophic, and tricuspid regurgitation develops. The interventricular septum can bulge into the left ventricle (LV), decreasing LV filling and cardiac output. Hypertrophic cardiomyopathy results in a small LV, making the patient preload-dependent. Left ventricular outflow tract obstruction worsens with inotropes or hypotension. Note that patients can have multiple or mixed types of cardiac pathology. LVOTO, left ventricular outflow tract obstruction; MR, mitral regurgitation; TR, tricuspid regurgitation.

history often identifies a diagnosis of coronary artery disease or previous cardiac surgery. If available, a prior echocardiogram and left and right heart catheterization data are valuable.

Although most patients in CS present with hypotension,[6] this is not universal. Patients with chronic heart failure develop long-standing neurohormonal compensation with chronic vasoconstriction.[1] These patients can have a normal blood pressure with high vasomotor tone, yet still can be hypoperfused because of poor cardiac output.[13,25] A narrow pulse pressure of less than 25% of the systolic blood pressure indicates low stroke volume.[26] Alternatively, systemic inflammation caused by cardiac injury and systemic hypoperfusion may induce vasoplegia. Given the potential variation in blood pressures, patients should be assessed for signs of perfusion, specifically focusing on cool extremities, poor capillary refill, and impaired mentation.[10] Placement of a urinary catheter to follow urine production is indicated.

Jugular venous pulse should be noted, because elevations in jugular venous pulse have been shown to correlate with increased mortality.[27] Although rales on pulmonary auscultation may be appreciated in acute left-sided failure with volume overload, they are often absent in patients with long-standing heart failure[26] because of chronic accommodation by the lymphatic system. Peripheral edema is neither sensitive nor specific for CS.[10]

Murmurs can indicate a variety of acute or chronic conditions leading to CS, as listed in **Table 1**. A third heart sound, or S3, is specific to heart failure in adults, because of rapid ventricular filling of a dilated ventricle. Louder in states of volume overload, an S3 has also been associated with increased mortality.[10,27]

Electrocardiogram

The electrocardiogram (ECG) should be checked promptly in all patients with shock,[24] because most CS arises from acute coronary syndrome. However, the ECG may or may not show acute changes, even in cases of CS. **Table 1** notes common ECG findings (**Fig. 4**).

Bedside Cardiac Ultrasound

Bedside cardiac ultrasound should be performed on all patients with undifferentiated shock in the ED. Protocols for shock assessment have shown to have clinical benefit.[28–30] Ultrasound can quickly rule out tamponade, and evaluate the left and RV function, inferior vena cava, and volume status. Beyond cardiac evaluations, ultrasonographic assessment can identify pulmonary edema or ascites caused by chronic heart failure. Comprehensive transthoracic echocardiography is indicated in all cases of CS to assess for potential etiologies and to follow hemodynamic evaluations (**Fig. 5**).[1,13]

Hemodynamic Monitoring

In addition to echocardiography, hemodynamic assessments are important for diagnosis and monitoring in all cases of shock presenting to the ED. An arterial catheter allows continuous blood pressure monitoring, tracking the patient's response to interventions, and repeated blood gas analysis.[13]

Historically, central venous catheters were placed to measure central venous pressure (CVP) to ensure adequate preload in shock.[13] In distributive shock, CVP does not correlate well with preload and does not indicate a volume-responsive state.[13,31] However, a CVP at the extremes, such as less than 6 or greater than 15 mm Hg,[31,32] can assist with determining the cause of shock and guide volume management.

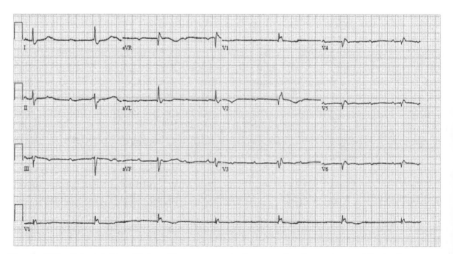

Fig. 4. ECG of a patient with baseline severe aortic stenosis who presented in CS from complete heart block. Unresponsive to chronotropes, emergency transvenous pacing wire placement was required.

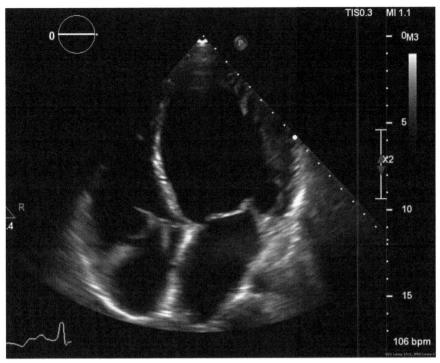

Fig. 5. Apical four-chamber view of an echocardiogram of a patient with idiopathic cardio-myopathy with an ejection fraction of 18%.

In CS, measurement of the central venous oxygen saturation ($ScvO_2$) is helpful, and reflects physiologic response to variations in cardiac output.[1,13]

Noninvasive Cardiac Output Monitors

Numerous brands of minimally invasive cardiac monitors are available, using proprietary technology to assess arterial line or pulse oximetry waveforms to monitor cardiac output.[33] These devices may hold promise in emergency medicine, but have not been sufficiently studied to integrate into routine practice.

Pulmonary Arterial Lines

Pulmonary arterial (PA) lines, or Swan-Ganz catheters measure and display pressures from the pulmonary artery and the pulmonary artery wedge pressure, serving as a surrogate for LV filling pressures. Additionally, PA catheters can measure mixed venous oxygen saturation (or SvO_2) and cardiac output using thermodilution.

Placement of PA lines used to be routine in critically ill patients, until several studies found no outcomes benefit with routine use.[10,34] The limitations of these studies were that they either included an overly heterogeneous group of patients[35,36] unlikely to benefit from this detailed hemodynamic monitoring, or they focused on patients with heart failure who were largely not in shock.[37] To date, only one small prospective study has evaluated PA lines in patients with CS, finding reduced short- and long-term mortality.[38] Risks of PA lines are consistent with the risks of any line placement, with infectious complications being the most common adverse event.[37]

Currently, guidelines[1,9,39,40] recommend placement of PA lines for patients with severe or refractory CS,[9,13] RV dysfunction,[2,9,13] an uncertain cause of shock,[1] or when the volume status is unclear.[9] Although PA lines are not placed in the ED, understanding potential indications are important, because ED clinicians have the opportunity to refer patients for early, invasive monitoring.

Laboratory Values

Troponin and natriuretic peptides can directly assess for cardiac injury. Checking troponin in cases of suspected CS is always indicated.[1] Natriuretic peptides are significantly elevated in CS and levels correlated with mortality.[1,41]

Additional laboratory values can provide markers of organ perfusion. Acute kidney injury, represented by elevated serum creatinine and decreased urine production, is associated with worse outcomes in CS.[42] Liver hypoperfusion results in a transaminitis, whereas hepatic congestion can lead to elevated alkaline phosphatase,[2,43] bilirubin, and international normalized ratio.[44]

Serum lactate levels are elevated in CS via several mechanisms, including inadequate peripheral tissue oxygen delivery, stress-induced hyperlactatemia, and impaired clearance.[45] Lactate levels in CS have been shown to correlate with mortality, similar to other etiologies of shock, and clearance of lactate is of similar prognostic value.[1,13,45,46]

MEDICAL MANAGEMENT

As with any patient in extremis, initial assessment and resuscitation occur simultaneously. Because of the relative infrequency of CS, especially outside of myocardial ischemia, clinicians must consider CS as part of the differential or risk missing the diagnosis. As opposed to the traditional "airway, breathing, circulation" survey used in most critically ill patients, considering "optimizing preload, contractility, and afterload" may be more useful in patients with CS.

When thinking of CS, one must consider RV failure differently than LV failure, because the two sides of the heart have important physiologic differences. The RV functions in a low-pressure, high-volume system and is therefore sensitive to changes in preload and afterload.[44] Specific resuscitation goals for RV failure are listed in **Table 2**.[44,47]

Preload

Assessing volume status is particularly difficult in patients with CS, especially with long-standing heart failure or pulmonary hypertension. Some patients may be volume responsive, especially in the setting of conditions causing volume depletion or concomitant vasoplegia. Guidelines recommend that in the absence of signs of acute volume overload, careful volume expansion in CS is appropriate.[13] Patients should be frequently reassessed to ensure that they remain volume responsive. Continued volume administration beyond responsiveness can increase organ congestion, lead to acute kidney injury,[48] and is associated with worsened outcomes.[49,50]

Some patients with chronic heart failure and CS are volume overloaded on presentation. Patients with CS and pulmonary edema may benefit from diuretics if intravascularly overloaded with an adequate blood pressure.[13] Diuresing a patient with volume overload can increase cardiac output and improve organ perfusion.[44] Similarly, high-volume fluid resuscitation can lead to worsened cardiac output. Although CVP measurements do not entirely reflect volume responsiveness, volume resuscitating a patient with an elevated CVP is more likely to be deleterious than a patient with a lower CVP.[31]

Table 2
Management of cardiogenic shock from right heart failure

Parameter	Pathophysiology	Management
Recognition	Often challenging to recognize; may be acute, such as RV infarct, or acute-on-chronic, such as with pulmonary hypertension	Management complex Consult pulmonary hypertension expert, usually pulmonologist or cardiologist, early in course
Preload	Acute RV dysfunction can be preload dependent May be volume depleted, based on history (eg, recent gastrointestinal illness) Pulmonary hypertension patients often chronically overloaded because of neurohormonal upregulation Volume status assessment challenging because of chronic adaptations	If patient needs volume from acute RV dysfunction or by history, provide in small aliquots Reassess frequently with vital signs, echocardiography, markers, or perfusion In cases of volume overload, may benefit from diuresis Often benefit from PA line placement
Contractility	Hypotension can lead to decreased coronary perfusion, leading to worse contractility Cannot tolerate arrhythmias	Provide early vasopressors to maintain coronary perfusion Add inotropes as able for RV support Manage arrhythmias aggressively
Afterload	Hypoxemic vasoconstriction, acidemia increase RV afterload Positive pressure ventilation can increase afterload Inhaled pulmonary vasodilators can dilate pulmonary vasculature	Avoid hypoxia and hypercapnia Support oxygenation with high-flow nasal cannulae Judicious noninvasive ventilation Avoid intubation if possible Prevent hypotension, hypoventilation/ hyperventilation with intubation Consider inhaled epoprostenol or nitric oxide

Contractility

Use of vasopressor and inotropic therapy is critical to restoring end-organ perfusion in CS.[51] It is critical to optimize contractility and coronary perfusion. Although there are no robust studies of mean arterial pressure (MAP) goals in CS, an initial MAP of 65 mm Hg is recommended.[13] Vasopressor or inotrope selection is guided by the patient's cause of CS and hemodynamics. Most inotropes are inodilators (**Table 3**), meaning that they often decrease MAP while increasing inotropy. Therefore, in patients with hypotension, vasopressors should be started first to support the blood pressure before starting an inotrope (**Fig. 6**).

Norepinephrine is the vasopressor of choice in CS.[1,13,52] Compared with dopamine, norepinephrine causes fewer arrhythmias and is associated with decreased mortality in patients with CS.[52] Vasopressin can be used to increase MAP,[53] especially in cases where norepinephrine leads to detrimental tachycardia (**Fig. 7**).

Patients in CS with a normal MAP should be started on inotropic therapy. Dobutamine is the first-line inotropic agent in CS.[10,13,52,54,55] Epinephrine has inotropic and vasopressor effects, but carries a higher risk of arrhythmias and is associated with increased lactate levels. As a result, epinephrine use can limit the interpretation of lactate as a marker of perfusion.[54] A recent large meta-analysis found epinephrine use was associated with higher mortality in CS, even when risk adjusted.[56] Thus, epinephrine use should be limited to patients with persistent hypotension despite adequate resuscitation.[9]

Table 3
Vasopressors and inotropes

Medication	Classification	Clinical Uses in Cardiogenic Shock
Phenylephrine	Vasopressor	Increased afterload of systemic and pulmonary circulations Generally not used in CS Useful in LVOTO to decrease gradient across outflow tract
Vasopressin	Vasopressor	Increased afterload of systemic but not pulmonary circulation Useful in isolated RV disease or vasoplegia with tachycardia
Norepinephrine	Vasopressor, mild inotrope	First-line vasopressor for CS in ED
Epinephrine	Inopressor	Increased risk of arrhythmias Recommended for symptomatic bradycardia or refractory hypotension
Dopamine	Inopressor	Increased risk of arrhythmias Only used in symptomatic bradycardia
Dobutamine	Inodilator	First-line inotrope for CS in ED Fast acting, easily titratable
Milrinone	Inodilator	Second-line agent, slower acting with 2.5 h half-life Renally cleared, can accumulate in AKI or CKD Less arrhythmogenic than other inotropes, better pulmonary vasodilation

Abbreviations: AKI, acute kidney injury; CKD, chronic kidney disease; LVOTO, left ventricular outflow tract obstruction.

Arrhythmia Management

Patients with CS often cannot tolerate loss of their atrial kick or the decreased ventricular filling times that occur with tachydysrhythmias. Cardioversion may be indicated to restore normal sinus rhythm.[13] Amiodarone, a class III antiarrhythmic, is appropriate for treating atrial and ventricular arrhythmias in CS, but can cause hypotension.[57] Negative inotropes, such as β-blockers and calcium channel blockers, are not recommended in the acute phase of CS.[1,13] Bradycardias should also be managed aggressively to improve cardiac output.

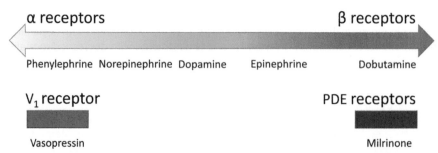

Fig. 6. Schematic representation of receptor activity of commonly used vasoactive medications. Note that vasopressin 1 (V$_1$) receptors are underneath α receptors, and phosphodiesterase-3 receptors are under β, because they have many similar effects, but are mechanistically distinct. PDE, phosphodiesterase.

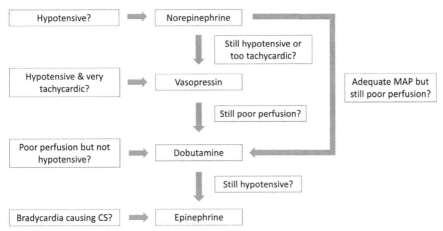

Fig. 7. Algorithm for selecting vasopressors and inotropes in known or suspected cardiogenic shock in the ED.

Afterload

One must consider the cause of CS before intubation. Positive pressure ventilation provides different effects for the RV and the LV, as illustrated in **Fig. 8.**[58] In cases of LV failure leading to CS, positive pressure ventilation may unload the LV by decreasing preload and afterload. However, if patients are preload dependent, or in RV failure, intubation may precipitate hemodynamic collapse. For patients in overt shock, intubation may be warranted to minimize work of breathing and oxygen consumption by respiratory muscles.

Many patients presenting with CS are hypotensive and require vasopressors, thereby preventing addition of vasodilators.[13] In these circumstances, blood pressure support should be prioritized. However, in patients with normal or elevated blood pressures and poor perfusion, decreasing afterload can improve cardiac output.

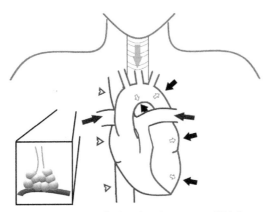

Fig. 8. Effects of positive pressure ventilation (PPV) can vary. PPV decreases preload (*open blue arrowheads*) for the interior vena cava, superior vena cava, and right heart. PPV can also lead to alveolar distention, crimping capillaries (*inset*), thereby increasing RV afterload, as indicated by the *large blue arrows*. PPV can also decrease afterload on the LV (*black arrows*) by decreasing the transmural gradient (*small red arrows*).

Intravenous nitroglycerin given as an infusion has a short half-life,[59] and therefore is reasonable to try in poorly perfused normotensive or hypertensive patients.

MECHANICAL CIRCULATORY SUPPORT

Because management of CS is complex and requires multidisciplinary support, many tertiary care centers have developed shock or mechanical circulatory support (MCS) management teams to rapidly assess patients and provide prompt management. The American Heart Association recommends establishing systems of care with high-volume hospitals used as hubs-with-spoke centers for early recognition and transfer.[1]

In addition to medical management, patients with CS often require procedural interventions. Those with ischemia need rapid cardiac catheterization,[1,13] and those with acute aortic insufficiency or mitral regurgitation require prompt surgical intervention.[13]

Table 4
Mechanical circulatory support options

Device	Support Offered	Advantages	Disadvantages
Intra-aortic balloon pump	0.5 L/min flow	Placement is straightforward, commonly available May assist coronary perfusion Decreases afterload	Offers lower flow Can migrate, become dislodged
Impella			
Impella 2.5	2.5 L/min flow	Can provide variable support, depending on device	Requires technical expertise
Impella CP	3.5 L/min flow		
Impella 5	5 L/min flow		
RP-Impella	Placed percutaneously across the AV, with inflow in LV and outflow in aorta	Decompress LV, reducing wall stress and oxygen consumption	Can migrate, become dislodged
	RP-Impella with inlet in IVC and output in pulmonary artery	RVADs are most commonly used in conjunction with LVADs	Impella 2.5 not recommended for CS
	Can be placed from axillary or femoral approach	May be used alone for RV infarcts	RP-Impella is a newer device, less clinical experience; not widely available
TandemHeart	Provides up to 4 L/min Placed percutaneously, left atrium to femoral artery	Decompress LV, reducing wall stress and oxygen consumption	Requires technical expertise Involves transseptal puncture
VA ECMO	Can provide 5–6 L/min flow Only mechanism with oxygenator in addition to pump	Provides total cardiopulmonary support Peripheral cannulation via femoral vessels can be rapid	Requires technical expertise Increase in afterload for native LV function

Abbreviations: AV, atrioventricular; IVC, inferior vena cava; LVAD, left ventricular assist device; RVAD, right ventricular assist device; VA ECMO, venoarterial extracorporeal membrane oxygenation.

Patients with persistent shock despite appropriate medical management may benefit from MCS. Although emergency medicine clinicians do not place MCS devices, understanding the available options is important for timely consultation or transfer. **Table 4** highlights key considerations in MCS.[12,60,61]

Types of MCS are classified as temporary or durable devices. Temporary MCS devices are those that are considered in patients with CS in the ED. These devices are inserted either percutaneously or surgically and are used as a bridge to recovery of cardiac function, bridge to a durable device, bridge to transplant, or bridge to a later decision.

The intra-aortic balloon pump used to be standard for mechanical support in CS.[62] However, the largest randomized trial in patients with acute myocardial infarction complicated by CS did not show a benefit with routine IABP in addition to revascularization,[63] resulting in a downgraded guideline recommendation.[1,64,65] Temporary LV assist device (LVAD) or extracorporeal membrane oxygenation (ECMO) should be used, if available, and temporary circulatory support is needed.[39] The Impella (Abiomed, Danvers, Massachusetts) and TandemHeart device (Cardiac Assist, Inc, Pittsburgh, PA) are small LVADs designed for temporary support. They have been shown in small studies[66–69] to improve hemodynamics but not change clinical outcomes. Surgically implanted intracorporeal LVADs are not used in the acute phase of CS.

Venoarterial ECMO is the preferred temporary circulatory support in many instances, especially in scenarios with poor oxygenation.[1,13] Although there are no randomized trials of ECMO for CS, clinical experience with venoarterial ECMO is increasing.[13] A recent study of more than 900 patients supported with ECMO for CS found a 51% survival rate.[70]

SUMMARY

Although CS is uncommon in the ED, it is associated with high mortality. Emergency medicine clinicians should assess for etiology, knowing that most CS is caused by myocardial infarction, but nonischemic etiologies are important to recognize. Once CS is suspected or identified, assessing volume status and perfusion are mandatory, because volume status can vary substantially. Hemodynamic monitoring including echocardiography, arterial lines, and even PA lines are important diagnostic tools and can guide clinical interventions.

Clinicians should optimize preload, contractility, and afterload for patients in CS. Patients who seem volume responsive should be given small aliquots of volume, with frequent reassessment for a favorable response. Some patients may require diuresis to improve cardiac output. Vasopressors are important to restore end-organ perfusion in hypotensive patients, and norepinephrine is the first-line agent. Inotropes can improve contractility, but may cause hypotension, and therefore should not be initiated until the blood pressure is adequate. Dobutamine is the first-line inotrope in the ED. Intubation and initiation of positive pressure ventilation decreases preload, which, depending on the patient's volume status, may be beneficial or deleterious. Positive pressure decreases LV afterload, but can also increase RV afterload. Although emergency medicine clinicians do not initiate MCS, knowing therapeutic options is important for timely consultation or transfer as indicated.

REFERENCES

1. van Diepen S, Katz JN, Albert NM, et al. Contemporary management of cardiogenic shock: a scientific statement from the American Heart Association. Circulation 2017;136(16):e232–68.

2. Mebazaa A, Tolppanen H, Mueller C, et al. Acute heart failure and cardiogenic shock: a multidisciplinary practical guidance. Intensive Care Med 2016;42(2): 147–63.

3. Lim HS. Cardiogenic Shock: Failure of Oxygen Delivery and Oxygen Utilization. Clin Cardiol 2016;39(8):477–83.

4. Gitz Holler J, Jensen HK, Henriksen DP, et al. Etiology of Shock in the Emergency Department: A 12-Year Population-Based Cohort Study. Shock 2019;51(1):60–7.

5. Nieminen MS, Brutsaert D, Dickstein K, et al. EuroHeart Failure Survey II (EHFS II): a survey on hospitalized acute heart failure patients: description of population. Eur Heart J 2006;27(22):2725–36.

6. Harjola V-PP, Lassus J, Sionis A, et al. Clinical picture and risk prediction of short-term mortality in cardiogenic shock. Eur J Heart Fail 2015;17(5):501–9.

7. Thiele H, Ohman EM, Desch S, et al. Management of cardiogenic shock. Eur Heart J 2015;36(20):1223–30.

8. French JK, Armstrong PW, Cohen E, et al. Cardiogenic shock and heart failure post–percutaneous coronary intervention in ST-elevation myocardial infarction: observations from "assessment of pexelizumab in acute myocardial infarction." Am Heart J 2011;162(1):89–97.

9. Ponikowski P, Voors AA, Anker SD, et al. 2016 ESC guidelines for the diagnosis and treatment of acute and chronic heart failure. Eur Heart J 2016;37(27): 2129–200.

10. Shah P, Cowger JA. Cardiogenic shock. Crit Care Clin 2014;30(3):391–412.

11. Klein T, Ramani GV. Assessment and management of cardiogenic shock in the emergency department. Cardiol Clin 2012;30(4):651–64.

12. Chakravarthy M, Tsukashita M, Murali S. A targeted management approach to cardiogenic shock. Crit Care Clin 2018;34(3):423–37.

13. Levy B, Bastien O, Karim B, et al. Experts' recommendations for the management of adult patients with cardiogenic shock. Ann Intensive Care 2015;5(1):52.

14. Babaev A, Frederick PD, Pasta DJ, et al. Trends in management and outcomes of patients with acute myocardial infarction complicated by cardiogenic shock. JAMA 2005;294(4):448–54.

15. Kar B, Gregoric ID, Basra SS, et al. The percutaneous ventricular assist device in severe refractory cardiogenic shock. J Am Coll Cardiol 2011;57(6):688–96.

16. Jacobs AK, Leopold JA, Bates E, et al. Cardiogenic shock caused by right ventricular infarction: a report from the SHOCK registry. J Am Coll Cardiol 2003;41(8): 1273–9.

17. Wilcox SR, Kabrhel C, Channick RN. Pulmonary hypertension and right ventricular failure in emergency medicine. Ann Emerg Med 2015;66(6):619–28.

18. Gardner M, Nair V, Hu D, et al. The evaluation and management of decompensated hypertrophic cardiomyopathy in the emergency department. Am J Emerg Med 2018;36(12):2286–8.

19. Medina De Chazal H, Giuseppe M, Buono D, et al. THE PRESENT AND FUTURE stress cardiomyopathy diagnosis and treatment JACC state-of-the-art review. 2018.

20. Elesber AA, Prasad A, Lennon RJ, et al. Four-year recurrence rate and prognosis of the apical ballooning syndrome. J Am Coll Cardiol 2007;50(5):448–52.

21. Burns DJP, Quantz MA. Use of the Impella 5.0 device as a bridge to recovery in adult fulminant viral myocarditis. Innovations (Phila) 2015;10(4):279–81.

22. Kindermann I, Barth C, Mahfoud F, et al. Update on myocarditis. J Am Coll Cardiol 2012;59(9):779–92.

23. Graudins A, Lee HM, Druda D. Calcium channel antagonist and beta-blocker overdose: antidotes and adjunct therapies. Br J Clin Pharmacol 2016;81(3): 453–61.

24. Henning DJ, Kearney KE, Hall MK, et al. Identification of hypotensive emergency department patients with cardiogenic etiologies. SHOCK 2018;49(2):131–6.

25. Menon V, Slater JN, White HD, et al. Acute myocardial infarction complicated by systemic hypoperfusion without hypotension: report of the SHOCK trial registry. Am J Med 2000;108(5):374–80. Available at: http://www.ncbi.nlm.nih.gov/pubmed/10759093. Accessed November 9, 2018.

26. Stevenson LW, Perloff JK. The limited reliability of physical signs for estimating hemodynamics in chronic heart failure. JAMA 1989;261(6):884–8. Available at: http://www.ncbi.nlm.nih.gov/pubmed/2913385. Accessed November 9, 2018.

27. Drazner MH, Rame JE, Stevenson LW, et al. Prognostic importance of elevated jugular venous pressure and a third heart sound in patients with heart failure. N Engl J Med 2001;345(8):574–81.

28. Volpicelli G, Lamorte A, Tullio M, et al. Point-of-care multiorgan ultrasonography for the evaluation of undifferentiated hypotension in the emergency department. Intensive Care Med 2013;39(7):1290–8.

29. Shokoohi H, Boniface KS, Pourmand A, et al. Bedside ultrasound reduces diagnostic uncertainty and guides resuscitation in patients with undifferentiated hypotension. Crit Care Med 2015;43(12):2562–9.

30. Shokoohi H, Boniface KS, Zaragoza M, et al. Point-of-care ultrasound leads to diagnostic shifts in patients with undifferentiated hypotension. Am J Emerg Med 2017;35(12):1984.e3–7.

31. De Backer D, Vincent J-L. Should we measure the central venous pressure to guide fluid management? Ten answers to 10 questions. Crit Care 2018;22(1):43.

32. Biais M, Ehrmann S, Mari A, et al. Clinical relevance of pulse pressure variations for predicting fluid responsiveness in mechanically ventilated intensive care unit patients: the grey zone approach. Crit Care 2014;18(6):587.

33. Sangkum L, Liu GL, Yu L, et al. Minimally invasive or noninvasive cardiac output measurement: an update. J Anesth 2016;30(3):461–80.

34. Tukey MH, Wiener RS. The current state of fellowship training in pulmonary artery catheter placement and data interpretation: a national survey of pulmonary and critical care fellowship program directors. J Crit Care 2013;28(5):857–61.

35. Shah MR, Hasselblad V, Stevenson LW, et al. Impact of the pulmonary artery catheter in critically ill patients: meta-analysis of randomized clinical trials. JAMA 2005;294(13):1664–70.

36. National Heart, Lung, and Blood Institute Acute Respiratory Distress Syndrome (ARDS) Clinical Trials Network, Wheeler AP, Bernard GR, Thompson BT, et al. Pulmonary-artery versus central venous catheter to guide treatment of acute lung injury. N Engl J Med 2006;354(21):2213–24.

37. Binanay C, Califf RM, Hasselblad V, et al. Evaluation study of congestive heart failure and pulmonary artery catheterization effectiveness: the ESCAPE trial. JAMA 2005;294(13):1625–33.

38. Rossello X, Vila M, Rivas-Lasarte M, et al. Impact of pulmonary artery catheter use on short- and long-term mortality in patients with cardiogenic shock. Cardiology 2017;136(1):61–9.

39. Yancy CW, Jessup M, Bozkurt B, et al. 2017 ACC/AHA/HFSA focused update of the 2013 ACCF/AHA guideline for the management of heart failure: a report of the American College of Cardiology/American Heart Association Task Force on

clinical practice guidelines and the Heart Failure Society of America. Circulation 2017;136(6):e137–61.

40. Lindenfeld J, Albert NM, Boehmer JP, et al. HFSA 2010 comprehensive heart failure practice guideline. J Card Fail 2010;16(6):e1–194.

41. Shah NR, Bieniarz MC, Basra SS, et al. Serum biomarkers in severe refractory cardiogenic shock. JACC Heart Fail 2013;1(3):200–6.

42. Fuernau G, Poenisch C, Eitel I, et al. Prognostic impact of established and novel renal function biomarkers in myocardial infarction with cardiogenic shock: a biomarker substudy of the IABP-SHOCK II-trial. Int J Cardiol 2015;191:159–66.

43. Nikolaou M, Parissis J, Yilmaz MB, et al. Liver function abnormalities, clinical profile, and outcome in acute decompensated heart failure. Eur Heart J 2013;34(10):742–9.

44. Konstam MA, Kiernan MS, Bernstein D, et al. Evaluation and management of right-sided heart failure: a scientific statement from the American Heart Association. Circulation 2018;137(20):e578–622.

45. Lazzeri C, Valente S, Chiostri M, et al. Clinical significance of lactate in acute cardiac patients. World J Cardiol 2015;7(8):483.

46. Cecconi M, De Backer D, Antonelli M, et al. Consensus on circulatory shock and hemodynamic monitoring. Task force of the European Society of Intensive Care Medicine. Intensive Care Med 2014;40(12):1795–815.

47. King C, May CW, Williams J, et al. Management of right heart failure in the critically ill. Crit Care Clin 2014;30(3):475–98.

48. Salahuddin N, Sammani M, Hamdan A, et al. Fluid overload is an independent risk factor for acute kidney injury in critically Ill patients: results of a cohort study. BMC Nephrol 2017;18(1):45.

49. Bouchard J, Soroko SB, Chertow GM, et al. Fluid accumulation, survival and recovery of kidney function in critically ill patients with acute kidney injury. Kidney Int 2009;76(4):422–7.

50. Zhang L, Chen Z, Diao Y, et al. Associations of fluid overload with mortality and kidney recovery in patients with acute kidney injury: a systematic review and meta-analysis. J Crit Care 2015;30(4):860.e7-13.

51. Yancy CW, Jessup M, Bozkurt B, et al. 2016 ACC/AHA/HFSA focused update on new pharmacological therapy for heart failure: an update of the 2013 ACCF/AHA guideline for the management of heart failure: a report of the American College of Cardiology/American Heart Association Task Force on Clinic. J Am Coll Cardiol 2016;68(13):1476–88.

52. De Backer D, Biston P, Devriendt J, et al. Comparison of dopamine and norepinephrine in the treatment of shock. N Engl J Med 2010;362(9):779–89.

53. Jolly S, Newton G, Horlick E, et al. Effect of vasopressin on hemodynamics in patients with refractory cardiogenic shock complicating acute myocardial infarction. Am J Cardiol 2005;96(12):1617–20.

54. Levy B, Perez P, Perny J, et al. Comparison of norepinephrine-dobutamine to epinephrine for hemodynamics, lactate metabolism, and organ function variables in cardiogenic shock. A prospective, randomized pilot study. Crit Care Med 2011;39(3):450–5.

55. Arrigo M, Mebazaa A. Understanding the differences among inotropes. Intensive Care Med 2015;41(5):912–5.

56. Léopold V, Gayat E, Pirracchio R, et al. Epinephrine and short-term survival in cardiogenic shock: an individual data meta-analysis of 2583 patients. Intensive Care Med 2018;44(6):847–56.

57. Saidi A, Akoum N, Bader F. Management of unstable arrhythmias in cardiogenic shock. Curr Treat Options Cardiovasc Med 2011;13(4):354–60.
58. Mahmood SS, Pinsky MR. Heart-lung interactions during mechanical ventilation: the basics. Ann Transl Med 2018;6(18):349.
59. Cohn PF, Gorlin R. Physiologic and clinical actions of nitroglycerin. Med Clin North Am 1974;58(2):407–15. Available at: http://www.ncbi.nlm.nih.gov/pubmed/4205472. Accessed November 10, 2018.
60. Touchan J, Guglin M. Temporary mechanical circulatory support for cardiogenic shock. Curr Treat Options Cardiovasc Med 2017;19(10):77.
61. van Nunen LX, Noc M, Kapur NK, et al. Usefulness of intra-aortic balloon pump counterpulsation. Am J Cardiol 2016;117(3):469–76.
62. Hochman JS, Sleeper LA, Webb JG, et al. Early revascularization in acute myocardial infarction complicated by cardiogenic shock. SHOCK Investigators. Should we emergently revascularize occluded coronaries for cardiogenic shock. N Engl J Med 1999;341(9):625–34.
63. Thiele H, Zeymer U, Neumann F-J, et al. Intra-aortic balloon counterpulsation in acute myocardial infarction complicated by cardiogenic shock (IABP-SHOCK II): final 12 month results of a randomised, open-label trial. Lancet 2013; 382(9905):1638–45, d.
64. Windecker S, Kolh P, Alfonso F, et al. 2014 ESC/EACTS guidelines on myocardial revascularization. EuroIntervention 2015;10(9):1024–94.
65. O'Gara PT, Kushner FG, Ascheim DD, et al. 2013 ACCF/AHA guideline for the management of ST-elevation myocardial infarction: executive summary: a report of the American College of Cardiology Foundation/American Heart Association Task Force on practice guidelines. Catheter Cardiovasc Interv 2013;82(1):E1–27.
66. Seyfarth M, Sibbing D, Bauer I, et al. A randomized clinical trial to evaluate the safety and efficacy of a percutaneous left ventricular assist device versus intra-aortic balloon pumping for treatment of cardiogenic shock caused by myocardial infarction. J Am Coll Cardiol 2008;52(19):1584–8.
67. Ouweneel DM, Eriksen E, Sjauw KD, et al. Percutaneous mechanical circulatory support versus intra-aortic balloon pump in cardiogenic shock after acute myocardial infarction. J Am Coll Cardiol 2017;69(3):278–87.
68. Thiele H, Sick P, Boudriot E, et al. Randomized comparison of intra-aortic balloon support with a percutaneous left ventricular assist device in patients with revascularized acute myocardial infarction complicated by cardiogenic shock. Eur Heart J 2005;26(13):1276–83.
69. Burkhoff D, Cohen H, Brunckhorst C, et al, TandemHeart Investigators Group. A randomized multicenter clinical study to evaluate the safety and efficacy of the TandemHeart percutaneous ventricular assist device versus conventional therapy with intraaortic balloon pumping for treatment of cardiogenic shock. Am Heart J 2006;152(3):469.e1-8.
70. El Sibai R, Bachir R, El Sayed M, et al. ECMO use and mortality in adult patients with cardiogenic shock: a retrospective observational study in U.S. hospitals. BMC Emerg Med 2018;18(1):20–8.

Critically Ill Patients with End-Stage Liver Disease

Sara Crager, MD[a,b,*]

KEYWORDS

- Complications of end-stage liver disease • Critical illness • Hepatic encephalopathy
- Gastrointestinal bleeding • Coagulopathy • Hepatorenal syndrome

KEY POINTS

- Patients with end-stage liver disease (ESLD) who require intensive care unit admission have high rates of mortality.
- Important complications encountered in critically ill ESLD patients include hepatic encephalopathy, gastrointestinal bleeding, bacterial peritonitis, hepatorenal syndrome, severe coagulopathy, and hepatic hydrothorax.
- Critically ill ESLD patients often present with multisystem organ dysfunction, and require prompt diagnosis of the underlying cause of acute decompensation and treatment initiation.

INTRODUCTION

Patients with end-stage liver disease (ESLD) who require intensive care unit (ICU) admission have high rates of mortality. Although less than 50% of these patients survive to hospital discharge, more than 90% of those patients who are successfully discharged from the hospital are still alive at 1 year.[1] This highlights the important role of high-quality critical care of these patients; if clinicians are able to get them through their hospital course, their intermediate-term mortality is surprisingly good.

Risk Stratification

The Model for End-Stage Liver Disease (MELD) score is probably the most useful scoring system for clinicians to rapidly obtain a gross estimate of baseline illness severity in ESLD patients.

- The MELD score was designed to predict 3-month survival, and examination of the curve reveals an inflection point in the curve between a score of 20 and 30 where mortality risk increases precipitously (**Fig. 1**).

Disclosure Statement: None.
[a] Department of Emergency Medicine, 924 Westwood Boulevard, Suite 300, Los Angeles, CA 90049, USA; [b] Division of Critical Care, Department of Anesthesia, University of California Los Angeles-David Geffen School of Medicine, Los Angeles, CA, USA
* 924 Westwood Boulevard, Suite 300, Los Angeles, CA 90095.
E-mail address: scrager@mednet.ucla.edu

Emerg Med Clin N Am 37 (2019) 511–527
https://doi.org/10.1016/j.emc.2019.03.008   emed.theclinics.com
0733-8627/19/© 2019 Elsevier Inc. All rights reserved.

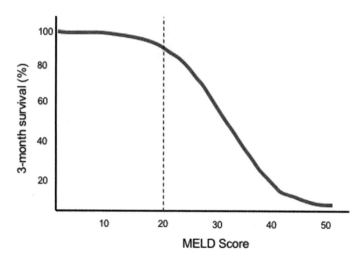

Fig. 1. The Model for End-Stage Liver Disease (MELD) system for clinicians. (*Adapted from* Teh SH, Nagorney DM, Stevens SR, et al. Risk factors for mortality after surgery in patients with cirrhosis. Gastroenterology 2007;132(4):1261 [Epub 2007 Jan 25]; with permission.)

- The variables used to calculate the score are readily available and include creatinine, international normalized ratio (INR), bilirubin, sodium, and renal replacement therapy.
- ESLD patients who are listed or being evaluated for transplant generally have previous MELD scores documented in the medical record, allowing the emergency clinician to easily obtain a global picture of the patient's overall trajectory.

Significance of Transplant Status

It is useful for the emergency provider to clarify the transplant status of a patient with ESLD. Transplant status may have implications for the approach taken in the acute care setting, as outlined in **Table 1**.

While the most common ICU-admitting diagnoses of ESLD patients are pneumonia, acute respiratory distress syndrome, and sepsis, this article focuses primarily on the most common complications specific to ESLD patients during critical illness.

Table 1 Significance of liver transplant status for the emergency provider	
Listed for liver transplantation	The goal of the emergency physician is to provide aggressive care to support the patient the preoperative period
Undergoing liver transplant candidacy evaluation	The goal of the emergency physician is immediate stabilization and prevention of further complications to provide time for candidacy evaluation
Not a liver transplant candidate	In this case, the focus of the emergency physician should be on identifying reversible causes of an acute decompensation, and clarification of a goal of care early on; carefully consider the appropriateness of initiation of aggressive measures, particularly in the case of conditions such as hepatorenal syndrome or hepatopulmonary syndrome, which are associated with extremely high mortality, and for which liver transplantation is the only definitive management

HEPATIC ENCEPHALOPATHY
Pathophysiology

It is becoming increasingly understood that the pathophysiology of hepatic encephalopathy (HE) is complex, involving a wide range of pathologic processes including astrocyte edema and dysfunction, increased GABAergic tone, inflammatory cytokines, and depletion of acetylcholine.[2] Despite the growing understanding of the multifactorial pathophysiology of this disease, ammonia continues to be thought to play a central role. In the brain, ammonia and glutamate are converted into glutamine and the resultant high levels of glutamine then act as an osmolyte, causing astrocyte edema and neuronal dysfunction.

Emergency Critical Care Assessment

The severity of HE is graded clinically:

- *Grade I*: personality and/or mood changes, mild confusion, slurred speech, disordered sleep
- *Grade II*: lethargy, moderate confusion
- *Grade III*: marked confusion, incoherent speech, depressed level of consciousness but remains arousable
- *Grade IV*: comatose, unresponsive to pain

On examination, patients with severe HE may exhibit hyporeflexia or hyperreflexia, rigidity, myoclonus, ataxia, dilated pupils, and even transient decerebrate posturing.

There are 2 key questions that need to be answered when an ESLD patient presents with altered mental status:

1. Is HE the primary cause of the altered mental status?
2. What has precipitated the HE?

Patients with ESLD are at high risk for numerous disease states that may cause altered mental status (eg, sepsis, uremia, alcohol withdrawal, intracerebral hemorrhage). As such, an ESLD patient with altered mental status should not be presumed to have HE until other causes have been systematically considered and ruled out.

Precipitants of hepatic encephalopathy

Key precipitants of HE that may require diagnosis and treatment in the emergency setting are listed in **Table 2**.

Ammonia levels in hepatic encephalopathy

Although ammonia is thought to play a central role in the pathogenesis of HE, interpretation of individual serum ammonia levels is not straightforward, and HE remains a primarily clinical diagnosis.

- A normal or modestly elevated blood ammonia level does not rule out the diagnosis of HE.[3]
- An elevated ammonia level is not necessarily diagnostic of HE. Nearly two-thirds of ESLD patients with elevated ammonia levels have no evidence of HE.[4]
- Although studies have shown that ammonia level may correlate to some extent with the severity of HE, absolute levels substantially overlap among patients with differing clinical grades of HE. As such, it is not possible to clearly identify a particular threshold cutoff value for ammonia that rules in or rules out HE in a given patient; ammonia levels must be interpreted in clinical context, and therefore there is limited clinical utility in obtaining ammonia levels in these patients.

Table 2
Precipitants of hepatic encephalopathy

Medication noncompliance	This is a frequent precipitant of hepatic encephalopathy. It is important to investigate the *reason* for medication noncompliance to rule out additional underlying pathology (ie, as altered mental status due to a distinct cause or intractable vomiting). Other precipitants that require specific treatment should be systematically considered even in cases when medication noncompliance is suspected as the primary precipitating cause
Gastrointestinal bleeding	Worsening hyperammonemia in this context is probably the result of a large blood protein load being broken down in the gastrointestinal tract
Hypokalemia	Hypokalemia causes potassium efflux from the intracellular space to the extracellular space with resultant intracellular influx of hydrogen; the ensuing intracellular acidosis in renal tubular cells increases the renal production of ammonia
Alkalosis	Alkalosis facilitates entry of ammonia into the central nervous system by increasing the conversion of ammonium (NH_4^+) into ammonia (NH_3), which, as an uncharged particle, can more easily cross the blood-brain barrier
Dehydration	This often occurs in the setting of aggressive diuresis in ESLD patients with ascites and peripheral edema; the resultant contraction alkalosis (often seen in conjunction with hypokalemia) is a common precipitant of hepatic encephalopathy
Sepsis	Inflammatory cytokines are thought to enhance ammonia-induced neurotoxicity
Constipation	Increasing the transit time through the gastrointestinal tract increases the amount of ammonia that may be absorbed
Alcohol or benzodiazepines	Short-term use of alcohol and benzodiazepines has been found to significantly increase the risk of acute development of hepatic encephalopathy

Emergency Critical Care Management

There are 3 key management principles for patients presenting with HE:

1. Airway management
2. Correct precipitating causes
3. Correct hyperammonemia

Airway management

Airway assessment should be performed immediately.

- Patients with grade IV HE often need intubation for airway protection.
- Even in patients who do not require immediate intubation for airway protection, it must be considered whether it is necessary to control the airway to initiate prompt treatment. The most important factor is whether the patient is alert and cooperative enough to safely take oral lactulose.
- Although there are some data showing that rectal lactulose is superior to tap water enemas in HE,[5] there are no high-quality data on the comparative efficacy of oral versus rectal lactulose, so it is unclear whether oral and rectal lactulose may be used interchangeably. Administering lactulose via a nasogastric tube is also an option, but it is unclear to what degree this truly mitigates the risk of aspiration.

Once intubated, sedation requirements in ESLD patients with severe HE tend to be relatively minimal.

- Propofol is a good choice because of its short duration of action, extrahepatic metabolism, and beneficial effects on intracranial pressure.
- Midazolam should be avoided given the potential for exacerbating the encephalopathy, as should large doses of opiates.
- Of note, even in patients without acute HE, both benzodiazepines and opiates should be administered at minimal doses or avoided altogether because their use in these patients is associated with significant morbidity in ESLD.

Correction of precipitating causes
Any precipitating causes that have been identified should be corrected.

- Dehydration-induced HE usually responds well to fluid resuscitation and correcting hypokalemia and hypomagnesemia. Albumin is the preferred resuscitation fluid, given recent evidence that it may improve outcomes in HE.[6]
- Gastrointestinal bleeding should be identified and treated, with blood product transfusion as needed.
- Patients with suspected sepsis should be administered broad-spectrum antibiotics, and their intravascular volume status optimized.

Correction of hyperammonemia
The final step in the treatment of HE is initiation of measures to correct hyperammonemia. Given the difficulty in identifying a single threshold cutoff value that may be generalized to rule out HE, these measures should be initiated in ESLD patients if there is a high clinical suspicion for HE regardless of ammonia levels (**Box 1**).

- Lactulose should be initiated at 20 g orally, and dosing should be titrated to achieve 3 to 4 soft stools per day. A 2016 Cochrane review concluded that there is moderate-quality evidence that lactulose reduces mortality as well as serious complications.[7]
- Rifaximin should be simultaneously initiated at 400 to 550 mg orally. A meta-analysis of 19 trials concluded that the addition of rifaximin appears to significantly reduce mortality in HE.[8]

Box 1
Key points: hepatic encephalopathy

Assessment

- Is HE the primary cause of altered mental status?
- If so, what has precipitated the HE?

Key precipitants of HE: gastrointestinal bleeding, sepsis, hypokalemia, dehydration (usually caused by overdiuresis), constipation, and alcohol/benzodiazepine use.

Blood ammonia levels cannot be used in a straightforward manner to rule in or rule out the diagnosis of HE.

Management

- Airway management
- Correct precipitating causes (correction of bleeding, volume resuscitation, electrolyte repletion, antibiotics, control of hemorrhage)
- Correct hyperammonemia (lactulose + rifaximin)

VARICEAL UPPER GASTROINTESTINAL BLEEDING
Pathophysiology

Among ESLD patients presenting with upper gastrointestinal bleeding (GIB), variceal bleeding is the underlying cause in approximately 60% of patients.[9] The outcomes for patients with variceal bleeding are closely correlated with the severity of liver disease, and mortality rates as high as 40% in patients with the most severe disease.[10]

Esophageal varices are a consequence of portal hypertension.

- Portal hypertension initially occurs in response to hepatic vascular bed distortion.
- Splanchnic vasodilatation occurs in response to increased resistance to portal blood flow, precipitating sodium and water retention, which further exacerbates portal hypertension.
- The development of portal-collateral circulation is a direct result of portal hypertension, with a minimum threshold hepatic venous pressure gradient of greater than 10 mm Hg for the development of esophageal varices.

Emergency Critical Care Assessment

Patients with variceal hemorrhage typically present with hematemesis and/or melena, but the clinician should be alert for occult bleeding episodes in patients presenting with altered mental status or shock. Large volumes of blood may collect in the upper gastrointestinal tract before the patient begins to have active hematemesis, and as such upper GIB should remain on the differential even in the absence of an overt history of bleeding. A disproportionately elevated blood urea nitrogen level may be a clue to an occult upper GIB.

Mortality resulting from acute massive hemorrhage has improved significantly with the advent of endoscopic variceal band ligation. A significant proportion of the mortality associated with variceal bleeding episodes is in fact due to complications that develop secondary to bleeding and massive transfusion as opposed to mortality caused by hemorrhagic shock during the acute bleeding episode. It is not unusual for multiple complications to develop simultaneously. Major complications include:

- Aspiration pneumonia
- Sepsis
- HE
- Renal failure

Emergency Critical Care Management

There are 3 primary goals of management during an acute episode of variceal bleeding:

1. Hemodynamic stabilization and blood product resuscitation
2. Treatment and prevention of complications
3. Hemorrhage control

Hemodynamic stabilization and blood product resuscitation

- In the setting of acute bleeding in the hemodynamically stable patient, a transfusion threshold of hemoglobin greater than 7 seems to be safe and is in fact associated with a lower risk of rebleeding than higher transfusion thresholds.[11]

- In the patient with evolving hemodynamic instability or massive exsanguinating bleeding, the patient's hemodynamics and ongoing assessment of end-organ perfusion should guide blood product resuscitation as opposed to a hemoglobin target.
- It is important to closely monitor these patients to avoid overtransfusion. Significant volume overload can be particularly problematic in the context of acute variceal bleeding because of the potential for rebound portal hypertension and resultant rebleeding.[12]

Treatment and prevention of complications

Although prophylactic intubation in a general population of patients with an upper GIB has not been shown to improve outcomes—and may in fact be associated with increased rates of hospital acquired pneumonia—early intubation should be pursued in patients with altered mental status and/or massive bleeding.

Bacterial infection is commonly found in the ESLD patient with acute variceal bleeding.[13] It remains unclear whether infection tends to precipitate bleeding or whether bleeding tends to precipitate infection, or both.

- Endotoxin released during bacterial infection can result in increased portal pressure via activation of endothelin activation and vasoconstrictive cyclooxygenases.[14]
- Increased bacterial translocation and complement deficiencies have been noted in ESLD patients during acute bleeding episodes.[13]

Irrespective of the direction of this effect, administration of prophylactic antibiotics in ESLD patients with variceal bleeding has been shown to significantly reduce the incidence of sepsis, rebleeding events, duration of hospitalization, and mortality.[15]

- Given the increasing rates of quinolone resistance, ceftriaxone 1 g is the preferred antibiotic choice, and should be initiated before endoscopy.

Hemorrhage control

Primary treatment of acute variceal bleeding is endoscopic variceal band ligation. Endoscopy should be done as soon as possible in a patient with clinically significant bleeding, and should not be delayed for more than 12 hours after presentation, as per the 2016 American Association for the Study of Liver Disease guidelines.[16]

There is also a supportive role for vasoactive medications to achieve hemostasis (**Box 2**).

- Use of octreotide or somatostatin has been associated with decreased length of stay in hospital and transfusion requirements,[17] and combination therapy with octreotide or somatostatin and band ligation has been shown to improve rates of successful hemorrhage control compared with band ligation alone, although no effect was found on mortality.[18]
- Octreotide (50 μg bolus followed by a drip at 50 μg/h) is the preferred vasoactive agent to potentiate hemorrhage control in ESLD patients with variceal bleeds. Given the high prevalence of nonvariceal bleeds in this population, it is reasonable to administer pantoprazole while awaiting endoscopy.
- Balloon tamponade can be performed as a temporizing measure, and the emergency physician should acquire familiarity with the equipment and the detailed steps required to successfully perform this relatively rare intervention in an emergent situation.

> **Box 2**
> **Key points: variceal bleeding**
>
> *Hemodynamic stabilization and blood product resuscitation*
> - Guided by hemodynamics and perfusion indices
> - Close monitoring to avoid overtransfusion
>
> *Treatment and prevention of complications*
> - Complications arising from bleeding and massive transfusion contribute significantly to mortality from active hemorrhage: aspiration pneumonia, sepsis, acute-on-chronic liver failure, HE, and renal failure
> - Early intubation, antibiotics
>
> *Hemorrhage control*
> - Octreotide
> - Endoscopic variceal ligation
> - Balloon tamponade as a temporizing measure

COAGULOPATHY AND HEMORRHAGE
Pathophysiology

Patients with ESLD are in a state of hemostasis disequilibrium whereby susceptibility to both bleeding and clotting may be increased, with the relative balance different for each patient.

- Patients with severe liver disease should not be assumed to be "autoanticoagulated" or at risk of bleeding based on standard coagulation testing, which does not give a full picture of the complex interplay of the simultaneously ongoing procoagulant and anticoagulant changes in these patients.

Coagulopathy in ESLD is multifactorial:

- *Decreased platelet number and function*. Thrombocytopenia results from a combination of splenic sequestration and decreased hepatic thrombopoietin production.
- *Decreased production of clotting factors*. The liver is responsible for production of almost all clotting factors, and ESLD patients may have severely diminished levels of clotting factors.
- *Increased fibrinolysis*. Systemic fibrinolysis occurs in up to 50% of patients with ESLD and corresponds to the degree of liver dysfunction. Hyperfibrinolysis promotes premature clot dissolution, and the associated consumption of clotting factors interferes with clot formation.
- *Poor nutritional status*. In a subset of patients with liver disease, particularly those actively using alcohol and/or with poor baseline nutritional status, vitamin K deficiency can further exacerbate deficiencies of vitamin K–dependent clotting factors.

Emergency Critical Care Assessment

Assessment of coagulopathy

The best way to assess coagulopathy in ESLD patients is viscoelastic testing, including thromboelastography (TEG) or thromboelastometry (ROTEM), which give a global picture of clot kinetics that represents the true state of their coagulopathy better than traditional measures such as INR.

- Numerous studies have shown that management of bleeding in ESLD patients guided by viscoelastic testing, as opposed to standard assays, significantly decreases the amount of product given without worsening outcomes, and in some cases has even been associated with improved outcomes.[19–21]

Emergency Critical Care Management

In any actively bleeding ESLD patient, the clinician should monitor platelets and fibrinogen levels, as well as following global assay of hemostasis such as TEG or ROTEM, when available.

- The decision of which products to administer should be based on the deficiencies identified on viscoelastic testing that are contributing to impaired clot formation rather than a single laboratory measurement.
- Management decisions should be unaffected by results of prothrombin time/ INR and activated partial thromboplastin time testing. If there is significant ongoing hemorrhage and the clinician does not have access to thromboelastography, a 1:1:1 transfusion strategy is reasonable.
- Cryoprecipitate should be administered to maintain a fibrinogen level ≥100 mg/dL.
- Platelets should be administered to maintain a platelet count greater than 50,000 for active, severe, or CNS bleeding.
- Platelet dysfunction may be evaluated to some degree by viscoelastic testing. If there is severe ongoing bleeding and platelet function is thought to be impaired, the clinician may consider platelet transfusion independent of platelet count.

Avoid overtransfusion

- The pathophysiology of hemorrhage in ESLD is complex. The increased propensity to bleeding is not fully explained by the various abnormalities of hemostasis seen on laboratory testing, and hemodynamic dysregulation consequent to portal hypertension may be at least as relevant as coagulopathy.[22]
- The clinician must carefully weigh the benefits of giving additional blood products in an attempt to optimize coagulopathy against the potential for increasing portal pressure, especially in a patient with varices, even if these are not the site of acute bleeding.

Prothrombin complex concentrate and recombinant factor VIIa PCC

Therapies such as PCC and rFVIIa should generally be avoided in ESLD patients.

- These products are quite costly and have not been shown to meaningfully affect outcomes.
- Recall that ESLD patients may also be expected to have prothrombotic tendencies. PCC and rFVII carry a greater thrombotic risk, and how that plays out in a given patient may be unpredictable.

Vitamin K

Vitamin K should be administered to patients at risk of vitamin K deficiency.

- Risks for vitamin K deficiency include poor nutritional status, active alcohol use, cholestatic disease, active diarrheal disease, or prolonged antibiotic use.
- If it is unknown whether the patient has any of these risk factors, it is reasonable to give vitamin K in the acutely bleeding patient.

- For major bleeding episodes, a single dose of 10 mg of vitamin K should be given as a slow infusion no faster than 1 mg/min.

Hypocalcemia

Hypocalcemia can become a significant problem during massive transfusion in ESLD patients (**Box 3**).

- In healthy patients, the half-life of citrate, which binds to calcium, is only a few minutes; however, in the setting of severe hepatic dysfunction compounded by hypotension, hypothermia, and acidosis, the metabolism of citrate can be fairly prolonged.
- It is important to trend ionized calcium levels and give adequate calcium repletion during massive transfusion.
- Evidence suggests that calcium gluconate does not require hepatic metabolism and is as effective as calcium chloride even in patients with absent liver function.[23]

SEPSIS AND BACTERIAL PERITONITIS
Pathophysiology

ESLD patients have greater susceptibility to bacterial infections than the general population and also have a higher risk of sepsis-associated mortality.

- The response to infection in patients with ESLD is often associated with dramatic cytokine imbalances characterized by a disproportionate inflammatory response, and consequent increased risk for the development of septic shock.
- In ESLD patients with sepsis, the resulting hemodynamic failure is more marked, partially because of the severe vasoplegia patients often exhibit at baseline.

Bacterial peritonitis is a frequent cause of sepsis in these patients that is not generally seen outside this population.

- ESLD predisposes to the development of bacterial peritonitis resulting from bacterial overgrowth and microbiome disturbances caused by altered intestinal motility, as well as increased intestinal permeability.

Emergency Critical Care Assessment

ESLD patients with bacterial infections may not present classically. Use of lactate to assess severity and trajectory of early sepsis may be challenging because of significant impairments in lactate clearance. However, acute increase in serum lactate level

---

Box 3
Key points: coagulopathy

- Pathologically rebalanced hemostasis → both bleeding and thrombosis are increased
- ESLD with or without coagulation abnormalities should not be assumed to be "autoanticoagulated"
- Risks of bleeding and thrombosis are not reflected in the conventional indices, and blood product administration should not be based on these indices, especially in the absence of acute bleeding
- Management of active bleeding in ESLD patients should ideally be guided by viscoelastic testing, which has been shown to significantly decrease the amount of product as well as improving outcomes
- Hypocalcemia can become a significant problem during massive transfusion in ESLD patients, and calcium should be closely monitored and aggressively repleted

is associated with very high mortality rates in the population,[24] and emergency physicians should *not* reflexively attribute an elevated lactate to underlying liver disease in the acute phase of care.

Bacterial peritonitis should be suspected in patients with ESLD who develop fever, abdominal pain, altered mental status, abdominal tenderness, or hypotension.

- The abdominal examination in patients with bacterial peritonitis can be deceptively benign. Ascites can prevent the development of classic peritoneal signs by creating a separation between the visceral and parietal peritoneum.

Primary versus secondary bacterial peritonitis

Although secondary bacterial peritonitis only represents approximately 5% of cases, it is critical to distinguish between the two as early as possible.

- The mortality of secondary bacterial peritonitis approaches 100% if treatment consists only of antibiotics without appropriate surgical intervention.[25]
- The mortality of primary bacterial peritonitis is approximately 80% if a patient receives an unnecessary exploratory laparotomy.[26]

Primary bacterial peritonitis is confirmed by a polymorphonuclear cell count in the ascitic fluid of ≥ 250 cells/mm³.

Secondary bacterial peritonitis may be associated with perforation peritonitis, but also with other processes such as an intra-abdominal abscess. Secondary spontaneous bacterial peritonitis (SBP) should be suspected when a least 2 of the following ascitic fluid findings are present:

- Total protein greater than 1 g/dL
- Glucose less than 50 mg/dL
- Lactate dehydrogenase greater than upper limit for serum

In addition, cultures showing a polymicrobial infection or a Gram stain demonstrating numerous different bacterial forms are strongly suggestive of intestinal perforation and secondary bacterial peritonitis.

Patients in whom there is a suspicion of secondary bacterial peritonitis should undergo an emergency computed tomography scan of the abdomen.

Emergency Critical Care Management

The vast majority of bacterial peritonitis cases are primary (**Box 4**).

Box 4
Key points: sepsis and bacterial peritonitis

- ESLD patients are more prone to infection and also more likely to have severe hemodynamic sequelae attributable to infection
- Initial diagnostic workup should focus on differentiating primary and secondary SBP
- Secondary SBP is only 5% of all SBP, but mortality approaches 100% if this diagnosis is missed
- Mortality is low if treatment was started before shock or acute renal failure

Treatment

- Cefotaxime 2 g intravenously every 8 hours
- Albumin (1.5 g/kg within 6 hours of diagnosis and 1 g/kg body weight on day 3)
- Pressor support ± octreotide if renal failure has already developed

Antibiotics

The infection-related mortality from SBP is relatively low with appropriate treatment, and mortality is close to zero for patients in whom treatment was initiated before the development of shock or renal failure.[27]

- In patients with fever, abdominal tenderness, or altered mental status, treatment should be started as soon as ascitic fluid and blood cultures have been obtained.
- In patients without these findings, it is reasonable to wait until the results of the ascitic fluid cell counts are available.
- Cefotaxime 2 g intravenously every 8 hours is the preferred treatment of SBP because it has been shown to produce excellent ascitic fluid levels. Ceftriaxone may also be used at 2 g every 24 hours.

Albumin

Renal failure develops in up to 40% of patients with SBP, and portends a significantly worse prognosis.[28]

- Albumin infusion in patients with SBP has been associated with a significant decrease in the incidence of renal impairment (8% vs 31%) and a significant reduction in mortality (16% vs 35%).[29]
- Albumin 1.5 g/kg should be given within 6 hours of diagnosis of SBP if any of the following criteria are met:
  ○ Creatinine is >1 mg/dL
  ○ Blood urea nitrogen is >30 mg/dL
  ○ Bilirubin is >4 mg/dL

HEPATIC HYDROTHORAX
Pathophysiology

Hepatic hydrothorax refers to a pleural effusion in a patient with decompensated liver failure that is not secondary to a cardiopulmonary, malignant, or other primary process.

- A hepatic hydrothorax is generated when negative intrathoracic pressure during inspiration promotes the passage of ascitic fluid from the abdominal cavity into the pleural space via small diaphragmatic defects.
- Diaphragmatic defects are frequently found in the right hemidiaphragm because the left hemidiaphragm is more muscular and thicker than the right. There have been case reports of patients with confirmed hepatic hydrothorax without the presence of clinically significant ascites,[30] presumably because most of the fluid ends up in the pleural space rather than the peritoneal space.

Similar to SBP in patients with abdominal ascites, approximately 15% of patients with hepatic hydrothorax may develop spontaneous bacterial empyema when the pleural effusion is seeded with bacteria spreading directly from the abdominal cavity.[31] Approximately one-half of cases of spontaneous bacterial empyema (SBEM) are associated with SBP, and the pathogens tend to be the same as those associated with SBP. Unlike SBP, SBEM is associated with high mortality rates, approaching 40%.[31]

Emergency Critical Care Assessment

Patients with hepatic hydrothorax can present with severe symptoms with relatively small volumes (~500 mL) present.

- Patients with hepatic hydrothorax commonly present with shortness of breath, pleuritic chest pain, cough, fatigue, and hypoxemia.
- Hepatic hydrothorax develops on the right in approximately 80% of patients, on the left in approximately 15% of patients and bilaterally in approximately 5% of patients.
- Occasionally patients may present with hemodynamic instability resulting from a tension hydrothorax.

SBEM should be suspected in patients with hepatic hydrothorax who also present with fever, encephalopathy, and/or unexplained acute kidney injury. Diagnostic criteria for SBEM include:

- Positive pleural fluid culture AND polymorphonuclear (PMN) cell count greater than 250 cells/mm^3
- Negative pleural fluid culture AND PMN count greater than 500 cells/mm^3
- No evidence of pneumonia on a chest imaging study

Emergency Critical Care Management

Patients who are severely symptomatic should undergo a therapeutic thoracentesis.

- Care should be taken to limit fluid removal to 1 to 2 L on initial thoracentesis, owing to concerns of precipitating negative pressure pulmonary edema, or even hepatorenal syndrome (HRS).

Patients presenting with SBEM should be administered ceftriaxone 2 g every 24 hours, with levofloxacin as an alternative agent in penicillin-allergic patients.

Occasionally chest tube placement may be necessary in patients with SBEM with frank pus or loculations; however, chest tubes should *not* be placed routinely for the treatment of hepatic hydrothorax (**Box 5**).

- Chest tube placement in these patients can result in massive protein and electrolyte losses, and there is no clear end point for chest tube removal because of continuous reaccumulation of fluid.
- Chest tube placement in ESLD patients with hepatic hydrothorax has been associated with numerous complications including infection, renal failure, empyema, bleeding, and an increased risk of mortality.

Box 5
Key points: hepatic hydrothorax

- Generally in the right hemithorax, but may also occur on the left or bilaterally
- Patients with hepatic hydrothorax may develop spontaneous bacterial empyema (SBEM), which is associated with a very high mortality rate
- Consider a diagnostic thoracentesis to rule out SBEM in patients with fever, encephalopathy, sepsis, and/or unexplained worsening renal function
- Treat SBEM with ceftriaxone 2 g every 24 hours
- Patients who are severely symptomatic should undergo therapeutic thoracentesis followed by diuretics
- Chest tubes should *not* be placed for the treatment of hepatic hydrothorax
- Placement of chest tubes in patients with hepatic hydrothorax → massive protein and electrolyte depletion, infection, renal failure, empyema, and bleeding, and is associated with increased mortality

HEPATORENAL SYNDROME
Pathophysiology

HRS arises from the progressive systemic vasodilation superimposed on profound renal vasoconstriction in patients with ESLD.

- Portal hypertension leads to profound splanchnic vasodilation, which ultimately leads to progressively worsening vasoplegia and a hyperdynamic circulation, thought to be predominantly mediated by nitric oxide dysregulation.
- These changes result in a decrease in effective arterial circulating volume, stimulating compensatory activation of the rennin-angiotensin-aldosterone system, ultimately leading to intense renal vasoconstriction and hypoperfusion.
- Resultant renal ischemia then increases production of intrarenal vasoconstrictors, further compromising renal hemodynamics and function.

Emergency Critical Care Assessment

HRS is just one of many possible causes of acute renal failure in patients with ESLD and is a diagnosis of exclusion that carries a very poor prognosis, with a 3-month mortality approaching 60%.[32]

- Mortality is significantly lower in ESLD patients with acute renal failure that is secondary to prerenal causes. Volume depletion, as may occur frequently in these patients with overly aggressive diuresis, can closely mimic HRS.

HRS is characterized by:

- Rising serum creatinine
- Oliguria
- Normal urine sediment
- Zero or minimal proteinuria
- Urine Na less than 10 mEq/L

Because HRS can be difficult to differentiate from prerenal causes of acute renal failure, the diagnosis also requires failure of improvement with fluid resuscitation and discontinuation of any nephrotoxic agents.

Emergency Critical Care Management

Critically ill patients with HRS should be treated with norepinephrine in combination with albumin.[33]

- Although the only definitive treatment of HRS is liver transplantation, vasopressors appear to improve rates of HRS reversal (34%–44% vs 9%–13%).[34] Previously, terlipressin was considered the vasopressor of choice; however, recent evidence has shown that norepinephrine has similar efficacy with fewer adverse events.[35] In patients who are critically ill, norepinephrine should be administered to elevate the mean arterial pressure to 10 to 15 mm Hg above baseline.
- In patients with HRS who are not critically ill and do not otherwise require ICU admission, octreotide plus midodrine should be initiated.
- Albumin is given for at least 3 days as an intravenous bolus (~ 1 g/kg per day). A recent meta-analysis found a dose-response relationship between 100-g increments of albumin dose and survival; over a cumulative dose range of 200 to 600 g, 30-day survival increased from 43% to 59%.[36]

ESLD patients who develop HRS and require dialysis have an extremely poor prognosis unless they are listed for liver transplantation.

Box 6
Key points: hepatorenal syndrome

- HRS is a diagnosis of exclusion
- Prognosis for acute kidney injury (AKI) caused by HRS is significantly worse than for other causes of AKI in ESLD patients

Renal replacement therapy (RRT) should be offered as a bridge to patients awaiting liver transplantation.

- Continuous RRT may be preferred in patients who are unlikely to hemodynamically tolerate intermittent hemodialysis and in patients with HE

Treatment of HRS

- Albumin 1 g/kg/d × 2 days PLUS either norepinephrine in patients who are critically ill OR octreotide and midodrine for patients who do not otherwise require ICU admission

---

- Provision of renal replacement therapy (RRT) should be offered as a bridge to patients awaiting liver transplantation or those undergoing liver transplant evaluation.
- Provision of long-term RRT is generally not indicated in ESLD except as a trial while awaiting return of renal function.

Hemodialysis is frequently difficult to perform in patients with HRS (**Box 6**).

- The combination of baseline vasoplegia and hypoalbuminemia makes ESLD patients poorly tolerant of rapid fluid shifts and, as such, continuous RRT may be a better tolerated modality, particularly in patients in whom HRS is precipitated by sepsis or upper GIB.

SUMMARY

Critically ill ESLD patients routinely and rapidly develop multiorgan system dysfunction. Although these patients are profoundly ill in the acute phase, they have relatively good intermediate-term outcomes if they can survive to hospital discharge. In the emergency department, clinicians should focus on identification and correction of underlying causes of acute decompensation while anticipating and preventing downstream complications. Pathophysiology and management pearls for critical illness specific to ESLD described in this article can help emergency department physicians achieve these goals.

REFERENCES

1. Warren A, Soulsby CR, Puxty A, et al. Long-term outcome of patients with liver cirrhosis admitted to a general intensive care unit. Ann Intensive Care 2017; 7(1):37.
2. Frederick RT. Current concepts in the pathophysiology and management of hepatic encephalopathy. Gastroenterol Hepatol (N Y) 2011;7(4):222–33.
3. Elgouhari HM, O'Shea R. What is the utility of measuring the serum ammonia level in patients with altered mental status? Cleve Clin J Med 2009;76(4):252–4.
4. Ong JP, Aggarwal A, Krieger D, et al. Correlation between ammonia levels and the severity of hepatic encephalopathy. Am J Med 2003;114(3):188–93.
5. Uribe M, Campollo O, Vargas F, et al. Acidifying enemas (lactitol and lactose) vs. nonacidifying enemas (tap water) to treat acute portal-systemic encephalopathy: a double-blind, randomized clinical trial. Hepatology 1987;7(4):639–43.

6. Sharma BC, Singh J, Srivastava S, et al. Randomized controlled trial comparing lactulose plus albumin versus lactulose alone for treatment of hepatic encephalopathy. J Gastroenterol Hepatol 2017;32(6):1234–9.

7. Gluud LL, Vilstrup H, Morgan MY. Non-absorbable disaccharides versus placebo/no intervention and lactulose versus lactitol for the prevention and treatment of hepatic encephalopathy in people with cirrhosis. Cochrane Database Syst Rev 2016;(5):CD003044.

8. Kimer N, Krag A, Møller S, et al. Systematic review with meta-analysis: the effects of rifaximin in hepatic encephalopathy. Aliment Pharmacol Ther 2014;40(2): 123–32.

9. Garcia-Tsao G, Sanyal AJ, Grace ND, et al. Prevention and management of gastroesophageal varices and variceal hemorrhage in cirrhosis. Hepatology 2007;46(3):922–38.

10. Abraldes JG, Villanueva C, Bañares R, et al, Spanish Cooperative Group for Portal Hypertension and Variceal Bleeding. Hepatic venous pressure gradient and prognosis in patients with acute variceal bleeding treated with pharmacologic and endoscopic therapy. J Hepatol 2008;48(2):229–36.

11. Villanueva C, Colomo A, Bosch A, et al. Transfusion strategies for acute upper gastrointestinal bleeding. N Engl J Med 2013;368(1):11–21.

12. Krige JE, Kotze UK, Distiller G, et al. Predictive factors for rebleeding and death in alcoholic cirrhotic patients with acute variceal bleeding: a multivariate analysis. World J Surg 2009;33(10):2127–35.

13. Lee YY, Tee HP, Mahadeva S. Role of prophylactic antibiotics in cirrhotic patients with variceal bleeding. World J Gastroenterol 2014;20(7):1790–6.

14. Goulis J, Patch D, Burroughs AK. Bacterial infection in the pathogenesis of variceal bleeding. Lancet 1999;353(9147):139–42.

15. Chavez-Tapia NC, Barrientos-Gutierrez T, Tellez-Avila FI, et al. Antibiotic prophylaxis for cirrhotic patients with upper gastrointestinal bleeding. Cochrane Database Syst Rev 2010;(9):CD002907.

16. Garcia-Tsao G, Abraldes JG, Berzigotti A, et al. Portal hypertensive bleeding in cirrhosis: Risk stratification, diagnosis, and management: 2016 practice guidance by the American Association for the study of liver diseases. Hepatology 2017;65(1):310–35.

17. Wells M, Chande N, Adams P, et al. Meta-analysis: vasoactive medications for the management of acute variceal bleeds. Aliment Pharmacol Ther 2012;35(11): 1267–78.

18. Bañares R, Albillos A, Rincón D, et al. Endoscopic treatment versus endoscopic plus pharmacologic treatment for acute variceal bleeding: a meta-analysis. Hepatology 2002;35(3):609–15.

19. Wang SC, Shieh JF, Chang KY, et al. Thromboelastography-guided transfusion decreases intraoperative blood transfusion during orthotopic liver transplantation: randomized clinical trial. Transplant Proc 2010;42(7):2590–3.

20. De Pietri L, Bianchini M, Montalti R, et al. Thrombelastography-guided blood product use before invasive procedures in cirrhosis with severe coagulopathy: a randomized, controlled trial. Hepatology 2016;63(2):566–73.

21. Leon-Justel A, Noval-Padillo JA, Alvarez-Rios AI, et al. Point-of-care haemostasis monitoring during liver transplantation reduces transfusion requirements and improves patient outcome. Clin Chim Acta 2015;446:277–83.

22. Mannucci PM, Tripodi A. Liver disease, coagulopathies and transfusion therapy. Blood Transfus 2013;11(1):32–6.

23. Martin TJ, Kang Y, Robertson KM, et al. Ionization and hemodynamic effects of calcium chloride and calcium gluconate in the absence of hepatic function. Anesthesiology 1990;73(1):62–5.
24. Drolz A, Horvatits T, Rutter K, et al. Lactate improves prediction of short-term mortality in critically ill patients with cirrhosis: a multinational study. Hepatology 2019;69(1):258–69.
25. Akriviadis EA, Runyon BA. Utility of an algorithm in differentiating spontaneous from secondary bacterial peritonitis. Gastroenterology 1990;98(1):127–33.
26. Garrison RN, Cryer HM, Howard DA, et al. Clarification of risk factors for abdominal operations in patients with hepatic cirrhosis. Ann Surg 1984;199(6):648–55.
27. Navasa M, Follo A, Llovet JM, et al. Randomized, comparative study of oral ofloxacin versus intravenous cefotaxime in spontaneous bacterial peritonitis. Gastroenterology 1996;111(4):1011–7.
28. Follo A, Llovet JM, Navasa M, et al. Renal impairment after spontaneous bacterial peritonitis in cirrhosis: incidence, clinical course, predictive factors and prognosis. Hepatology 1994;20(6):1495–501.
29. Salerno F, Navickis RJ, Wilkes MM. Albumin infusion improves outcomes of patients with spontaneous bacterial peritonitis: a meta-analysis of randomized trials. Clin Gastroenterol Hepatol 2013;11(2):123–30.e1.
30. Kirsch CM, Chui DW, Yenokida GG, et al. Case report: hepatic hydrothorax without ascites. Am J Med Sci 1991;302(2):103–6.
31. Chen CH, Shih CM, Chou JW, et al. Outcome predictors of cirrhotic patients with spontaneous bacterial empyema. Liver Int 2011;31(3):417–24.
32. Allegretti AS, Ortiz G, Wenger J, et al. Prognosis of acute kidney injury and hepatorenal syndrome in patients with cirrhosis: a prospective cohort study. Int J Nephrol 2015;2015:108139.
33. Duvoux C, Zanditenas D, Hézode C, et al. Effects of noradrenalin and albumin in patients with type I hepatorenal syndrome: a pilot study. Hepatology 2002;36(2):374–80.
34. Sanyal AJ, Boyer T, Garcia-Tsao G, et al. A randomized, prospective, double-blind, placebo-controlled trial of terlipressin for type 1 hepatorenal syndrome. Gastroenterology 2008;134(5):1360–8.
35. Nassar Junior AP, Farias AQ, D' Albuquerque LA, et al. Terlipressin versus norepinephrine in the treatment of hepatorenal syndrome: a systematic review and meta-analysis. PLoS One 2014;9(9):e107466.
36. Salerno F, Navickis RJ, Wilkes MM. Albumin treatment regimen for type 1 hepatorenal syndrome: a dose-response meta-analysis. BMC Gastroenterol 2015;15:167.

Intracranial Hemorrhage and Intracranial Hypertension

Evie Marcolini, MD[a,b,]*, Christoph Stretz, MD[c],
Kyle M. DeWitt, PharmD[d]

KEYWORDS

- Intracerebral hemorrhage • Subarachnoid hemorrhage • Traumatic brain injury
- Blood pressure • Anticoagulation • Intracranial hypertension • Herniation
- ICP monitoring

KEY POINTS

- Intracranial hemorrhage is a heterogeneous disease and includes intracerebral hemorrhage, subarachnoid hemorrhage, and traumatic brain injury.
- Optimal blood pressure management depends on many factors, including the type of hemorrhage.
- Anticoagulation reversal is a critical component of mitigating risk for intracranial hemorrhage of all types and depends on the type of anticoagulant.
- Intracranial hypertension and brain herniation may occur jointly or independently as a result of various traumatic and nontraumatic brain injuries.
- Therapeutic interventions include baseline measures, osmotherapy, sedation and analgesia, neuromuscular paralysis, therapeutic hypothermia, barbiturates, and neurosurgical interventions.

INTRODUCTION

Neurologic hemorrhage, a life-changing event for patients and loved ones, presents a challenge for emergency physicians to diagnose accurately and work efficiently to improve patient outcome. The primary injury is irrevocable, but accurate diagnosis and aggressive therapeutic action do much to improve a patient's chances of

Disclosure Statement: The authors have no disclosures to report.
[a] Department of Surgery, Division of Emergency Medicine, University of Vermont College of Medicine, 111 Colchester Avenue, Burlington, VT 05401, USA; [b] Department of Neurology, Division of Neurocritical Care, University of Vermont College of Medicine, 111 Colchester Avenue, Burlington, VT 05401, USA; [c] Division of Vascular Neurology, Yale School of Medicine, 15 York Street, LLCI Building Suite 1004, New Haven, CT 06510, USA; [d] Department of Pharmacy, The University of Vermont Medical Center, 111 Colchester Avenue, Mailstop 272 BA1, Burlington, VT 05401, USA
* Corresponding author. 111 Colchester Avenue, Burlington, VT 05401, USA.
E-mail address: emarcolini@gmail.com

meaningful recovery. As with much in the neurosciences, the science continues to evolve. This article presents the latest of what is known about managing patients with neurologic hemorrhage, especially with respect to management of blood pressure, reversal of antithrombotic agents, and treatment of increased intracranial pressure (ICP) for traumatic brain injury (TBI), intracerebral hemorrhage (ICH), and subarachnoid hemorrhage (SAH).

TYPES OF CENTRAL NERVOUS SYSTEM HEMORRHAGE

Central nervous system hemorrhage has multiple pathophysiologic etiologies. Intracranial hemorrhage refers to any bleeding within the skull. SAH originates in the subarachnoid space from a ruptured cerebral aneurysm; in this context the bleeding also can extend into the intraventricular system (intraventricular hemorrhage) and/or the brain parenchyma. ICH originates from the parenchymal vessels within the brain and also can extend into the ventricular system. The most common etiology of ICH is longstanding hypertension that leads to small vessel lipohyalinosis and rupture where hemorrhages typically are located within deep cerebral structures.

Spontaneous ICH also can occur in the setting of vascular malformations (eg, cavernous malformations, arteriovenous malformation, and dural arteriovenous fistula), amyloid angiopathy, venous infarction, and tumor. TBI can be associated with multicompartmental hemorrhage in any or all of these areas (subarachnoid, intraventricular, and parenchymal) or extra-axial bleeding in the subdural or epidural space.

Resuscitation strategies vary significantly, depending on type of hemorrhage and patient characteristics. Initial assessment mandates diligence in synthesizing history, physical examination, and vital signs to determine first steps, even before diagnosis can be obtained, usually by imaging. Clues in the history help with diagnosis. A history of trauma can point toward TBI, with different physiologic manifestations, as described later. Sudden onset of headache, altered mental status, or neurologic deficit may accompany SAH, ICH, or acute ischemic stroke. Subtle mental status changes, dizziness, nausea, vomiting, or unsteadiness can present in the case of a posterior acute ischemic stroke or ICH.

The adage, "intubate for Glasgow Coma Scale (GCS) score less than 8," may not strictly apply to patients with central nervous system hemorrhage, because a patient may still be able to protect the airway despite other neurologic deficits. The process of intubation decreases the ability to perform a thorough and repeated neurologic examination, which is the most important and accurate method of monitoring for deterioration. A change in neurologic status may portend an SAH rebleed, ICH volume expansion, development of intracerebral edema, or herniation, any of which requires immediate and aggressive attention.

The injured brain is highly vulnerable to blood pressure changes. Specific targets for each etiologic entity must be managed with tight accuracy to optimize cerebral blood flow (CBF) and perfusion. The hemodynamic effects of rapid sequence intubation medications, laryngoscopy, and mechanical ventilation can affect outcome. In most cases, a diagnosis is made with CT or MRI, but if a patient's examination seems worse than the imaging would indicate, possibility of edema, increased ICP, or subclinical seizure activity should be considered.

HEMODYNAMIC TARGETS FOR THE PATIENT WITH A CENTRAL NERVOUS SYSTEM HEMORRHAGE
Traumatic Brain Injury

TBI is a heterogeneous disease that can result in several different types of hemorrhage. Brain perfusion, indirectly measured by cerebral perfusion pressure (CPP), is dependent on CBF and cerebral vascular resistance. The brain's autoregulatory mechanisms maintain a constant CBF through vasoconstriction and vasodilation in response to multiple variables, including Pa_{CO_2} and the brain's metabolic rate of oxygen and glucose. CBF usually is maintained throughout the range of systolic blood pressure (SBP) between 60 mm Hg and 150 mm Hg and outside of those parameters becomes passively dependent on mean arterial pressure (MAP).

In the setting of TBI, autoregulatory mechanisms can be disrupted throughout the brain in a heterogeneous distribution due to various mechanisms, such as breakdown of the blood brain barrier. Unfortunately, each TBI etiology has different effects on the brain, which are challenging to measure directly. Although manipulation of blood pressure is a simple method of preserving CPP, specific targets are difficult to establish in the setting of heterogeneous injury, unknown proportion of healthy versus damaged tissue, and unknown condition of CBF autoregulation. Inadequate CPP is associated with ischemia, and overaggressive CPP targets can result in secondary injury, such as acute lung injury, as a result of fluid and vasopressor use to maintain higher CPP levels.[1]

A single episode of hypotension, or SBP less than 90 mm Hg, has been associated with a 150% increase in mortality in patients with severe head injury, establishing a long-held standard.[2] Subsequent studies have shown the threshold for hypotension and mortality is actually higher,[3–6] may be represented by a U-shaped curve, and warrants more prospectively derived data. Age-specific blood pressure thresholds for patients with moderate to severe TBI include

- SBP greater than 100 mm Hg for ages 50 to 69
- SBP greater than 110 mm Hg for ages 15 to 49 and ages greater than 69

These thresholds are associated with lower mortality and are supported by current Brain Trauma Foundation guidelines.[7,8]

Intracerebral Hemorrhage

A majority of patients with ICH present with an elevated SBP in the first hours post-bleed due to increased ICP, physical and psychological stress, pain, autonomic dysfunction, and premorbid hypertension.[9,10] An elevated SBP is associated with hematoma volume expansion in up to 38% of ICH patients, with 25% of patients who do experience expansion occurring in the first hour. Every 1-cm^3 increase in hematoma growth may increase death/disability by 7%.[11]

Blood pressure control is a critical intervention to reduce the risk of neurologic deterioration, disability, and mortality.[12] Intriguingly, many studies show worse outcomes with higher SBP after ICH, but none has been able to show improved functional outcome with lowering of SBP.[13] This raises the question of whether acute BP lowering is safe and, if so, what is the optimal target.

Specific blood pressure goals have been studied extensively but have not been definitively established. The 2 largest randomized trials evaluating acute blood pressure targets in patients with ICH determined that acutely lowering SBP to less than 140 mm Hg is safe.[14,15] A meta-analysis of 6 randomized controlled trials found improved patient outcomes with earlier and a more aggressive SBP management.[11,16] A subgroup analysis of younger patients (<60 years old), with ICH volume <15 ml, receiving SBP management within 6 hours showed reduced hematoma growth. Current guidelines recommend lowering SBP if between 150 mm Hg and 220 mm Hg, with a lower limit of 140 mm Hg for optimal outcome.[9] An SBP greater than 220 mm Hg may require more aggressive reduction and close monitoring.

One important clinical question that remains to be answered is, "How low should the SBP be pushed?" Overly aggressive blood pressure control has the potential to reduce

CBF to vulnerable perihematomal areas, which can cause parenchymal ischemia. A recent study using CT perfusion scans to evaluate perihematomal CBF found no differences in blood flow between an SBP target of less than 150 mm Hg versus less than 180 mm Hg.[17] Although local CBF may not be significantly impacted by different SBP targets, MRI has revealed significant vasogenic edema and inflammatory changes,[17–19] in studies of patients with an SBP less than 130 mm Hg, which also was associated with worse clinical outcomes.[20] In light of these findings, a maximal benefit may be seen with a tight systolic goal, targeting an SBP of 130 mm Hg to 139 mm Hg.[16]

Subarachnoid Hemorrhage

Early management, during the first 6 hours to 12 hours of care, is the most critical for a patient with an acute SAH. Rapid blood pressure control should be an early resuscitative target because it can reduce the incidence of secondary hemorrhage (or rebleeding) and may reduce morbidity and mortality. Patients at particular risk for SAH rebleeding include those who have a history of hypertension or present with sentinel headache, syncope, seizure, altered mental status, or multiple or complex aneurysms.[21]

Most leading authorities agree that early blood pressure control prior to surgical aneurysm interventions reduces the risk of secondary bleed, but specific blood pressure targets have not been prospectively evaluated.[22–24] Guidelines recommend maintaining SBP between 100 mm Hg and 160 mm Hg or MAP less than 110 mm Hg.[23] Many institutions have pushed the target further, aiming for an SBP less than 140 mm Hg[25] until the aneurysm is secured. This usually is accomplished by endovascular coiling (preferred) or open surgical clipping, which may be necessary if the aneurysm is anatomically not amenable to safe and effective coiling.

MEDICAL MANAGEMENT FOR THE PATIENT WITH A CENTRAL NERVOUS SYSTEM HEMORRHAGE
Antihypertensive and Vasoactive Therapy

The optimal medication choice for blood pressure management in neurologic emergencies is short acting, easily titratable, and accessible. The most commonly used medications are nicardipine, labetalol, and esmolol. Clevidipine, fenoldopam, and enalaprilat also are possible choices. Agents, such as nitroprusside or nitroglycerin, have the side effect of increasing CBF through vasodilation and may increase ICP. Nitroprusside carries a risk of thiocyanate toxicity. Irrespective of agent used, arterial blood pressure and the neurologic examination should be followed closely if blood pressure is being lowered.

Oral Anti Thrombotic Reversal in Intracranial Hemorrhage

Compared to patients with spontaneous ICH not anticoagulated, those on antithrombotics are more likely to experience secondary hematoma expansion, poor functional outcome, and death.[26–28] Pooled data from four large trials of 84,540 patients comparing direct oral anticoagulants (DOACs) with warfarin demonstrate that rates of ICH are significantly lower in those treated with DOACs compared to warfarin with a median relative risk reduction of 58%.[29] This may be attributed to the notion that DOACs inhibit less local factors Xa and IIa generated in response to cerebral vascular injury compared to warfarin. Nonetheless, ICH with concomitant oral anticoagulant use is associated with 30-day mortality rates approaching 50%[30] and rapid reversal of coagulopathy is often necessary to slow hemorrhage expansion and improve outcomes.

Significant life-threatening ICH may require general supportive measures such as endotracheal intubation, hemodynamic resuscitation, and neurosurgical decompression or drainage. The anticoagulant should be immediately discontinued and specific reversal agents, when available, are preferred over general hemostatic agents (**Fig. 1**). Several important factors must be taken into consideration in the setting of antithrombotic-induced ICH:

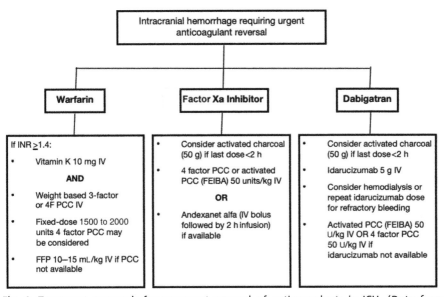

Fig. 1. Treatment approach for emergent reversal of anticoagulants in ICH. (*Data from* Refs.[34–36])

- Anticoagulant pharmacokinetics (**Table 1**)
- Indication (eg mechanical heart valve, stroke prevention, etc.)
- Time of last dose
- Renal and/or hepatic dysfunction
- Drug-drug interactions

Table 1
Pharmacokinetic properties or oral anticoagulants

Drug	Mechanism	Time to Peak (h)	Half-life (h)	Renal Excretion (%)	Protein Binding (%)	Dialyzable
Warfarin	Vitamin K antagonist	72–120	Up to 168	92	99	No
Apixaban	Factor Xa inhibitor	3	9–14	25	87	Minimal
Rivaroxaban	Factor Xa inhibitor	3	9	66	92–95	No
Edoxaban	Factor Xa inhibitor	1–2	11	35	55	No
Dabigatran	Direct thrombin inhibitor	2	14–17	80	35	Yes

Data form Frontera JA, Lewin JJ, 3rd, Rabinstein AA, et al. Guideline for Reversal of Antithrombotics in Intracranial Hemorrhage: A Statement for Healthcare Professionals from the Neurocritical Care Society and Society of Critical Care Medicine. Neurocrit Care. 2016;24(1):6-46, and Lip GYH, Banerjee A, Boriani G, et al. Antithrombotic Therapy for Atrial Fibrillation: CHEST Guideline and Expert Panel Report. Chest. 2018;154(5):1121-1201.

Oftentimes, an accurate history and time of last dose cannot be reliably obtained in the emergency department setting. Coagulation assays may provide clinicians with a better understanding of the patient's serum drug concentrations and help to guide treatment decisions (**Table 2**). Treatment with a reversal agent should not be delayed while waiting for assay results in a patient with life threatening ICH presumed to be on a DOAC.

Table 2		
Suggestions for laboratory measurement of direct oral anticoagulants		
Drug	**Suggested Test**	**Interpretation**
Apixaban Rivaroxaban Edoxaban	Anti–factor Xa	Absent anti–factor Xa assay activity likely excludes clinically relevant[a] drug concentrations
Dabigatran	dTT ECT Ecarin chromogenic assay	Normal result likely excludes clinically relevant[b] drug concentrations

[a] Normal PT, INR, and aPTT do not exclude clinically relevant concentrations.
[b] Normal aPTT may not exclude on-therapy concentrations.
Courtesy of CSL Behring, King of Prussia, PA.

Warfarin

Prothrombin time (PT) and international normalized ratio (INR) are readily available and can accurately determine the extent of anticoagulation induced by warfarin (given no underlying hepatic dysfunction). The Neurocritical Care Society recommends reversal of warfarin in the setting of ICH for patients with an INR greater than 1.4.[31]

4 factor prothrombin complex concentrate (4F-PCC) is preferred for emergent reversal of warfarin-induced coagulopathy in the setting of life-threatening ICH due to its rapid onset of action, small volume of infusion, and relatively short preparation time.[31–33] In a randomized open-label trial, 4F-PCC was noninferior to plasma for effective hemostasis and was more likely to correct INR to less than or equal to 1.3 within 30 minutes after infusion. Thrombotic events were similar between groups, with an occurrence of 7.8% and 6.4% in the 4F-PCC and fresh frozen plasma groups, respectively.[34] Prothrombin complex concentrate (human) and factor IX complex, should be considered in patients with a known history of heparin-induced thrombocytopenia.[31]

The Food and Drug Administration–approved dose of Kcentra is determined by body weight and INR.[34] More recently, a fixed-dose strategy has emerged as a potential alternative for emergent reversal of warfarin. Multiple studies have evaluated a fixed-dose regimen in the ICH population with promising results; however, methodology and outcome measures are highly variable.[35,36] The 2017 American College of Cardiology Task Force consensus statement has proposed that a fixed-dose of 1500 units of PCC may be considered, as an alternative to weight-based dosing, for warfarin reversal in patients with ICH. Interestingly, the document does not provide citations or further discussion to support this recommendation.[33] Additional well-designed trials are needed prior to global adoption of this practice, but it may be considered on a case-by-case basis.

Vitamin K (phytonadione) 5–10 mg should be administered intravenously in combination with PCC as the duration of action of PCC is short lived (6–8 hours).[31–33] Intravenous vitamin K will begin to increase the production of clotting factors within 1-

2 hours and reach peak effect at 12 hours. When administered orally, peak effect is delayed to 24 hours and is therefore not preferred in the setting of life threatening hemorrhage. Hypersensitivity reactions are extremely rare with an estimated incidence of 3 per 10,000 doses.[37]

Factor Xa Inhibitors

Anti-factor Xa activity is linear over a wide range of drug levels and may be used for quantification. An undetectable anti-factor Xa activity likely excludes clinically relevant drug concentrations. Billoir and colleagues evaluated a low-molecular-weight heparin (LMWH) calibrated anti-factor Xa assay for the quantification of rivaroxaban and apixaban plasma concentration in the emergency department. The authors demonstrated a significant linear correlation between LMWH anti-factor Xa activity and rivaroxaban and apixaban plasma concentrations.[38] Although further validation of LMWH anti-factor Xa assays in the setting of ICH is needed, it may serve as a useful marker of anticoagulation when an accurate history cannot be obtained from the patient or caregiver. PT, INR, and activated partial thromboplastin time (aPTT) lack both specificity and sensitivity (especially for apixaban) for detection of factor Xa inhibitor serum concentration and a result within normal range may not exclude clinically relevant concentrations.[39]

Historically, 50 units/kg of activated PCC factor eight inhibitor bypassing activity (FEIBA) or 4F-PCC has been suggested as a nonspecific reversal strategy based on limited evidence.[31,33] Lower doses of 25 units/kg have achieved effective hemostasis in patients with intracranial hemorrhage.[40,41] Andexanet alfa, A factor Xa decoy that binds and sequesters factor Xa inhibitors, was approved in 2018 for rapidreversal of apixaban and rivaroxaban in the setting of acute major bleeding. ANNEXA-4 was an open-label, single-arm trial that included 352 patients (64% with ICH) who received andexanet for acute major bleeding within 18 hours of factor Xa inhibitor administration.[42] A bolus and subsequent 2-hour infusion of andexanet provided excellent or good hemostasis in 80% of patients with ICH who could be evaluated. Anti- factor Xa activity returned to 68% and 58% of baseline at 4 hours post-infusion among patients receiving apixaban and rivaroxaban, respectively.Reduction in anti- factor Xa activity was not predictive of hemostatic efficacy. Thrombosis occurred in10% of patients, which may be attributed to the drug directly interacting with tissue factor pathway inhibitor (TFPI).[43] An ongoing randomized controlled trial is expected to provide more data on the efficacy and safety of andexanet compared to standard of care.[44]

Ciraparantag (PER977) is a small synthetic molecule that binds factor Xa inhibitors, direct thrombin inhibitors, low-molecular weight heparin, and unfractionated heparin. Ongoing clinical trials have demonstrated a rapid onset of action and reversal effects that are maintained at 24 hours.[45] Although ciraparantag is still in the early phases of development, preliminary results indicate this novel agent may be a viable option for the reversal of multiple anticoagulants.

Dabigatran

Diluted thrombin time (dTT), ecarin clotting time (ECT), and ecarin chromogenic assay (ECA) are the preferred assays for detection of serum dabigatran concentrations; however, these tests are not commonly available in the emergency department setting. An elevated aPTT confirms on-therapy or above on-therapy concentrations of dabigatran; however, because it is less sensitive, a normal aPTT cannot exclude clinically relevant drug concentrations.[39]

Idarucizumab is a humanized monoclonal antibody fragment that neutralizes the anticoagulant effect of dabigatran by binding to both dabigatran and its metabolites. The binding affinity for idarucizumab is approximately 350-fold higher than that of dabigatran to thrombin.[46] In the Idarucizumab for Dabigatran Reversal — Full Cohort Analysis (RE-VERSE AD) trial, 5 g (as two 2.5 g doses administered within 15 minutes) of idarucizumab provided rapid and complete reversal of dabigatran (based on dTT or ECT assays) in patients with acute major bleeding and non-bleeding patients who required urgent surgery or intervention.[47] ICH accounted for 32.6% of patients who presented with major bleeding. Although all patients achieved complete reversal laboratory assays within 4 hours, the time to cessation of bleeding could not to be assessed in any patient with ICH. Rates of thrombosis at 90 days were 6.3% among patients with acute bleeding and 7.4% among patients who required reversal to facilitate surgical intervention.

Antiplatelet Agents

Data is conflicting with regard to reversing antiplatelet agents (e.g. cyclooxegenase and P2Y12 inhibitors) in the setting of ICH. Two systematic reviews of lower quality, heterogeneous studies found no benefit of platelet infusions for spontaneous or traumatic ICH.[48,49] Furthermore, the platelet transfusion versus standard care after acute stroke due to spontaneous cerebral hemorrhage associated with antiplatelet activity (PATCH) trial demonstrated that patients administered platelet infusions were 2.5× more likely to experience death or disability compared to placebo.[50] Based on these findings, routine infusion of platelets is not recommended and the decision to administer should be made on a case-bycase basis for patients that require neurosurgical intervention.[31,33] The PATCH trial did not include patients with SAH or TBI.[50]

Desmopressin (DDAVP) has been shown to increase the release of von Willebrand factor and promote endothelial platelet adhesion, which may reduce further hemorrhage in patients on antiplatelets. Two small studies suggest that DDAVP improves platelet function assays and limits hematoma expansion in ICH patients exposed to antiplatelet therapy.[51,52] Despite a paucity of literature, DDAVP, 0.4 μg/kg IV, may be considered in ICH patients on antiplatelet agents, given its potential benefit, low cost, and safety profile.

INTRACRANIAL HYPERTENSION

All intracranial hemorrhage puts patients at risk for intracranial hypertension (IH), typically from mass effect or edema. The pathophysiology of IH and best practices to diagnose and manage this complication in an emergency department are reviewed.

Definitions and Pathophysiology

Normal ICP ranges between 5 mm Hg and 15 mm Hg.[53] According to the Monroe-Kellie doctrine,[54,55] the total intracranial volume consisting of brain, blood, and cerebrospinal fluid (CSF) must remain constant. Any increase in volume of 1 component must be accommodated by a reciprocal change in another. Common conditions that can increase ICP include a space-occupying fourth component (such as extra-axial or intra-axial hemorrhage, brain tumors, or abscesses), increases in brain volume (eg, edema after an ischemic stroke or hypoxic-ischemic injury), increases in both brain and blood volume (ie, TBI, meningoencephalitis, and SAH), and increases in CSF volume (eg, hydrocephalus and choroid plexus papilloma).[56] IH is defined by persistent (>5 minutes) elevation of ICP above 20 mm Hg.[57]

Brain herniation and IH can occur together or independently.[58] Both IH and brain herniation constitute neurologic emergencies warranting prompt recognition and management (**Table 3**).

The absolute value of ICP in itself has limited significance. Clinical interpretation is often dependent on other factors, such as CPP (CPP) and brain compliance.[56] CPP is defined as MAP–ICP and can be used as a marker for CBF. Brain compliance is defined as change in volume divided by change in pressure. The relationship between volume and pressure initially is linear but eventually becomes exponential when small increases in volume may manifest with a clinically significant rise in ICP.[56]

Table 3
Common brain herniation syndromes

Syndrome	Clinical Features	Etiologies
Uncal (lateral transtentorial)	Ipsilateral CN III palsy Contralateral or bilateral motor posturing	Temporal mass lesions
Central transtentorial	Bilateral decorticate progresses to decerebrate posturing Rostral to caudal loss of brainstem reflexes	Global cerebral edema Hydrocephalus
Subfalcine	Asymmetric motor posturing Oculocephalic reflex preserved	Convexity (frontal/parietal) mass lesion
Cerebellar (upward or downward)	Progression to coma with motor posturing Cerebellar signs	Cerebellar mass lesion

Adapted from Lee K, Mayer SA. Management of increased intracranial pressure. In: Lee K. (Ed)The NeuroICU Book 2nd edition. New York, NY: McGraw Hill, 2017; with permission.

Diagnosis

Clinical signs and symptoms of elevated ICP include headache, diplopia, nausea, vomiting, papilledema, and cranial nerve (CN) VI palsy. These may be accompanied by hypertension, bradycardia, irregular respiratory pattern (Cushing triad),[59] or changes in mental status.[53,58] Recognizing clinical signs of IH is particularly important in an emergency department, because direct measurement of ICP is invasive and infrequently available.[53,58,60]

In patients with TBI, ICP monitor placement is recommended for patients with a GCS less than 8 after initial resuscitation who

1. Have an abnormal head CT (or)
2. Exhibit 2 of 3 criteria: age greater than 40 years, SBP less than 90 mm Hg, or abnormal posturing[7,57]

In nontraumatic coma, ICP and CPP monitoring may be performed in patients at increased risk for IH in capable ICUs.[61] An external ventricular drain (EVD) is both diagnostic and therapeutic for patients with SAH, intraventricular hemorrhage, and/or obstructive hydrocephalus.

Management

The management of IH should follow a tiered approach, such as that outlined in the *Emergency Neurological Life Support* protocol of the Neurocritical Care Society.[58] The following adapted therapeutic algorithm is further illustrated in **Fig. 2** and in **Table 4**.

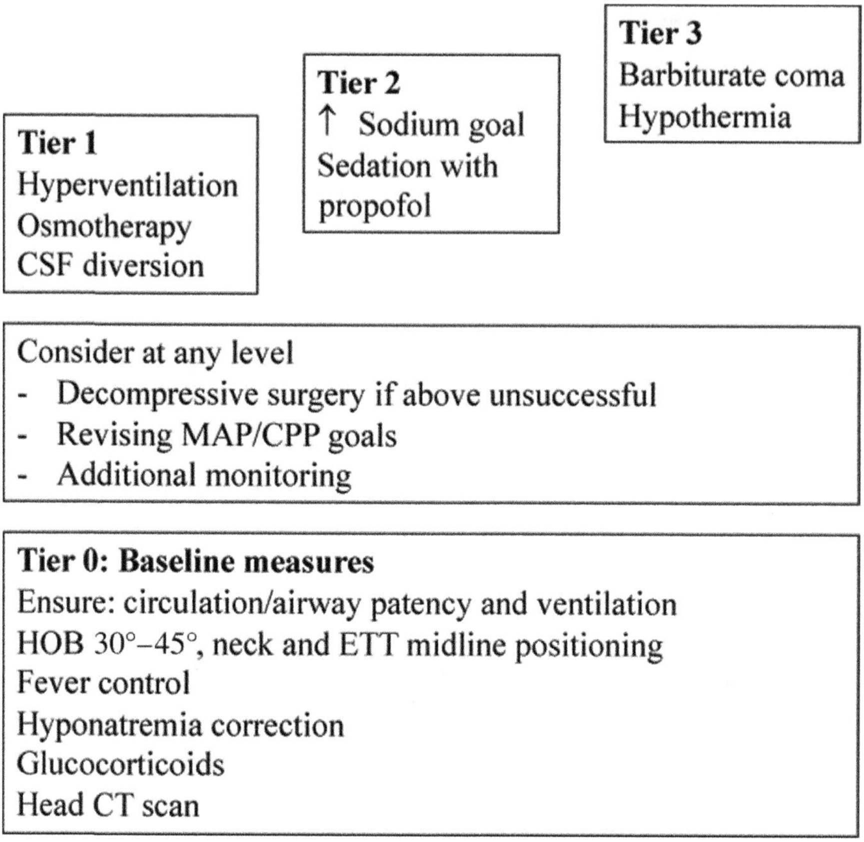

Tier 1
Hyperventilation
Osmotherapy
CSF diversion

Tier 2
↑ Sodium goal
Sedation with
propofol

Tier 3
Barbiturate coma
Hypothermia

Consider at any level
- Decompressive surgery if above unsuccessful
- Revising MAP/CPP goals
- Additional monitoring

Tier 0: Baseline measures
Ensure: circulation/airway patency and ventilation
HOB 30°–45°, neck and ETT midline positioning
Fever control
Hyponatremia correction
Glucocorticoids
Head CT scan

Fig. 2. A tiered approach to IH. HOB, head of bed. (*Data from* Cadena R, Shoykhet M, Ratcliff JJ. Emergency Neurological Life Support: Intracranial Hypertension and Herniation. Neurocrit Care. 2017;27(Suppl 1):82-88.)

During the initial phase of IH treatment in an emergency department, the airway must be assessed and secured if needed. It is important to recognize that even with a lower GCS, a patient may be able to protect the airway, unlike in other pathologies, where GCS less than 8 typically triggers intubation. Elevating the head of bed to 30° to 45° with a midline neck position can improve venous drainage and mitigate rising ICP. Treating fever, maintaining normal sodium levels, and choosing iso-osmotic or hyperosmotic fluids all are neuroprotective.[53,56] Steroids are useful only in cases of tumor-related vasogenic edema or other neuroinflammatory conditions.[62,63]

Osmolar therapy should be given in bolus dosing to maximize the osmolar effect.[64] Recommended mannitol dosing is 0.25 g/kg to 1.5 g/kg by a peripheral IV line, typically repeated every 4 hours to 6 hours as determined by monitoring serum osmolality.[53,58] Hypertonic saline (HTS) can be bolused over 5 minutes to 15 minutes and can be given in concentrations ranging from 1.5% to 23.4%. These agents can be given in combination and should be reserved for changes in neurologic examination suggesting an increase in ICP. The highest concentration of HTS typically is reserved for life-threatening ICP crisis and should be given through a central line if possible due

Table 4
Overview of management options for elevated intracranial pressure

Intervention	Mechanism	Pearls/Pitfalls
Baseline measures		
• HOB 30°–45° • Neck midline • ETT positioning	Promotion of venous drainage	• Reduction of CPP if HOB >45°
Neurosurgical procedures		
CSF diversion	Reduction of CSF volume	• EVD allows for ICP monitoring and CSF diversion • Infection, SDH, and tract hemorrhage may occur
Craniectomy/craniotomy	Evacuation allows room for swelling	• Potential causal treatment • Risk of surgery/anesthesia • Reduces mortality, not morbidity
Sedation, analgesia	Reduction of CBF ASM effect	• Titratable effect • Hypotension, respiratory depression, loss of neurologic examination, PRIS
Neuromuscular paralysis	Prevention of ICP spikes	• Facilitates mechanical ventilation • Loss of neurologic examination • Requires: intubation, mechanical ventilation, sedation, TOF monitoring
Barbiturate coma	Reduction of CBF ASM effect	• Titrate to EEG burst suppression or normal ICP • Loss of neurologic examination, respiratory depression, hypotension, immunosuppression, ileus
Hyperventilation	Cerebral vasoconstriction	• $Paco_2$ goal of 30–35 mm Hg for <2 h • Cerebral ischemia and worse outcomes in TBI may occur
Osmotherapy		

HTS common doses
  1.5% or 3% infusion
  14.6% bolus
  23.4% bolus
	Water removal from the brain	• Monitor serum sodium every 4–6 h, hold if >160 mEq, central access needed if concentration ≥3%
		• Can cause CHF, hypernatremia, acidosis, CPM

Mannitol 20%, 0.25–1.5 g/kg	Water removal from the brain Increase in CPP	• Holding parameters as with HTS and if OSM >320, peripheral administration • Can cause hypotension, acute renal failure, electrolyte depletion
Hypothermia	Reduction in cerebral metabolism	• Set goal temperature • Shivering, arrhythmias, infection, electrolyte abnormalities, delay in drug clearance can occur.

Abbreviations: ASM, antiseizure medications; CHF, congestive heart failure; CPM, central pontine myelinolysis; ETT, endotracheal tube; HOB, head of bed; OSM, osmolarity; SDH, subdural hemorrhage; TOF, train-of-four.
Data from Freeman WD. Management of Intracranial Pressure. Continuum (Minneap Minn). 2015;21(5 Neurocritical Care):1299-1323.

to the risk of infiltration and tissue necrosis but can be given peripherally in a crisis situation with risk-benefit consideration[65] (see **Table 4**).

Draining CSF via EVD is a quick method of reducing ICP. In TBI patients, this should be done in small increments, with a target CPP of 60 mm Hg to 70 mm Hg.[7] There is no comparable evidence for CPP goals in nontraumatic IH.[58]

Hyperventilation is a potent measure to reduce ICP but is contraindicated in the first 24 hours of brain injury due to the brain's heightened sensitivity to lower perfusion and risk of inducing stroke. In general, hyperventilation should be reserved for extreme crisis preceding decompressive therapy, because the initial effect is cerebral vaso-constriction followed by vasodilation as the brain compensates for respiratory alkalosis.[57,66]

Deep sedation with propofol, midazolam, or dexmedetomidine can mitigate IH. If using propofol, surveillance laboratory tests should be monitored to anticipate and screen for signs of propofol infusion syndrome, which can be life threatening, and is more common with larger doses or longer duration of treatment. Monitoring for meta-bolic acidosis, rhabdomyolysis, cardiac dysfunction, and elevated triglycerides is an accepted monitoring method for propofol-related infusion syndrome (PRIS).[58,67,68]

The most aggressive interventions for IH have the most side effects and are less studied.[58] Barbiturate-induced coma with pentobarbital titrated to continuous EEG burst suppression can be achieved with a bolus dose of 10 mg/kg over 30 minutes to 2 hours, then 5 mg/kg/h $\times$ 3 h, with maintenance infusion of 1 mg/kg/h to 4 mg/kg/h titrated to ICP goal.[58,69] Targeted temperature management to a core temperature of 32C to 34C has been shown to reduce ICP, although evidence of improved outcome is lacking.[70] Either surface cooling devices or intravascular cooling catheters can be used.[56]

Surgical decompression is the procedure of last resort to relieve IH (excluding epidural/subdural hemorrhage) and should be considered in concert with neurosur-gical, neurocritical care colleagues as well as the family to explain prognostic expectations.

Many of these interventions are not implemented in an emergency department but are considered in the first 24 hours for patients with severe IH. Other monitoring de-vices include jugular venous oximetry, brain tissue oxygenation, and cerebral micro-dialysis. Other monitoring devices are utilized to measure jugular venous oxygen saturation, brain tissue oxygenation and brain tissue biochemistry.[55]

Aggressive management of intracranial hemorrhage, including TBI, ICH and SAH will optimize patient outcome in the setting of a potentially devastating injury. Under-standing the nuances of blood pressure management, anticoagulation or antiplatelet reversal and intracranial hypertension treatment is key to managing these patients.

REFERENCES

1. White H, Venkatesh B. Cerebral perfusion pressure in neurotrauma: a review. Anesth Analg 2008;107(3):979–88.
2. Chesnut RM, Marshall LF, Klauber MR, et al. The role of secondary brain injury in determining outcome from severe head injury. J Trauma 1993;34(2):216–22.
3. Brenner M, Stein DM, Hu PF, et al. Traditional systolic blood pressure targets un-derestimate hypotension-induced secondary brain injury. J Trauma Acute Care Surg 2012;72(5):1135–9.
4. Fuller G, Hasler RM, Mealing N, et al. The association between admission systolic blood pressure and mortality in significant traumatic brain injury: a multi-centre cohort study. Injury 2014;45(3):612–7.
5. Shibahashi K, Sugiyama K, Okura Y, et al. Defining hypotension in patients with severe traumatic brain injury. World Neurosurg 2018;120:e667–74.
6. Spaite DW, Hu C, Bobrow BJ, et al. Mortality and prehospital blood pressure in patients with major traumatic brain injury: implications for the hypotension threshold. JAMA Surg 2017;152(4):360–8.

7. Carney N, Totten AM, O'Reilly C, et al. Guidelines for the management of severe traumatic brain injury, fourth edition. Neurosurgery 2017;80(1):6–15.
8. Berry C, Ley EJ, Bukur M, et al. Redefining hypotension in traumatic brain injury. Injury 2012;43(11):1833–7.
9. Hemphill JC 3rd, Greenberg SM, Anderson CS, et al. Guidelines for the management of spontaneous intracerebral hemorrhage: a guideline for healthcare professionals from the American Heart Association/American Stroke Association. Stroke 2015;46(7):2032–60.
10. Qureshi AI, Ezzeddine MA, Nasar A, et al. Prevalence of elevated blood pressure in 563,704 adult patients with stroke presenting to the ED in the United States. Am J Emerg Med 2007;25(1):32–8.
11. Shi L, Xu S, Zheng J, et al. Blood pressure management for acute intracerebral hemorrhage: a meta-analysis. Sci Rep 2017;7(1):14345.
12. Zhang Y, Reilly KH, Tong W, et al. Blood pressure and clinical outcome among patients with acute stroke in Inner Mongolia, China. J Hypertens 2008;26(7): 1446–52.
13. Boulouis G, Morotti A, Goldstein JN, et al. Intensive blood pressure lowering in patients with acute intracerebral haemorrhage: clinical outcomes and haemorrhage expansion. Systematic review and meta-analysis of randomised trials. J Neurol Neurosurg Psychiatry 2017;88(4):339–45.
14. Anderson CS, Heeley E, Huang Y, et al. Rapid blood-pressure lowering in patients with acute intracerebral hemorrhage. N Engl J Med 2013;368(25):2355–65.
15. Qureshi AI, Palesch YY, Barsan WG, et al. Intensive blood-pressure lowering in patients with acute cerebral hemorrhage. N Engl J Med 2016;375(11):1033–43.
16. Arima H, Heeley E, Delcourt C, et al. Optimal achieved blood pressure in acute intracerebral hemorrhage: INTERACT2. Neurology 2015;84(5):464–71.
17. Butcher KS, Baird T, MacGregor L, et al. Perihematomal edema in primary intracerebral hemorrhage is plasma derived. Stroke 2004;35(8):1879–85.
18. Butcher KS, Jeerakathil T, Hill M, et al. The intracerebral hemorrhage acutely decreasing arterial pressure trial. Stroke 2013;44(3):620–6.
19. Olivot JM, Mlynash M, Kleinman JT, et al. MRI profile of the perihematomal region in acute intracerebral hemorrhage. Stroke 2010;41(11):2681–3.
20. Buletko AB, Thacker T, Cho SM, et al. Cerebral ischemia and deterioration with lower blood pressure target in intracerebral hemorrhage. Neurology 2018; 91(11):e1058–66.
21. Solanki C, Pandey P, Rao KV. Predictors of aneurysmal rebleed before definitive surgical or endovascular management. Acta Neurochir (Wien) 2016;158(6): 1037–44.
22. Alfotih GT, Li F, Xu X, et al. Risk factors for re-bleeding of aneurysmal subarachnoid hemorrhage: meta-analysis of observational studies. Neurol Neurochir Pol 2014;48(5):346–55.
23. Connolly ES Jr, Rabinstein AA, Carhuapoma JR, et al. Guidelines for the management of aneurysmal subarachnoid hemorrhage: a guideline for healthcare professionals from the American Heart Association/American Stroke Association. Stroke 2012;43(6):1711–37.
24. Tang C, Zhang TS, Zhou LF. Risk factors for rebleeding of aneurysmal subarachnoid hemorrhage: a meta-analysis. PLoS One 2014;9(6):e99536.
25. Rose JC, Mayer SA. Optimizing blood pressure in neurological emergencies. Neurocrit Care 2006;4(1):98.
26. Flibotte JJ, Hagan N, O'Donnell J, et al. Warfarin, hematoma expansion, and outcome of intracerebral hemorrhage. Neurology 2004;63(6):1059–64.

27. Franke CL, de Jonge J, van Swieten JC, et al. Intracerebral hematomas during anticoagulant treatment. Stroke 1990;21(5):726–30.
28. Rosand J, Eckman MH, Knudsen KA, et al. The effect of warfarin and intensity of anticoagulation on outcome of intracerebral hemorrhage. Arch Intern Med 2004; 164(8):880–4.
29. Vanassche T, Hirsh J, Eikelboom JW, et al. Organ-specific bleeding patterns of anticoagulant therapy: lessons from clinical trials. Thromb Haemost 2014; 112(5):918–23.
30. Cervera A, Amaro S, Chamorro A. Oral anticoagulant-associated intracerebral hemorrhage. J Neurol 2012;259(2):212–24.
31. Frontera JA, Lewin JJ 3rd, Rabinstein AA, et al. Guideline for reversal of antithrombotics in intracranial hemorrhage: a statement for healthcare professionals from the Neurocritical Care Society and Society of Critical Care Medicine. Neurocrit Care 2016;24(1):6–46.
32. Lip GYH, Banerjee A, Boriani G, et al. Antithrombotic therapy for atrial fibrillation: CHEST guideline and expert panel report. Chest 2018;154(5):1121–201.
33. Tomaselli GF, Mahaffey KW, Cuker A, et al. 2017 ACC expert consensus decision pathway on management of bleeding in patients on oral anticoagulants: a report of the American College of Cardiology Task Force on expert consensus decision pathways. J Am Coll Cardiol 2017;70(24):3042–67.
34. Sarode R, Milling TJ Jr, Refaai MA, et al. Efficacy and safety of a 4-factor prothrombin complex concentrate in patients on vitamin K antagonists presenting with major bleeding: a randomized, plasma-controlled, phase IIIb study. Circulation 2013;128(11):1234–43.
35. Hall ST, Molina KC. Fixed-dose 4-factor prothrombin complex concentrate: we don't know where we're going if we don't know how to get there. J Thromb Thrombolysis 2018;46(1):50–7.
36. Scott R, Kersten B, Basior J, et al. Evaluation of fixed-dose four-factor prothrombin complex concentrate for emergent warfarin reversal in patients with intracranial hemorrhage. J Emerg Med 2018;54(6):861–6.
37. Britt RB, Brown JN. Characterizing the severe reactions of parenteral vitamin K1. Clin Appl Thromb Hemost 2018;24(1):5–12.
38. Billoir P, Barbay V, Joly LM, et al. Anti-factor Xa oral anticoagulant plasma concentration assay in real life: rivaroxaban and apixaban quantification in emergency with LMWH calibrator. Ann Pharmacother 2018;53(4):341–7.
39. Cuker A, Siegal DM, Crowther MA, et al. Laboratory measurement of the anticoagulant activity of the non-vitamin K oral anticoagulants. J Am Coll Cardiol 2014; 64(11):1128–39.
40. Smith MN, Deloney L, Carter C, et al. Safety, efficacy, and cost of four-factor prothrombin complex concentrate (4F-PCC) in patients with factor Xa inhibitor-related bleeding: a retrospective study. J Thromb Thrombolysis 2019. [Epub ahead of print].
41. Berger K, Santibanez M, Lin L, et al. A Low-Dose 4F-PCC Protocol for DOAC-Associated Intracranial Hemorrhage. J Intensive Care Med 2019. [Epub ahead of print].
42. Connolly SJ, Milling TJ Jr, Eikelboom JW, et al. Andexanet Alfa for acute major bleeding associated with factor Xa inhibitors. N Engl J Med 2016;375(12): 1131–41.
43. Lu G, Lin JP, Curnutte JT, et al. Effect of andexanet-TFPI interaction on in vitro thrombin formation and coagulation markers in the TF-pathway. Blood 2017; 130(Suppl 1):629.

44. ClinicalTrials.gov number, NCT03661528.
45. Ansell JE, Bakhru SH, Laulicht BE, et al. Use of PER977 to reverse the anticoagulant effect of edoxaban. N Engl J Med 2014;371(22):2141–2.
46. Schiele F, van Ryn J, Canada K, et al. A specific antidote for dabigatran: functional and structural characterization. Blood 2013;121(18):3554–62.
47. Pollack CV Jr, Reilly PA, van Ryn J, et al. Idarucizumab for dabigatran reversal - full cohort analysis. N Engl J Med 2017;377(5):431–41.
48. Batchelor JS, Grayson A. A meta-analysis to determine the effect on survival of platelet transfusions in patients with either spontaneous or traumatic antiplatelet medication-associated intracranial haemorrhage. BMJ Open 2012;2(2):e000588.
49. Nishijima DK, Zehtabchi S, Berrong J, et al. Utility of platelet transfusion in adult patients with traumatic intracranial hemorrhage and preinjury antiplatelet use: a systematic review. J Trauma Acute Care Surg 2012;72(6):1658–63.
50. Baharoglu MI, Cordonnier C, Al-Shahi Salman R, et al. Platelet transfusion versus standard care after acute stroke due to spontaneous cerebral haemorrhage associated with antiplatelet therapy (PATCH): a randomised, open-label, phase 3 trial. Lancet 2016;387(10038):2605–13.
51. Kapapa T, Rohrer S, Struve S, et al. Desmopressin acetate in intracranial haemorrhage. Neurol Res Int 2014;2014:298767.
52. Naidech AM, Maas MB, Levasseur-Franklin KE, et al. Desmopressin improves platelet activity in acute intracerebral hemorrhage. Stroke 2014;45(8):2451–3.
53. Freeman WD. Management of intracranial pressure. Continuum (Minneap Minn) 2015;21(5 Neurocritical Care):1299–323.
54. Kellie G. An account of the appearances observed in the dissection of two of three individuals presumed to have perished in the storm of the 3d, and whose bodies were discovered in the vicinity of Leith on the morning of the 4th, November 1821; with some reflections on the pathology of the brain: part I. Trans Med Chir Soc Edinb 1824;1:84–122.
55. Monro A. Observations on the structure and functions of the nervous system 1783.
56. KL. Management of intracranial pressure. In: KL, editor. The NeuroICU book. 2nd edition. McGraw Hill; 2017.
57. Carney N, Totten AM, O'Reilly C, et al. Guidelines for the management of severe traumatic brain injury, fourth edition. Neurosurgery 2017;80(1):6–15.
58. Cadena R, Shoykhet M, Ratcliff JJ. Emergency neurological life support: intracranial hypertension and herniation. Neurocrit Care 2017;27(Suppl 1):82–8.
59. Cushing H. Concerning a definite regulatory mechanism of the vasomotor centers which controls blood pressure during cerebral compression. Bull Johns Hopkins Hosp 1901;12.
60. Keegan J, Hwang DY. Principles of neurocritical care. In: Salardini A, Biller J, editors. The Hospital Neurology Book. New York: Mc Graw Hill; 2015. p. 339–41.
61. Le Roux P, Menon DK, Citerio G, et al. Consensus summary statement of the International Multidisciplinary Consensus Conference on Multimodality Monitoring in Neurocritical Care : a statement for healthcare professionals from the Neurocritical Care Society and the European Society of Intensive Care Medicine. Intensive Care Med 2014;40(9):1189–209.
62. Rangel-Castilla L, Gopinath S, Robertson CS. Management of intracranial hypertension. Neurol Clin 2008;26(2):521–41, x.
63. Mayer SA. Brain edema and disorders of intracranial pressure. In: Louis ED, Mayer SA, Rowland LP, editors. Merritt's Neurology. 13th edition. Philadelphia: Wolters Kluwer; 2016. p. 933–6.

64. Ropper AH. Hyperosmolar therapy for raised intracranial pressure. N Engl J Med 2012;367(8):746–52.
65. Bulger EM, May S, Brasel KJ, et al. Out-of-hospital hypertonic resuscitation following severe traumatic brain injury: a randomized controlled trial. JAMA 2010;304(13):1455–64.
66. Heffner JE, Sahn SA. Controlled hyperventilation in patients with intracranial hypertension. Application and management. Arch Intern Med 1983;143(4):765–9.
67. Kelly DF, Goodale DB, Williams J, et al. Propofol in the treatment of moderate and severe head injury: a randomized, prospective double-blinded pilot trial. J Neurosurg 1999;90(6):1042–52.
68. Roberts RJ, Barletta JF, Fong JJ, et al. Incidence of propofol-related infusion syndrome in critically ill adults: a prospective, multicenter study. Crit Care 2009; 13(5):R169.
69. The use of barbiturates in the control of intracranial hypertension. Brain Trauma Foundation. J Neurotrauma 1996;13(11):711–4.
70. Polderman KH. Induced hypothermia and fever control for prevention and treatment of neurological injuries. Lancet 2008;371(9628):1955–69.

Sedation and Analgesia for Mechanically Ventilated Patients in the Emergency Department

Christopher Noel, MD[a],*, Haney Mallemat, MD[b]

KEYWORDS

- Sedation • Analgesia • Mechanical ventilation • Emergency medicine • Critically ill

KEY POINTS

- Provide immediate analgosedation after rapid sequence intubation to avoid discomfort during paralysis.
- Treat pain aggressively, using medications for sedation as a supplement to adequate analgesia, not as a substitute for it.
- Use objective scoring systems to frequently assess patients' levels of pain and sedation, and adjust medications based on these assessments.
- Whenever possible, target lighter levels of sedation over deep sedation.
- Aim to standardize patient assessment and medication protocols across the ED and ICU.

INTRODUCTION

Hospital crowding has led to critically ill patients increasingly spending more time boarding in the emergency department (ED). A large number of these patients are mechanically ventilated and experience pain, anxiety, and agitation associated with their care.[1,2] Managing these symptoms requires a structured approach. This article reviews pain control and sedation (analgosedation) strategies for mechanically ventilated patients in the ED, including goals, specific agents, targets, special scenarios, and restraints as adjuncts to pharmacologic management.

Disclosure Statement: The authors do not have any disclosures.
[a] Critical Care Medicine, Cooper University Hospital, One Cooper Plaza, D427C, Camden, NJ 08103, USA; [b] Cooper University Hospital, Camden, NJ 08103, USA
* Corresponding author.
E-mail address: christopher.b.noel@gmail.com

GOALS AND GENERAL PRINCIPLES OF ANALGOSEDATION

Mechanically ventilated, critically ill patients can experience significant discomfort and anxiety associated with their care. On the other hand, early deep sedation has been independently associated with mortality in patients in the ED and intensive care unit (ICU) requiring mechanical ventilation.[3–5] Therefore, the analgosedation goal should be to use the lowest dose possible to control symptoms, ensure patient safety, and address any specific needs associated with their condition.

The first step of analgosedation for mechanically ventilated patients is to control pain. Endotracheal tubes, indwelling catheters, routine care (eg, decubitus ulcer care), and invasive procedures are all potential sources of pain for the critically ill. Pain has been associated with anxiety and post-traumatic stress disorder.[2,6] Furthermore, patients in pain may simply appear to be agitated owing to difficulties in communicating. Therefore, an analgesia-first or analgesia-only strategy is currently recommended by the Society of Critical Care Medicine, with dosing guided by validated pain-assessment tools.[7] Prophylactic doses of analgesics should also be considered before procedures.[8]

If patients remain anxious or agitated despite adequate analgesia, sedatives should be added to supplement the analgesia. However, sedatives should not be used as a substitute for adequate pain control.

A basic algorithm for analgesia and sedation for mechanically ventilated, critically ill patients in the ED is shown in **Fig. 1**.[9]

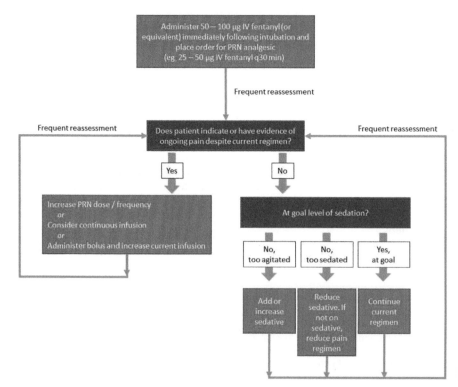

Fig. 1. Basic algorithm for management of analgesia and sedation for mechanically ventilated, critically ill ED patients.

TIMING

The sedative medications typically used for rapid sequence intubation (RSI) are short acting. Therefore, symptom management with adequate provision of analgosedation should begin immediately following intubation.

The early administration of analgosedation is particularly important for patients who receive longer-acting paralytics because the clinical effects far outlast typical sedatives (eg, ketamine or etomidate) used for RSI. Alarmingly, patients receiving rocuronium for RSI can experience significant delays in initiation of sedation and underdosing of analgesics.[10,11] Therefore, the authors recommend empirically administering a minimum of a 50 to 100 μg bolus of intravenous (IV) fentanyl immediately after intubation followed by further analgosedation as needed.

AGENTS

The ideal medication to treat symptoms associated with critical illness would be rapid in onset, would adequately control symptoms, be short acting, and have no adverse immediate or longer-term effects on a patient's clinical condition or cognition; unfortunately, no such medication exists. Given the goals of controlling pain first and addressing persistent anxiety and agitation second, medications are typically divided into classes of those for analgesia and those for sedation.

Analgesia

Opiates form the backbone of pain management for mechanically ventilated patients. Common intravenous agents include fentanyl, hydromorphone, morphine, and remifentanil. The preferred agent will depend on patient factors, pharmacokinetic profile, cost, and institutional availability. Fentanyl or hydromorphone are typically well tolerated. General dosing regimens and pharmacokinetics are shown in **Table 1**.[9] A patient's specific need for an agent may vary widely and should be based on validated pain-assessment scores (see later discussion). The choice between intermittent dosing and an infusion will depend on a patient's needs and feasibility with respect to dosing intervals. Consider starting with intermittent doses as needed and escalating to a continuous infusion only when needed. Also consider administering an intermittent dose before painful procedures or when an increase in an infusion is needed.

Although opiates are often necessary to control pain in mechanically ventilated patients, their side-effect profile warrants consideration of a multimodal approach to pain management. Common adjuncts that may reduce opiate requirements include acetaminophen[7,12,13] and ketamine,[14–16] and neuropathic agents (eg, gabapentin, pregabalin, carbamazepine) in patients with neuropathic pain.[7,17,18] Regional anesthesia can also be considered, and has been used successfully in long bone fractures to reduce pain levels, time to pain control, and opiate requirements when compared with management with medication alone.[19–21]

Sedation

Many patients will achieve symptom control with analgesia alone. Other patients will experience anxiety and agitation that persists despite adequate pain control and will also require sedative medications. There are multiple sedative agents available that can be administered as a bolus for acute episodes of anxiety and agitation, although they are typically administered as continuous infusions.

General dosing regimens and pharmacokinetics are shown in **Table 2**.[9,15,16,22,23] As with analgesics, patient needs can vary widely and should be based on validated

Table 1
Common opiates for analgesia in mechanically ventilated patients

Medication	IV Bolus/Intermittent	IV Infusion	Time of Onset (min)	Elimination Half-Life	Notes
Fentanyl	0.35–0.5 µg/kg intravenous (IV) every 0.5–1 h (50–100 µg boluses are typically well tolerated)	0.7–10 µg/kg/h (infusions >200–300 µg/h are generally not required)	1–2	2–4 h	Can accumulate with hepatic impairment. Relatively hemodynamically stable. Consider as first-line agent
Hydromorphone	0.2–0.6 mg IV every 1–2 h	0.5–3 mg/h	5–15	2–3 h	Can accumulate with renal/hepatic impairment. Consider as first-line agent
Morphine	2–4 mg IV every 1–2 h	2–30 mg/h	5–10	3–4 h	Can accumulate with renal/hepatic impairment. Histamine release. Not recommended in patients with renal impairment or as first-line agent
Remifentanil	Not applicable	Loading dose: 1.5 µg/kg IV; maintenance dose: 0.5–15 µg/kg/h IV	1–3	3–10 min	Does not accumulate with renal/hepatic impairment. Ideal body weight (IBW) recommended if patient >130% IBW

Table 2
Common agents for sedation in mechanically ventilated patients

Medication	IV Bolus	IV Infusion	Time of Onset (min)	Elimination Half-Life	Adverse Effects/Notes
Dexmedetomidine	1 μg/kg over 10 min	0.2–1.5 μg/kg/h	5–10	1.8–3.1 h	Can cause bradycardia and hypotension. Should not be used in scenarios where deep sedation (eg, continuous paralysis) is needed. Otherwise consider as first-line agent
Propofol	5 μg/kg/min over 5 min	5–50 μg/kg/min	1–2	3–12 h in short-term use	Can cause respiratory depression, hypotension, hypertriglyceridemia, propofol infusion syndrome. Consider as first-line agent
Midazolam	0.01–0.05 mg/kg loading over several minutes	0.02–0.1 mg/kg/h	2–5	3–11 h	Can cause respiratory depression and hypotension
Ketamine	0.5–1 mg/kg over 1–2 min	1–2 μg/kg/min titrating up as needed to 10–20 μg/kg/min	<5	Alpha: 5–17 min; beta: 300 min	Also has analgesic effects

sedation-assessment scores targeting a provider-specified sedation level (see later discussion).

Historically, infusions of benzodiazepine (eg, lorazepam or midazolam) were used in conjunction with opiates; however, benzodiazepine infusions are associated with prolonged durations of effect and have been associated with higher rates of delirium and worse outcomes in critically ill patients.[23] Therefore, benzodiazepines are no longer agents of choice.

Current guidelines recommend the use of propofol or dexmedetomidine as first-line agents in critically ill and mechanically ventilated patients.[7] This conditional recommendation is based on literature showing shorter times to achieve light sedation[24] and shorter times to extubation[25] with propofol versus benzodiazepines, and shorter times to extubation and reduced delirium with dexmedetomidine versus benzodiazepines.[26]

The literature directly comparing the clinical outcomes of propofol with dexmedetomidine is limited. Dexmedetomidine may carry a lower risk of delirium[27,28] and may be more cost-effective when compared with other sedatives (eg, reduction in ICU length of stay).[29] Whether propofol or dexmedetomidine is a superior agent is an area for which future research is needed.

Ketamine is not commonly used as a continuous sedative in mechanically ventilated critically ill patients, but is an option for use as an adjunct or sole agent for symptoms that are difficult to control.[15,16]

Sedation Depth

The desired level of sedation for a patient depends on the clinical scenario. Early deep sedation has been associated with increased mortality and prolonged mechanical ventilation in both ED and ICU patients.[3–5,30,31] Therefore, although deeper levels of sedation are sometimes warranted (ie, during pharmacologic paralysis for acute respiratory distress syndrome), lighter levels of sedation should be targeted whenever possible.[7]

ANALGOSEDATION TARGET

The continuous use of analgesic and sedative agents requires frequent reassessment. A patient's pain and anxiety can change often during their ED stay, and the underuse or overuse of these medications can have negative adverse effects on patients. For these reasons, pain and sedation-scoring scales are often used in critically ill patients. Among the variety of scales in the literature, the focus here is on the most commonly used. An important point to highlight is that there is no reference standard with which to compare these scoring scales.[32] Nevertheless, these tools are vital to managing critically ill patients.

Pain-Scoring Scales

A major challenge when managing pain in critically ill patients is that many are unable to effectively communicate and cannot self-report pain. Scales that rely on nonverbal factors must therefore be used. The 2 most commonly recommended scores are the Critical-Care Pain Observation Tool (CPOT)[33] and the Behavioral Pain Scale (BPS).[34,35] These scales use nonverbal cues such as body movement, facial expressions, and compliance with the ventilator to determine the need for analgesia. Both BPS and CPOT are simple to use, have been widely validated in trials of critically ill patients, and are recommended in current guidelines.[7]

Sedation Scoring

The goal for sedation in most critically ill patients is to achieve a state whereby the patient is spontaneously alert and arousable or can be aroused with verbal stimuli. Having objective scoring systems are helpful to standardize the level of a patient's consciousness. Various scales are available and have been validated in the literature. The most common are the Richmond Agitation-Sedation Scale (RASS)[36] and the Riker Sedation-Agitation Scale.[37] The goal for sedation using the RASS scale has historically been between a score of 0 and −2. However, the current guidelines state that even lighter levels of sedation should be targeted, so a goal of +1 to −2 should be considered in patients who do not need deeper sedation for uncomfortable procedures or certain clinical conditions (eg, elevated intracranial pressure or status epilepticus).[7,38] Irrespective of the goal, sedation-scoring scales can help standardize communication between providers and specify targets for medication titration.

Protocols to Minimize Sedation and Analgesia

Several strategies have been studied to minimize the risk of oversedation, but the 2 most favorable approaches are the daily interruption of sedation and nursing-driven protocols for analgosedation.

Daily interruption of sedation involves turning off continuous infusions of analgesia and sedatives at specific times and allowing the patient to wake up.[39] These infusions are restarted as needed when the patient follows commands or appears uncomfortable, but typically at lower rates than were administered before the interruption. Daily interruption allows for ongoing patient assessment and can help ensure that the lowest possible doses of medications are used to achieve a desired level of sedation, often specified by one of the sedation scales described (eg, RASS). One problem with daily interruption of sedation is that it requires careful observation by nurses and staff because there is an increased risk of self-harm by the patient (eg, self-extubation).[40]

Nursing-driven protocols allow nursing to either continuously or intermittently administer medications to keep patients at specific sedation and pain scores without the need to fully wake the patient as in the protocols already described.[41,42] Several studies have compared the 2 methods, and no significant difference has been found favoring one approach over another.[40,43] In fact, guidelines state that either method is a viable means to achieve light sedation for patients who are mechanically ventilated.[7] As awakening trials are unlikely to be practical in many ED settings, we recommend the use of a nurse-driven protocol targeting light sedation on mechanically ventilated patients in the ED.

There are no prospectively validated protocols specifically for analgosedation in the ED. Therefore, the decision to select a protocol should involve a multidisciplinary discussion with the ED team, nursing team, and critical care team. We suggest using a protocol in the ED that is similar, if not identical, to the protocol used in the ICU to promote simplicity and uniformity in the sedation and analgesia goals for critically ill patients.

SPECIAL SCENARIOS
Hypotension with Sedation

Hypotension is common in mechanically ventilated patients. There are several reasons for hypotension including patient pathology, positive pressure ventilation, and medications. A challenge to managing these patients is that several medications commonly used for pain and sedation can cause or exacerbate hypotension. A stepwise approach to these patients is recommended, and the following should be considered:

1. Is the patient fully resuscitated? Patients will often need further treatment of the original condition (eg, additional blood product resuscitation in hemorrhagic shock). Do not assume that a patient's hemodynamic insult is medication related before evaluating and addressing other life-threatening causes.
2. Is the patient being overmedicated with sedatives? Reduce dose or discontinue sedative if the patient's level of sedation is at or below goal.
3. Is the patient being overmedicated with analgesics? Reduce dose or discontinue analgesic if patient denies or has no clinical evidence of pain.
4. If the aforementioned have been addressed or do not apply, continue appropriate analgosedation and support hemodynamics. Treatment should not be withheld in hypotensive patients who are in pain or agitated, even if further resuscitation or hemodynamic support is needed.

Studies that compare the hemodynamic effects of various sedating agents in the critically ill are limited. However, 2 recent studies found no difference in hemodynamic events between propofol and dexmedetomidine in patients with septic shock[44] and following abdominal surgery.[45]

Importantly, sedatives should not be used as antihypertensives. For example, a propofol infusion should not be increased to lower blood pressure when pain and agitation are already well controlled.

Persistently Agitated Patient

Some patients remain persistently agitated despite aggressive pain management and sedation. These patients can pose a danger both to themselves and to staff and are challenging to manage. High medication tolerance (eg, opioid dependence), delirium, acute substance use or withdrawal, psychiatric illness, and pre-existing cognitive impairment can play a role in this agitation. Important points to consider in these patients are to:

1. Aggressively seek and treat the underlying cause for the patient's agitation (eg, persistent pain, alcohol withdrawal, head injury)
2. Consider a one-time bolus dose to control acute, severe symptoms and when increasing infusion rates to achieve a new steady state more rapidly. Titrating the infusion without a bolus may lead to overshoot and excessive drip rates owing to a delay in achieving steady-state drug levels.
3. Consider switching to an alternative sedating agent or adding an additional agent if necessary (eg, ketamine). Antipsychotics can be considered, similar to when used for severely agitated patients who are not intubated. Keep in mind that benzodiazepines can worsen agitation and delirium and should be avoided when possible.[7]

Paralyzed Patient

Neuromuscular blocking agents should not be routinely administered following intubation itself. There are patients, however, who may remain paralyzed long after RSI, arrive after receiving long-acting neuromuscular blocking agents by transporting services, or benefit from ongoing paralysis, such as in severe acute respiratory distress syndrome.[46,47] As traditional pain-scoring systems cannot be performed in these patients, analgesic and sedative drugs should be continuously administered with the goal of deep sedation until the paralytic is withdrawn and an assessment can be made.[47] Boluses of 250 μg/kg propofol and 1 mg of hydromorphone followed by continuous infusion rates of 20 μg/kg/min and 1 mg/h, respectively, are reasonable starting points for deep sedation with doses adjusted based on patient needs (eg, pain being manifested as hypertension and tachycardia). Once a patient is no longer paralyzed, light sedation should again be targeted whenever possible.[7]

Status Epilepticus

Patients with status epilepticus (SE) are often intubated for airway protection or for additional antiepileptic therapy if refractory to antiepileptic medications. Patients with SE should be deeply sedated until there is clinical or electroencephalograph (EEG) evidence to support cessation of seizures. When there is concern for ongoing seizure activity, Neurocritical Care Society (NCS) guidelines recommend a continuous infusion of antiepileptic drugs such as midazolam, propofol, or pentobarbital.[38] Suggested dosing regimens have been noted previously in various studies,[9,38,48-50] titrating to continuous EEG. NCS guidelines note that there is insufficient evidence to recommend one agent over another, and that therapy should be guided by continuous EEG findings rather than specific drug levels.[38]

PHYSICAL RESTRAINTS

Physical restraints (PR) are often used to prevent patients from removing essential devices, injuring staff, and inflicting self-harm.[51,52] However, their use is controversial and varies widely, with opponents citing increased unplanned extubations, medication use, musculoskeletal injuries, psychological trauma, and length of stay.[53-56] Therefore, the decision to use PR should be tailored to patient and staff-specific factors. The need for their use should be continuously reassessed and they should be removed once it is safe to do so. Furthermore, the authors recommend that PR only be used as a bridge to adequate chemical restraints.

SUMMARY

Mechanically ventilated patients experience significant pain and anxiety associated with their care. These symptoms should be aggressively treated, but can be challenging to manage without a systematic approach. This article reviewed recent literature, current guidelines, and best practices in managing pain, agitation, and anxiety in mechanically ventilated patients in the ED. Providers should:

- Begin appropriate analgosedation immediately following intubation or patient arrival
- Treat pain aggressively using medications for sedation as a supplement to adequate analgesia, not as a substitute for it
- Use objective scoring systems to frequently assess patients' levels of pain and sedation and adjust medications based on these assessments
- Whenever possible, target lighter levels of sedation over deep sedation
- Aim to standardize patient assessment and medication protocols across the ED and ICU

REFERENCES

1. Payen J-F, Chanques G, Mantz J, et al. Current practices in sedation and analgesia for mechanically ventilated critically Ill patientsA prospective multicenter patient-based study. Anesthesiology 2007;106(4):687–95.
2. Turner JS, Briggs SJ, Springhorn HE, et al. Patients' recollection of intensive care unit experience. Crit Care Med 1990;18(9):966–8.

3. Stephens RJ, Ablordeppey E, Drewry AM, et al. Analgosedation practices and the impact of sedation depth on clinical outcomes among patients requiring mechanical ventilation in the ED: a cohort study. Chest 2017;152(5):963–71.

4. Shehabi Y, Bellomo R, Reade MC, et al. Early intensive care sedation predicts long-term mortality in ventilated critically ill patients. Am J Respir Crit Care Med 2012;186(8):724–31.

5. Tanaka LMS, Azevedo LCP, Park M, et al. Early sedation and clinical outcomes of mechanically ventilated patients: a prospective multicenter cohort study. Crit Care 2014;18(4):R156.

6. Davydow DS, Gifford JM, Desai SV, et al. Posttraumatic stress disorder in general intensive care unit survivors: a systematic review. Gen Hosp Psychiatry 2008; 30(5):421–34.

7. Devlin JW, Skrobik Y, Gélinas C, et al. Clinical practice guidelines for the prevention and management of pain, agitation/sedation, delirium, immobility, and sleep disruption in adult patients in the ICU. Crit Care Med 2018;46(9):e825–73.

8. Marra A, Ely EW, Pandharipande PP, et al. The ABCDEF bundle in critical care. Crit Care Clin 2017;33(2):225–43.

9. Barr J, Fraser GL, Puntillo K, et al. Clinical practice guidelines for the management of pain, agitation, and delirium in adult patients in the intensive care unit. Crit Care Med 2013;41(1):263–306.

10. Watt JM, Amini A, Traylor BR, et al. Effect of paralytic type on time to postintubation sedative use in the emergency department. Emerg Med J 2013; 30(11):893–5.

11. Korinek JD, Thomas RM, Goddard LA, et al. Comparison of rocuronium and succinylcholine on postintubation sedative and analgesic dosing in the emergency department. Eur J Emerg Med 2014;21(3):206–11.

12. Memis D, Inal MT, Kavalci G, et al. Intravenous paracetamol reduced the use of opioids, extubation time, and opioid-related adverse effects after major surgery in intensive care unit. J Crit Care 2010;25(3):458–62.

13. Cattabriga I, Pacini D, Lamazza G, et al. Intravenous paracetamol as adjunctive treatment for postoperative pain after cardiac surgery: a double blind randomized controlled trial. Eur J Cardiothorac Surg 2007;32(3):527–31.

14. Guillou N, Tanguy M, Seguin P, et al. The effects of small-dose ketamine on morphine consumption in surgical intensive care unit patients after major abdominal surgery. Anesth Analg 2003;97(3):843–7.

15. Erstad BL, Patanwala AE. Ketamine for analgosedation in critically ill patients. J Crit Care 2016;35:145–9.

16. Patanwala AE, Martin JR, Erstad BL. Ketamine for analgosedation in the intensive care unit: a systematic review. J Intensive Care Med 2017;32(6):387–95.

17. Pandey CK, Bose N, Garg G, et al. Gabapentin for the treatment of pain in Guillain-Barré syndrome: a double-blinded, placebo-controlled, crossover study. Anesth Analg 2002;95(6):1719–23.

18. Pandey CK, Raza M, Tripathi M, et al. The comparative evaluation of gabapentin and carbamazepine for pain management in Guillain-Barré syndrome patients in the intensive care unit. Anesth Analg 2005;101(1):220–5.

19. Beaudoin FL, Haran JP, Liebmann O. A comparison of ultrasound-guided three-in-one femoral nerve block versus parenteral opioids alone for analgesia in emergency department patients with hip fractures: a randomized controlled trial. Acad Emerg Med 2013;20(6):584–91.

20. Fletcher AK, Rigby AS, Heyes FL. Three-in-one femoral nerve block as analgesia for fractured neck of femur in the emergency department: a randomized, controlled trial. Ann Emerg Med 2003;41(2):227–33.
21. Mutty CE, Jensen EJ, Manka MA Jr, et al. Femoral nerve block for diaphyseal and distal femoral fractures in the emergency department. J Bone Joint Surg Am 2007;89(12):2599–603.
22. Pandharipande PP, Pun BT, Herr DL, et al. Effect of sedation with dexmedetomidine vs lorazepam on acute brain dysfunction in mechanically ventilated patients: the MENDS randomized controlled trial. JAMA 2007;298(22):2644–53.
23. Riker RR, Shehabi Y, Bokesch PM, et al. Dexmedetomidine vs midazolam for sedation of critically ill patients: a randomized trial. JAMA 2009;301(5):489–99.
24. Chamorro C, de Latorre FJ, Montero A, et al. Comparative study of propofol versus midazolam in the sedation of critically ill patients: results of a prospective, randomized, multicenter trial. Crit Care Med 1996;24(6):932–9.
25. Barrientos-Vega R, Sanchez-Soria MM, Morales-Garcia C, et al. Prolonged sedation of critically ill patients with midazolam or propofol: impact on weaning and costs. Crit Care Med 1997;25(1):33–40.
26. Riker R, SEDCOM (Safety and Efficacy of Dexmedetomidine Compared With Midazolam) Study Group. Dexmedetomidine vs midazolam for sedation of critically ill patients: a randomized trial. JAMA 2009;301:489–99.
27. Liu X, Xie G, Zhang K, et al. Dexmedetomidine vs propofol sedation reduces delirium in patients after cardiac surgery: a meta-analysis with trial sequential analysis of randomized controlled trials. J Crit Care 2017;38:190–6.
28. Skrobik Y, Duprey MS, Hill NS, et al. Low-dose nocturnal dexmedetomidine prevents ICU delirium. A randomized, placebo-controlled trial. Am J Respir Crit Care Med 2018;197(9):1147–56.
29. Turunen H, Jakob SM, Ruokonen E, et al. Dexmedetomidine versus standard care sedation with propofol or midazolam in intensive care: an economic evaluation. Crit Care 2015;19(1):67.
30. Stephens RJ, Dettmer MR, Roberts BW, et al. Practice patterns and outcomes associated with early sedation depth in mechanically ventilated patients: a systematic review and meta-analysis. Crit Care Med 2018;46(3):471–9.
31. Shehabi Y, Chan L, Kadiman S, et al. Sedation depth and long-term mortality in mechanically ventilated critically ill adults: a prospective longitudinal multicentre cohort study. Intensive Care Med 2013;39(5):910–8.
32. Wittbrodt ET. The ideal sedation assessment tool: an elusive instrument. Crit Care Med 1999;27(7):1384–5.
33. Gélinas C, Fillion L, Puntillo KA, et al. Validation of the critical-care pain observation tool in adult patients. Am J Crit Care 2006;15(4):420–7.
34. Gélinas C, Fortier M, Viens C, et al. Pain assessment and management in critically ill intubated patients: a retrospective study. Am J Crit Care 2004;13(2):126–36.
35. Payen J-F, Bru O, Bosson J-L, et al. Assessing pain in critically ill sedated patients by using a behavioral pain scale. Crit Care Med 2001;29(12):2258–63.
36. Sessler CN, Grap MJ, Brophy GM. Multidisciplinary management of sedation and analgesia in critical care. Semin Respir Crit Care Med 2001;22(2):211–26.
37. Riker RR, Picard JT, Fraser GL. Prospective evaluation of the sedation-agitation scale for adult critically ill patients. Crit Care Med 1999;27(7):1325–9.
38. Brophy GM, Bell R, Claassen J, et al. Guidelines for the evaluation and management of status epilepticus. Neurocrit Care 2012;17(1):3–23.

39. Girard TD, Kress JP, Fuchs BD, et al. Efficacy and safety of a paired sedation and ventilator weaning protocol for mechanically ventilated patients in intensive care (awakening and breathing controlled trial): a randomised controlled trial. Lancet 2008;371(9607):126–34.
40. Nassar Junior AP, Park M. Sedation protocols versus daily sedation interruption: a systematic review and meta-analysis. Rev Bras Ter Intensiva 2016;28(4):444–51.
41. Brook AD, Ahrens TS, Schaiff R, et al. Effect of a nursing-implemented sedation protocol on the duration of mechanical ventilation. Crit Care Med 1999;27(12): 2609–15.
42. Arias-Rivera S, del Mar Sánchez-Sánchez M, Santos-Díaz R, et al. Effect of a nursing-implemented sedation protocol on weaning outcome. Crit Care Med 2008;36(7):2054–60.
43. Mehta S, Burry L, Cook D, et al. Daily sedation interruption in mechanically ventilated critically ill patients cared for with a sedation protocol: a randomized controlled trial. JAMA 2012;308(19):1985–92.
44. Nelson KM, Patel GP, Hammond DA. Effects from continuous infusions of dexmedetomidine and propofol on hemodynamic stability in critically ill adult patients with septic shock. J Intensive Care Med 2018. https://doi.org/10.1177/0885066618802269.
45. Chang Y-F, Chao A, Shih P-Y, et al. Comparison of dexmedetomidine versus propofol on hemodynamics in surgical critically ill patients. J Surg Res 2018;228: 194–200.
46. Papazian L, Forel J-M, Gacouin A, et al. Neuromuscular blockers in early acute respiratory distress syndrome. N Engl J Med 2010;363(12):1107–16.
47. Murray MJ, DeBlock H, Erstad B, et al. Clinical practice guidelines for sustained neuromuscular blockade in the adult critically ill patient. Crit Care Med 2016; 44(11):2079–103.
48. Kam P, Cardone D. Propofol infusion syndrome. Anaesthesia 2007;62(7): 690–701.
49. Krauss B, Green SM. Procedural sedation and analgesia in children. Lancet 2006;367(9512):766–80.
50. Ehrnebo M. Pharmacokinetics and distribution properties of pentobarbital in humans following oral and intravenous administration. J Pharm Sci 1974;63(7): 1114–8.
51. Benbenbishty J, Adam S, Endacott R. Physical restraint use in intensive care units across Europe: the PRICE study. Intensive Crit Care Nurs 2010;26(5):241–5.
52. Leith B. Canadian critical care nurses and physical restraints. Off J Can Assoc Crit Care Nurs 1999;10(1):10–4.
53. Rose L, Burry L, Mallick R, et al. Prevalence, risk factors, and outcomes associated with physical restraint use in mechanically ventilated adults. J Crit Care 2016;31(1):31–5.
54. Kandeel NA, Attia AK. Physical restraints practice in adult intensive care units in Egypt. Nurs Health Sci 2013;15(1):79–85.
55. Warlan H, Howland L. Posttraumatic stress syndrome associated with stays in the intensive care unit: importance of nurses' involvement. Crit Care Nurse 2015; 35(3):44–52.
56. Fink RM, Makic MBF, Poteet AW, et al. The ventilated patient's experience. Dimens Crit Care Nurs 2015;34(5):301–8.

Extubation in the Emergency Department and Resuscitative Unit Setting

Chidinma C. Nwakanma, MD[a],*, Brian Joseph Wright, MD, MPH[b,c]

KEYWORDS

- ED Extubation • Resuscitation • Emergency Department Critical Care

KEY POINTS

- A subset of intubated patients can be extubated in the emergency department (ED).
- Appropriate physician and nurse monitoring is required for ED extubation to detect and manage potential complications and extubation failure.
- The disease process that led to intubation should be reversed before considering extubation in the ED.
- ED physicians should select patients with a low probability of extubation failure for ED extubation.

INTRODUCTION

Patients are placed on invasive mechanical ventilation (IMV) for many different reasons. The common goal is to safely protect the airway while maintaining adequate oxygenation and ventilation until the underlying disease process is reversed. Patients should be on IMV for the shortest amount of time that is medically necessary. Endotracheal Intubation (ETI) and IMV are life-saving interventions, but are associated with complications like ventilator-associated pneumonia, lung injury, venous thromboembolism, delirium, and acquired weakness. IMV also requires expensive and scarce critical care resources, including high-intensity nursing and intensive care unit (ICU) beds. Finally, ETI and IMV can be uncomfortable and painful.

Disclosure Statement: I have no financial disclosures to report.
^a Department of Emergency Medicine, Perelman School of Medicine at the Hospital of University of Pennsylvania, 3400 Spruce Street, Philadelphia, PA 19104, USA; ^b Department of Emergency Medicine, Renaissance School of Medicine, Stony Brook University, 101 Nicolls Road, Health Sciences Center, Level 4, Stony Brook, NY 11794, USA; ^c Department of Neurosurgery, Renaissance School of Medicine, Stony Brook University, 101 Nicolls Road, Health Sciences Center, Level 4, Stony Brook, NY 11794, USA
* Corresponding author.
E-mail address: chidi776@gmail.com

Emerg Med Clin N Am 37 (2019) 557–568
https://doi.org/10.1016/j.emc.2019.03.004   emed.theclinics.com
0733-8627/19/© 2019 Elsevier Inc. All rights reserved.

Resuscitation and critical care specialists should have expertise in both initiation and cessation of IMV.

Extubation is not a common emergency department (ED) practice. With the development of ED-ICUs and resuscitation units, and the increased boarding of critically ill patients managed by emergency medicine providers, ED extubation (EDEx) may become a more common practice. This article provides a framework for determining appropriate patients for EDEx and a practical approach on how to safely perform the procedure.

DIFFERENCES BETWEEN EXTUBATION IN THE EMERGENCY DEPARTMENT VERSUS INTENSIVE CARE UNIT

There is a paucity of published literature on EDEx. Weingart and colleagues[1] examined the safety of extubation in a cohort of 50 ED trauma patients cared for in a highly specialized ED with ICU-level nurse-patient ratios (1:2 or 1:3) and run by trauma and critical care specialists experienced in extubation. Selected patients were intoxicated, had no significant injury after the initial trauma workup was completed, or had injuries that required temporary deep sedation only. In carefully selected patients they found that EDEx was safe with no unplanned reintubations. Sixteen percent of their patients were discharged from the ED. The application of this and similar extubation studies from the ICU or Post Anesthesia Care Unit should be applied with caution to the general ED setting. EDEx is safe and feasible provided that certain unit logistic and patient features are met.[1,2]

Close monitoring after extubation is the biggest obstacle to EDEx. The clinical environment must provide intensive monitoring by clinicians and nurses who can recognize and manage extubation failure and reintubate if necessary. Continuous pulse oximetry, telemetry, and blood pressure monitoring are a minimum. End-tidal carbon dioxide monitoring is not standard practice but may be helpful in determining the presence of apnea, airway obstruction, hypoventilation, or hypercapnia. Dedicated staff (1:1 or 1:2 nurse:patient) must continuously monitor a newly extubated patient, similar to recovering a patient after procedural sedation.

There is debate in extubation literature regarding acceptable reintubation or extubation failure rates.[3,4] Extubation failure is associated with significant morbidity and mortality, even after correcting for the underlying disease process that led to extubation failure.[4] ED patients are early in their disease process. If there is question or concern about extubation readiness and whether a particular disease process is resolved, then the patient should be extubated in a traditional ICU setting.

Patients with a low risk of reintubation should be selected (excluding elective reintubations) and the ED unit should have a goal of a near zero rate of reintubation. Patients should be monitored closely for an appropriate amount of time after extubation. Based on existing evidence, 1 hour should be the minimum duration for intensive monitoring and specific patient characteristics should also be considered after EDEx.[1] Patients with cardiac or lung disease may need to be observed for longer than 1 hour in a monitored setting. Further evidence is needed to determine optimal length of monitoring after EDEx.

SELECTION OF PATIENTS FOR EXTUBATION IN THE EMERGENCY DEPARTMENT AND RESUSCITATIVE UNIT

Patient selection for EDEx is highly dependent on the original indication for intubation, and should be more stringent than in the ICU (**Table 1**). For most patients intubated in the ED, a prolonged ventilatory course and ICU admission are necessary. A subset of patients may require only transient IMV.

Table 1
Suggested clinical presentations for emergency department extubation (EDEx) consideration/ avoidance

EDEx Can be Safely Attempted[a]	EDEx Can be Considered with Caution[a]	EDEx Should Not be Considered
• Intoxicated or drug overdose with clinical sobriety • Airway protection for procedural sedation (ie, endoscopy) • Head trauma with improving mental status and negative neuroimaging • Palliative/Terminal extubation[b]	• Anaphylaxis/laryngeal edema with improved symptoms and resolution of airway edema[c] • Severe asthma/chronic obstructive pulmonary disease with significant improvement • Undifferentiated altered mental status[d] • Cardiogenic pulmonary edema with significant improvement and resolved hypoxia/hypercarbia after aggressive management (eg, diuresis, afterload reduction)	• Hemodynamically unstable • Need for high ventilatory support • Expected prolonged clinical course (eg, drowning, pneumonia) • Expected need for repeated invasive procedures, transfer or surgery • Significant neuromuscular disease (eg, myasthenia gravis, multiple sclerosis) • Trauma/Injury to cervical spine, oropharynx, larynx or lung • Cerebrovascular Accident (pons or brainstem lesions can affect airway maintenance)

[a] Assuming all extubation criteria are achieved.
[b] Extubation in this setting can be performed without meeting criteria.
[c] Anaphylaxis may have biphasic distribution, thus despite initial improvement a secondary phase may occur even up to 24 h after primary presentation.
[d] Undifferentiated altered mental status is a clinical challenge, as prediction of clinical course is difficult.

Indications for IMV must be resolved in the ideal EDEx candidate. Selected patients should meet ALL of the following criteria before consideration (**Box 1**).[2]

Resolution of Initial Indication for Intubation

Ventilator liberation will rely on the resolution of the condition that led to necessitation of IMV. This should be the first consideration of EDEx candidacy. The clinician should have

Box 1
Suggested inclusion criteria for emergency department extubation

• Resolution of initial indication for intubation

• Able to oxygenate and ventilate on minimal ventilator settings

• Awake and able to follow commands

• Hemodynamically stable

• Uncomplicated initial intubation

• Expected to maintain airway patency postextubation

• Anticipated hospital course does not require mechanical ventilation

From Gray SH, Ross JA, Green RS. How to safely extubate a patient in the emergency department: a user's guide to critical care. CJEM 2013;15(5):303–306; with permission.

a definitive understanding of the initial indication for IMV. This will indicate the likelihood of extubation failure. For example, the intoxicated patient (with no significant trauma) that is now exhibiting clinical sobriety is an ideal candidate for extubation. A drowning victim who may worsen in the next 24 hours would not be a good candidate (see **Table 1**).

Pulmonary Assessment: Ability to Oxygenate and Ventilate on Low Ventilator Settings

A patient's ability to oxygenate and ventilate on minimal ventilatory settings (continuous positive airway pressor [CPAP] alone or minimal pressure support [PS]) may be able to risk stratify the patient as low-risk for a failed extubation. Generally, a spontaneously breathing patient should be able to generate a tidal volume ≥ 5 mL/kg on CPAP or minimal PS and adequate oxygenation with a Fio_2 less than 40% on a positive end-expiratory pressure (PEEP) ≤ 8.[5] An arterial blood gas on minimal ventilator settings can support the decision to extubate in patients with cardiac or pulmonary pathology but may not be necessary in patients without cardiovascular or pulmonary pathology. Adequate oxygenation can be defined as oxygen saturation greater than 92% and Pao_2 greater than 70 mm Hg. Adequate ventilation can be defined as a $Paco_2$ between 38 and 42 mm Hg.[2,5]

A spontaneous breathing trial (SBT) can be helpful for clinicians to determine extubation readiness, especially if the patient was intubated for pulmonary or cardiovascular pathology. SBTs have been studied heavily and implemented in most ICU ventilator weaning strategies. Patients should be clinically and hemodynamically stable for an SBT. There are 3 potential approaches to an SBT (**Box 2**).[4,6]

PS provides the most ventilatory assistance during the SBT and the T-piece provides the least.[4] Current extubation guidelines recommend that a PS SBT is an acceptable screening for extubation readiness and may be more sensitive than the other methods.[7–9] A CPAP-only or T-piece strategy may be more specific, but can incorrectly classify patients as SBT failures that may otherwise be extubated safely.[4,10] CHEST and the American Thoracic Society[7] recommend using a PS strategy in patients who have been on the ventilator for more than 24 hours.

Patients extubated in the ED setting should have an exceedingly low rate of reintubation. As a result, we recommend using a low PS trial or CPAP-only trial as it provides a good estimation of extubation readiness and does not require additional equipment. The SBT should be conducted for at least 30 minutes and no longer than 120 minutes.[4,6] **Box 3** includes successful SBT criteria.[2]

The rapid shallow breathing index (RSBI) is a dynamic measurement that can be used *during an SBT* to determine extubation preparedness.[9,11] RBSI is defined as follows:

Box 2
Ventilator setting options for spontaneous breathing trial

- Pressure support spontaneous breathing trial: pressure support (PS) of 5 cm H_2O (to overcome the resistance of the endotracheal tube [ETT]) with positive end-expiratory pressure (PEEP) ≤ 5 cm H_2O

- Continuous positive airway pressure only: PEEP ≤ 5 cm H_2O, no PS

- T-piece trial: Supplemental oxygen only through the ETT

Data from Thille AW, Richard JCM, Brochard L. The decision to extubate in the intensive care unit. Am J Respir Crit Care Med 2013;187(12):1294–1302. http://doi.org/10.1164/rccm.201208-1523CI; and Zein H, Baratloo A, Negida A, Safari S. Ventilator weaning and spontaneous breathing trials; an educational review. Emergency 2016;4(2):65–71. https://www.ncbi.nlm.nih.gov/pmc/articles/PMC4893753/pdf/emerg-4-065.pdf.

Box 3
Predictors of a successful spontaneous breathing trial

- Respiratory rate <30 breaths per minute and more than 8 breaths per minute

- Heart rate <140 beats per minute and more than 60 beats per minute

- Systolic blood pressure less than 200 mm Hg and more than 90 mm Hg or less than 20% change from baseline

- Oxygen saturation greater than 92%, Pao_2 greater than 70 mm Hg (on Fio_2 <0.4 and PEEP ≤8 cm H_2O)

- Spontaneous tidal volume >5 mL/kg

- No signs of increased work of breathing, severe anxiety, or altered mental status

Data from Weingart SD, Menaker J, Truong H, Bochicchio K, Scalea TM. Trauma patients can be safely extubated in the emergency department. J Emerg Med 2011;40(2):235–239. http://doi.org/10.1016/j.jemermed.2009.05.033; and Gray SH, Ross JA, Green RS. How to safely extubate a patient in the emergency department: a user's guide to critical care. CJEM 2013;15(5):303–306.

Respiratory Rate (breaths per minute)/tidal volume (L)

Optimal breathing is slow and deep with a low RSBI. A patient with an inability to tolerate independent breathing will tend to breath fast and shallow generating a high RSBI. A threshold RSBI of less than 75 breaths per min/L (on PS ventilation) or less than 100 breaths per min/L (with T-piece) predict successful weaning and are more accurate than other accepted RSBI values.[12] RSBI less than 105 is wildly cited as an acceptable criterion for extubation success.[4,12] We recommend using an RSBI of less than 75 breaths per min/L using the PS or CPAP trial technique in the ED. A lower RSBI cutoff is more specific and will potentially reduce the risk of extubating borderline patients.

Despite the common use of RSBI, it is important to remember that extubation evaluation is a global assessment and RSBI should not be used as a singular benchmark for success. In addition to the RSBI formula, the interpretation of SBT failure/success should also consider work of breathing, ability to clear secretions, and clinical appearance. Blood gas analysis is not always necessary to make this determination, especially if the patient was intubated for nonpulmonary indications. An arterial blood gas may be helpful for borderline cases or patients who were intubated for pulmonary indications, particularly if the clinician is concerned about effective oxygenation and ventilation at the end of the trial. If the SBT is successful, proceeding with extubation is encouraged as long as airway, hemodynamic, and neurologic criteria are met. In the setting of SBT failure, the patient should remain on full ventilatory support and the EDEx attempt should be aborted and deferred to the ICU.

Neurologic Assessment: Awake and Able to Follow Commands

When assessing a patient for extubation, it is important to ensure that the patient is fully awake and able to participate in independent breathing. Sedation should be weaned and time should be given to allow the patient to regain full consciousness. Small doses of analgesia or anxiolytic agents may be necessary to maintain patient comfort while sedation is discontinued. Dexmedetomidine (DMT) is an excellent anxiolytic that does not affect respiratory drive and may facilitate extubation in patients with agitation from pain or discomfort due to the endotracheal tube. DMT should not be given in bolus doses, as this is associated with significant bradycardia. The onset of therapeutic effect is usually reached in 15 to 40 minutes.[13] DMT use to facilitate safe extubation should be used only if the clinician is certain that the increased respiratory rate is from agitation due to the endotracheal tube and not from a respiratory or cardiovascular derangement. Clinically, the patient should spontaneously achieve normal or high tidal volumes. A blood gas may help discriminate tachypnea due to agitation versus ventilatory insufficiency. A high respiratory rate secondary to agitation will be associated with a respiratory alkalosis and low Pco_2. A normal or elevated Pco_2 with a high respiratory rate should trigger the clinician to consider that the patient's agitation and tachypnea is a compensatory mechanism. Once the patient is awake, he or she should have a consistent neurologic examination, and be able to follow commands. Asking a patient to lift his or her head should always be included in the neurologic assessment, as cervical mobility and strength are vital for clearing secretions and maintaining a patent airway.

Cardiovascular Assessment: Hemodynamic Stability

Ensuring hemodynamic stability before extubation is a critical component of assessing readiness for extubation. An extubation candidate should be liberated from the use of inotropes and vasopressors. One suggested criterion for hemodynamic stability includes the following[2,5]:

1. Oxygen saturation greater than 92% (on Fio_2 <0.4)
2. Heart rate less than 100 beats per minute
3. Respiratory rate less than 30/min
4. Systolic blood pressure greater than 90 mm Hg unassisted by vasopressors
5. No active cardiac ischemia or unstable arrhythmia

Good clinical judgment would likely include these recommendations, along with the patient's hemodynamic baseline. Weaning-induced cardiovascular dysfunction is a well-described phenomenon, and a common cause for extubation failure.[4,14,15] Risk factors include volume overload, depressed left ventricular dysfunction, diastolic dysfunction, structural heart disease, obesity, and chronic obstructive lung disease.[14]

Procedural Considerations

It is important to review initial airway assessment and documentation before extubation. Airway trauma may increase the risk of postintubation stridor and respiratory failure from airway compromise. Aspiration can lead to delayed airway compromise and progressive hypoxemia. Knowledge of a difficult airway, multiple ETI attempts, and airway trauma should lead to a more comprehensive assessment of airway patency. A cuff leak (CL) test may be indicated in certain patients.[9]

Maintenance of Airway Patency Postextubation

The ability to cough and adequately clear secretions is paramount in maintaining airway patency. Moderate to copious secretion volume is an independent predictor of extubation failure.[16] The patient should be able to generate enough strength to lift his or her head off of the bed and produce a strong cough before extubation.

It is important to avoid extubation in patients with suspected ongoing laryngeal edema.[17,18] Patients with brainstem strokes and cervical spine injuries have a high risk for reintubation.[19] Extreme caution should be used in these patients and they are probably better served to be extubated in an ICU.

Anticipated Hospital Course Does Not Require Mechanical Ventilation

It is important to anticipate the patient's hospital course before considering extubation. Additional need for high-risk diagnostic testing where limited monitoring is available (ie, MRI), interhospital transfer, or need for future procedural sedation/general anesthesia should be considered. Patients with diseases that classically get worse during the early hospital stay, drowning, acute respiratory distress syndrome, pneumonia, spinal cord injury, ischemic and hemorrhagic cerebrovascular accidents, should remain intubated.

PHYSIOLOGICAL ASPECTS OF EXTUBATION AND MANAGEMENT OF CLINICAL COMPLICATIONS
Postextubation Hypoxemia

The transition from positive pressure ventilation (PPV) to negative-pressure ventilation can lead to significant physiologic cardiopulmonary challenges. Postextubation cardiac dysfunction is one of these well-described complications. Significant increases in left ventricular transmural pressure and afterload can occur after extubation. This can clinically present as an increased work of breathing, hypertension, pulmonary edema, hypoxemia, and progressive recurrent respiratory failure. Postextubation hypertension and new B-lines on lung ultrasound are both concerning signs of postextubation cardiac dysfunction. Myocardial ischemia, arrhythmias, and sudden cardiac death are rare but potential events that require clinical vigilance.[15]

Postextubation hypoxemia can also be the result of compromised pulmonary function and gas exchange. Significant de-recruitment, atelectasis, changes in work of breathing, increased airway resistance and shunt can all contribute to new onset hypoxemia or recurrent respiratory dysfunction after extubation. Soummer and colleagues[20] prospectively evaluated 86 ICU patients with lung ultrasound before extubation after a successful SBT. Of the patients who developed postextubation respiratory distress (more than 30%), there was a higher incidence of loss of lung aeration (indicated by development of new B-lines or consolidation on lung ultrasound) during their SBT. Lung ultrasound may be a clinically useful tool in assessing patients during SBT or after extubation with respiratory distress.

Management of postextubation cardiac dysfunction is similar to management of a patient with sympathetic crashing pulmonary edema. Intravenous nitroglycerin is an excellent agent to reduce cardiac preload and afterload. Diuretics also may be helpful, as negative fluid balance is associated with less extravascular lung water, better pulmonary function, and decreased ventilator time.[21] The reinstitution of PPV with a trial of noninvasive ventilation (NIV) may be a valuable temporary intervention to allow time for aggressive medical management. However, similar to the use of NIV for other causes of acute respiratory failure, reintubation should not be delayed if the patient is not rapidly improving with these interventions.

Altered Mental Status and Agitation

The standard approach to extubation assessment includes pausing sedation to assess mental status and perform a neurologic examination. Agitation and delirium are common conditions in critical illness and may be either secondary to the primary underlying pathology or the clinical interventions (ie, intubation, sedative agents).

Delirium is characterized as fluctuating alteration in consciousness with impaired cognition. It can present as hyperactive, hypoactive, or mixed. Delirium in ICU patients is associated with prolonged mechanical ventilation, extended hospitalization, and increased risk of mortality.[22] Delirium in the ED is usually a result of the underlying presenting condition given the relatively short in-hospital time and ventilator duration compared with an inpatient ICU. Given the fluctuating course of delirium, if present, these patients should not be extubated in the ED.

Airway Assessment and Management of Postextubation Stridor

Careful airway assessment and management is paramount for anticipated extubation success. Often the clinician considering extubation was not present during the patient's initial presentation. Before proceeding with any extubation, all initial intubation documentation and airway evaluations should be reviewed to prepare for potential postextubation complications. For example, documentation of the presence of edema before intubation informs the clinician that this condition was not a result of the presence of the endotracheal tube (ET) tube. Resolution of preexisting edema should occur before extubation. Of note, ET-induced laryngeal edema usually occurs after the first 36 hours[8,17,18] and this is usually greater than the average length of stay in an ED.

The CL test is used to predict postextubation stridor and is a surrogate marker of laryngeal edema.[8] To perform a CL test, first document the patient's inspiratory and expiratory tidal volumes (TV) before ET tube cuff deflation on Volume Control IMV. While on Volume Control IMV, TV should *temporarily* be up titrated to 8 to 10 mL/kg ideal body weight, as lower TV may fail to show a CL when one is present.[23,24] After the ET tube cuff is deflated, the difference between the inhaled and exhaled tidal volume represents the CL, or volume lost around the tube. The volume of air lost should be >110 mL.[18,23,24] The CL can also be measured by an audible leak or volume loss approximately more than 24% tidal volume.[24] A small or absent CL (volume <110 mL) suggests laryngeal edema and is associated with an increased risk of postextubation stridor and respiratory distress.

Risk factors for postintubation laryngeal edema include traumatic intubation, intubation more than 6 days, large ET, female sex, and reintubation after unplanned extubation.[8,24] Without these factors, a patient can be deemed low risk and extubated without a CL assessment.[8,24] Higher-risk patients may benefit from a CL test, and if present likely safe to extubate. If CL is absent, initiation of intravenous (IV) glucocorticoid therapy may reduce edema and reduce risk for postextubation stridor. It is important to note that absence of a CL does not necessarily diagnose laryngeal edema. An oversized ET relative to the cross-sectional area of the patient's trachea or secretions around the deflated cuff can also cause a negative CL.

Ultimately, EDEx should be avoided in patients with suspected laryngeal edema or airway trauma. Peri-intubation laryngeal injuries should be viewed with great caution and avoided when selecting for EDEx. If a difficult airway was noted on the initial intubation, the patient may not be appropriate for EDEx. If the decision is made to proceed with extubation, appropriate difficult airway equipment should be readily available at the bedside along with a detailed reintubation plan that is discussed with the ED team before extubation.

Postextubation Stridor Management

Unfortunately, even low-risk patients may experience postextubation stridor.[8,24] Prompt assessment and management is necessary to avoid additional morbidity. First, all equipment (including difficult airway equipment) and medications for potential reintubation should be readily available for all extubations. Stridor management generally involves administration of nebulized epinephrine and IV steroids (**Box 4**).[17] The combination of steroids and epinephrine can reduce laryngeal edema by anti-inflammatory and vasoconstriction mechanisms, respectively. Consider emergent

---

Box 4
Recommended pharmacologic treatment for postextubation stridor

- Steroids:
  - Methylprednisolone: 40 to 125 mg intravenous (IV) every 6 to 8 hours
  - Dexamethasone 5 mg IV every 6 hours
- Nebulized epinephrine:
  - 5 to 10 mL of undiluted "code epinephrine" (0.1 mg/mL, 1:10,000)
  - 0.5 mL of a 2.25% racemic epinephrine diluted in a volume of 2 to 4 mL

Data from Lee CH, Peng MJ, Wu CL. Dexamethasone to prevent postextubation airway obstruction in adults: a prospective, randomized, double-blind, placebo-controlled study. Crit Care 2007;11(4):R72. https://doi.org/10.1186/cc5957; and Pluijms WA, van Mook WN, Wittekamp BH, Bergmans DC. Postextubation laryngeal edema and stridor resulting in respiratory failure in critically ill adult patients: updated review. Crit Care 2015;19(1):295. https://doi.org/10.1186/s13054-015-1018-2.

---

reintubation if the patient is in severe respiratory distress, or if the stridor does not improve after 1 to 2 hours after treatment.

Before reintubation, direct airway assessment via nasopharyngolaryngoscopy may identify cause for airway obstruction; however, this may be difficult in a patient with significant respiratory distress. Potential etiologies that are refractory to steroids and epinephrine (eg, vocal cord paralysis, laryngeal lesions) can be identified and reintubation can be reconsidered based on the findings.

Palliative Extubation

Palliative extubation refers to the intentional cessation of ventilatory support to limit patient and family suffering. Usually palliative extubation is performed on the patient who is unknowingly intubated against his or her prior expressed desires, or diagnosed with a nonsurvivable medical condition after intubation that would not be consistent with his or her goals of care or desired quality of life (ie, devastating neurologic injury). These patients are ideal candidates for EDEx; however, extubation must be performed in an organized and well-communicated manner.

Initially, the patient's end-of-life wishes should be confirmed with the patient's health care proxy. This discussion should include a family meeting that details the patient's current clinical status, prognosis, expected outcome, postextubation protocol, and an offer of clergy or social work support if needed. The act of withdrawal of life support and extubation can be emotionally and ethically taxing for a patient's loved ones in many instances. It is important that communication is compassionate, yet informed and direct. If extubation is ultimately decided by the family and clinical team, it must be accomplished in a controlled manner to avoid patient and caregiver discomfort.

Providing comfort, alleviating patient or family distress, and effective team communication should be the cornerstone of any palliative extubation. First, the treatment plan should be thoroughly discussed with the patient's nurse and respiratory therapist. Nursing staff must perform frequent patient reassessments to guide medication titration after extubation. Turning off patient alarms can reduce unnecessary patient stimulation and family distress. Allow time for any paralytic to wear off (by identifying spontaneous breaths on the ventilator) so that the clinicians and nurses can assess for nonverbal cues of discomfort (eg, grimacing, tearing, sweating). Medications aimed at managing dyspnea and pain should be initiated before extubation. An opioid infusion, with additional as-needed boluses available for nursing, should be titrated for signs of pain or respiratory distress. Anxiety can be managed with IV boluses of lorazepam or midazolam. Glycopyrrolate can be used to control copious oral secretions. These medications should be part of a standard comfort care order set available for use in the ED.

Once optimal comfort is achieved, the respiratory therapist may deflate the ET tube cuff and remove the tube. As the patient coughs or exhales, oral secretions should be suctioned. Room air is generally preferred, to avoid any unnecessary patient tubing that may cause discomfort. Supplemental oxygen may unnecessarily prolong the dying process, but more importantly seeing their loved ones unencumbered with medical devices may be more comforting to family members. Patients may expire minutes after extubation; however, admission to a general medical floor or other private area where palliative care can continue may be warranted in instances in which the patient does not immediately die.

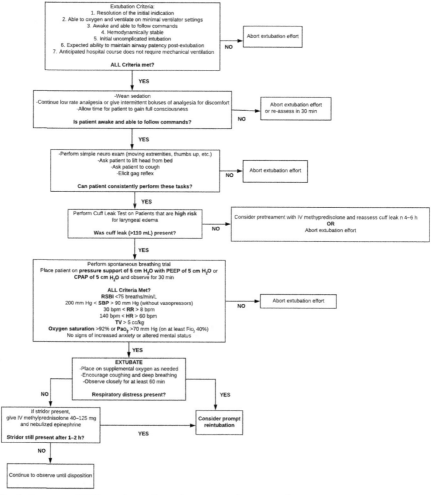

Fig. 1. Suggested EDEx pathway. bpm, beats per minute; HR, heart rate; RR, respiratory rate; SBP, systolic blood pressure.

One of the most discomforting experiences for families is to watch their loved one experience agonal respirations, gasping, or "death rattles." It is often helpful to assess the patient for these issues after extubation and before bringing the family back to the bedside. Additional analgesia and anxiolytics are often helpful. Repositioning the airway with pillows under the shoulders and/or head may improve respiratory mechanics.

SUMMARY

A subset of patients can safely be extubated in the ED. There is a paucity of data on EDEx, but early extubation of carefully selected ED patients has the potential to minimize the risk of preventable ventilator complications and can also save scarce inpatient ICU resources. More objective data and published research in the ED setting would be helpful to prove or disprove these assertions.

EDEx should be done with diligence and attention to detail. The ED provider should be prepared for both common and life-threatening complications. Patients selected for EDEx should be low-risk for complications with a unit goal of a near zero reintubation rate. Intensive nursing care, monitoring, and reintubation equipment must be readily available. **Fig. 1** provides a suggested EDEx pathway. Unfortunately, there is no perfect predictor of extubation success, but objective risk stratification tools such as the RSBI during an SBT trial and CL test can improve the patient selection process.

REFERENCES

1. Weingart SD, Menaker J, Truong H, et al. Trauma patients can be safely extubated in the emergency department. J Emerg Med 2011;40(2):235–9.
2. Gray SH, Ross JA, Green RS. How to safely extubate a patient in the emergency department: a user's guide to critical care. CJEM 2013;15(5):303–6.
3. Krinsley JS, Reddy PK, Iqbal A. What is the optimal rate of failed extubation? Crit Care 2012;16(1):111.
4. Thille AW, Richard J-CM, Brochard L. The decision to extubate in the intensive care unit. Am J Respir Crit Care Med 2013;187(12):1294–302.
5. Boles J-M, Bion J, Connors A, et al. Weaning from mechanical ventilation. Eur Respir J 2007;29:1033–56.
6. Zein H, Baratloo A, Negida A, et al. Ventilator weaning and spontaneous breathing trials; an educational review. Emergency 2016;4(2):65–71. https://www.ncbi.nlm.nih.gov/pmc/articles/PMC4893753/pdf/emerg-4-065.pdf.
7. Ouellette DR, Patel S, Girard TD, et al. Liberation from mechanical ventilation in critically ill adults: an official American College of Chest Physicians/American Thoracic Society clinical practice guideline. Chest 2017;151(1):166–80.
8. Girard DTD, Alhazzani DW, Kress DJP, et al. An official American Thoracic Society/American College of Chest Physicians clinical practice guideline: liberation from mechanical ventilation in critically ill adults. Rehabilitation protocols, ventilator liberation protocols, and cuff leak tests. Am J Respir Crit Care Med 2016; 195(1):120–33.
9. Schmidt GA, Girard TD, Kress JP, et al. Official executive summary of an American Thoracic Society/American College of Chest Physicians clinical practice guideline: liberation from mechanical ventilation in critically ill adults. Am J Respir Crit Care Med 2016;195(1):115–9.
10. Pellegrini J, Moraes R, Maccari J, et al. Spontaneous breathing trials with T-piece or pressure support ventilation. Respir Care 2016;61(12):1693–703.

11. Baptistella AR, Sarmento FJ, da Silva KR, et al. Predictive factors of weaning from mechanical ventilation and extubation outcome: a systematic review. J Crit Care 2018;48:56–62.

12. Zhang B, Qin YZ. Comparison of pressure support ventilation and T-piece in determining rapid shallow breathing index in spontaneous breathing trials. Am J Med Sci 2014;348(4):300–5.

13. Yu S-B. Dexmedetomidine sedation in ICU. Korean J Anesthesiol 2012;62(5): 405–11.

14. Liu J, Shen F, Teboul JL, et al. Cardiac dysfunction induced by weaning from mechanical ventilation: incidence, risk factors, and effects of fluid removal. Crit Care 2016;20(1):369.

15. Tobin MJ. Extubation and the myth of "minimal ventilator settings." Am J Respir Crit Care Med 2012;185(4):349–50.

16. Mokhlesi B, Tulaimat A, Gluckman TJ, et al. Predicting extubation failure after successful completion of a spontaneous breathing trial. Respir Care 2007;52: 1710–7.

17. Pluijms WA, van Mook WN, Wittekamp BH, et al. Postextubation laryngeal edema and stridor resulting in respiratory failure in critically ill adult patients: updated review. Crit Care 2015;19(1):295.

18. Wittekamp B, Van Mook W, Tjan D, et al. Clinical review: post-extubation laryngeal edema and extubation failure in critically ill adult patients. Crit Care 2009;13:233.

19. Asehnoune K, Roquilly A, Cinotti R. Respiratory management in patients with severe brain injury. Crit Care 2018;22(1):76.

20. Soummer A, Perbet S, Brisson H, et al. Ultrasound assessment of lung aeration loss during a successful weaning trial predicts postextubation distress*. Crit Care Med 2012;40(7):2064–72.

21. National Heart, Lung, and Blood Institute Acute Respiratory Distress Syndrome (ARDS) Clinical Trials Network, Wiedemann HP, Wheeler AP, Bernard GR, et al. Comparison of two fluid-management strategies in acute lung injury. N Engl J Med 2006;354(24):2564–75.

22. Arumugam S, El-Menyar A, Al-Hassani A, et al. Delirium in the intensive care unit. J Emerg Trauma Shock 2017;10(1):37–46.

23. Lee CH, Peng MJ, Wu CL. Dexamethasone to prevent postextubation airway obstruction in adults: a prospective, randomized, double-blind, placebo-controlled study. Crit Care 2007;11(4):R72.

24. Farkas J. PulmCrit- Liberating the patient with no cuff leak. EMCrit Blog; 2017. Available at: http://emcrit.org/pulmcrit/cuff-leak/. Accessed January 29, 2019.

Resuscitating the Critically Ill Geriatric Emergency Department Patient

Danya Khoujah, MBBS[a],*, Ashley N. Martinelli, PharmD, BCCCP[b],
Michael E. Winters, MD, MBA[a]

KEYWORDS

• Sepsis • Trauma • Cardiopulmonary resuscitation • Triage • End of life • Airway

KEY POINTS

• Older adults are being treated in emergency departments and intensive care units in increasing numbers, so it is prudent for emergency medicine providers to understand the unique care considerations for this patient population.

• Several key historical and examination findings, such as fever, tachycardia, and hypotension, are not reliable in detecting critical illness in older adults.

• Older adults should be assumed to have a "difficult airway" due to the anatomic and physiologic changes that occur with aging.

• Elderly adults with sepsis should be treated with fluids and vasopressors as generously as their younger counterparts, with more frequent reassessments to prevent iatrogenic morbidity.

• A leading cause of death among older adults is trauma, which has more subtle presentations that require liberal imaging, aggressive resuscitation, and the use of massive transfusion when warranted.

INTRODUCTION

The world's population is aging rapidly. In the United States, 15% of the population is older than 65 years, the category defined by the Centers for Disease Control and Prevention as "older adults."[1] That percentage is expected to increase to 20% by 2030, making the elderly the fastest growing segment of the population.[2] Medical care delivered to these vulnerable patients tends to be complex, as they tend to have more underlying comorbidities and to be on more chronic medications.[3,4] Specifically, 61% of

Disclosure Statement: The authors have no financial conflicts of interest to disclose.
[a] Department of Emergency Medicine, University of Maryland School of Medicine, 110 South Paca Street, 6th Floor, Suite 200, Baltimore, MD 21201, USA; [b] Emergency Medicine, University of Maryland Medical Center, 22 South Greene Street, Baltimore, MD 21201, USA
* Corresponding author.
E-mail address: dkhoujah@gmail.com

older adults have 2 or more chronic conditions,[5] and when these underlying diseases are geriatric syndromes, such as functional decline and delirium, they are underrecognized.[6]

Although older patients represent only 15% of the population, they account for 20% of emergency department (ED) visits and 30% to 50% of hospital admissions.[4] When they are hospitalized, they are more likely than their younger counterparts to have morbidity related to their acute illness and to require an intensive care unit bed.[3]

Early and aggressive treatment improves outcomes in critically ill geriatric patients.[7,8] Unfortunately, geriatric patients are often treated differently than younger patients with similar disease processes,[7,9] with fewer life-saving therapies and less compliance with guidelines. This approach raises concern about age-related treatment bias and lack of knowledge and comfort with the evaluation and resuscitation of older patients in the ED.[10,11] Chronologic age alone should not be used to predict outcome or as a reason to dampen resuscitation efforts, as several other factors play a role as well.[7]

COMMON AGE-RELATED PHYSIOLOGIC CHANGES
Immunosenescence

Immunosenescence, the impaired ability to react to immunologic insults, is a normal part of aging and occurs due to a decrease in both humoral and cellular immunity. In addition, physical barriers in older adults against infection are impaired, as the motility of respiratory cilia decreases, skin fragility increases, and the prevalence of indwelling catheters and hardware increases. Collectively, these changes increase susceptibility to infection, increase the likelihood of atypical presentation, and decrease the ability to mount leukocytosis in response to infection.[12]

Cognitive Impairment

Cognitive impairment in the form of acute or chronic altered mental status is common in older adults, affecting 25% of those who come to EDs.[13] This is a major contributor to the challenges in caring for older adults, as it leads to delayed presentation and difficulty in obtaining a history. Cognitive impairment should not be assumed to be due to age alone. Delirium, an acute confusional state, is a sign of acute illness in the elderly and is frequently missed.[6] It should be considered a sign of critical illness until proved otherwise.[14]

Frailty and Impaired Mobility

Frailty, defined as age-associated decline in physiologic reserves and resistance to stressors, has a stronger correlation to poor outcomes than age itself.[15] Although definitive diagnosis is too complex for the ED setting, as it include evaluating elements such as grip strength, walking speed, and weight loss, frailty can be estimated with simple clinical tools, such as the Canadian Study of Health and Aging Clinical Frailty Scale (http://www.managingmds.com/content/Clinical_Frailty_Scale.pdf) using baseline functional status.[16] Frailty, combined with impaired mobility, increases the older adult's risk of falls and significant trauma and leads to worsened outcome in the setting of acute illness.

Respiratory Physiology

Older adults have increased chest wall rigidity, worsened kyphosis, decreased respiratory muscle strength, and decreased elastic recoil of the lung, leading to decreased vital capacity.[7,17,18] They are also more likely to have underlying lung disease, such as fibrosis, lung scarring, and chronic obstructive pulmonary disease. Additional changes in the geriatric patient include loss of the protective cough mechanism, decreased mucociliary clearance, decreased diffusion capacity, increased ventilation/perfusion heterogeneity, and dysfunction of the central and peripheral chemoreceptors.[7,17,18] These changes lead to reduced respiratory reserve[18] and increased risk of uncompensated hypoxia and hypercarbia.

Cardiovascular Physiology

As one ages, there is progressive stiffening of both the arterial vasculature and the myocardium.[7,17] Stiffening of the vasculature leads to higher baseline blood pressure and a more precipitous drop in blood pressure with exposure to a stressor.[17] Progressive stiffening of the myocardium ultimately leads to diastolic cardiac dysfunction and decreased cardiac output.[7,19]

Renal Function and Fluid Balance

Kidney mass and the number of glomeruli decrease with age, which may lead to decreased renal function, especially in patients with hypertension and chronic heart disease,[20] and a decreased ability to retain sodium and water.[21]

Serum creatinine should not be used in the geriatric population to estimate renal function, as creatinine levels normally decrease with age in the setting of lower lean body mass and malnutrition. Therefore, it is prudent to calculate either the glomerular filtration rate (GFR) or creatinine clearance (CrCl) to determine overall renal function. The Cockroft-Gault equation for CrCl is the basis for manufacturer-recommended medication dose adjustments.[22] It is estimated that the GFR decreases by 10% per decade after the age of 40 in most of the older adults.[23]

The decreased ability to retain fluids and sodium places this population at increased risk of dehydration, especially when combined with their frequently impaired thirst response and compounded by poor oral intake resulting from decreased mobility. Small reductions in total body water, as little as a 2% decrease, can lead to significant physical, visual, motor, psychological, and cognitive impairment.[24]

Pharmacokinetics and Pharmacodynamics

Pharmacokinetic and pharmacodynamic responses to medications change with aging. Total body water and circulating plasma proteins decrease but total body fat concentration increases,[25] altering the volume of distribution and total plasma levels of hydrophilic, lipophilic, and highly protein-bound medications. In addition, it is important to take into account the physiologic decrease in renal function, which may be compounded in the critically ill and might fluctuate during an acute resuscitation.

CLINICAL MANIFESTATIONS OF THE CRITICALLY ILL GERIATRIC PATIENT

Recognition of critical illness among older adults can be challenging, as their clinical presentations may be atypical,[26] their complaints nonspecific,[27] and the normal parameters of their vital signs different. This subtlety in presentation may lead to inappropriate or delayed ED evaluation and subsequently worsened outcomes[28] and necessitates higher vigilance when triaging this vulnerable population.

Physical Examination

Vital signs

Because physiologic changes affect older patients' vital signs (**Table 1**), different thresholds for tachycardia, hypotension, and fever must be considered. Tachypnea

Table 1
Vital signs in geriatric patients compared with average adult

Vital Sign	Physiologic Change	Underlying Mechanism	Proposed Concerning Threshold
Heart rate (HR)	Blunting of tachycardic response[7]	• Impaired catecholamine release in response to insults • Medications (eg, ß-blockers, calcium channel blockers)	HR >90 beats per minute
Blood pressure (BP)	Higher baseline BP	Stiffening of vascular wall	• SBP <100 mm Hg • Decrease of SBP >40 mm Hg from baseline
Temperature	• Lower baseline temperature by 0.15°C per decade[62] • Increased differential between core and surface temperature[63]	• Immunosenescence • Medications (eg, steroids, acetaminophen, aspirin, NSAIDs)	• Fever: persistent oral temperature $\geq$37.2°C or rectal temperature $\geq$37.5°C[64] • Use of core temperature instead of tympanic or oral temperature

Abbreviations: NSAIDs, nonsteroidal antiinflammatory drugs; SBP, systolic blood pressure.

is the most sensitive vital sign for critical illness in older patients[29]; therefore, it must be measured accurately.

Skin examination

Capillary refill is normally longer in older patients, at 4.5 seconds compared with less than 3 seconds in the average adult.[30] Other signs classically used to assess perfusion, such as skin turgor, moist mucous membranes, and axillary moisture are not reliable measures of perfusion and hydration status in this population.[31]

Impact of Medications on Clinical Manifestation of Critical Illness

Adverse drug events (ADEs) are a leading cause of hospitalization and death in the older population, estimated to cause approximately 10% of hospitalizations.[32] Resources such as the Beers Criteria for Potentially Inappropriate Medication Use in Adults can be used to evaluate high-risk medications.[33] Those that are most prone to ADEs in the elderly include diuretics, analgesics, cardiovascular agents, diabetic agents, and anticoagulants.[34] Older adults are especially susceptible to ADEs, as polypharmacy (being prescribed 5 or more medications) is common, affecting 30% of older adults.[35] In addition, changes in pharmacokinetics and pharmacodynamics in the elderly increase the risk for ADEs, especially in the presence of reduced renal function and subsequently prolonged medication half-life.[34] For example, a patient on lisinopril may present with hypotension in the setting of acute kidney injury due to impaired renal elimination and drug accumulation.

The "Domino" Effect

In older patients, a small initial insult can precipitate other conditions and a disabling cascade of adverse effects, called the "domino effect," which can severely worsen the outcome. For example, a urinary tract infection can decompensate underlying heart failure and precipitate demand myocardial ischemia. This sequence of events is even more common in frail patients and those with an initial life-threatening insult.[36]

RESUSCITATING THE UNDIFFERENTIATED CRITICALLY ILL GERIATRIC PATIENT IN THE EMERGENCY DEPARTMENT

Resuscitation of the critically ill geriatric patient in the ED is challenging. Decisions regarding the extent of resuscitation efforts should not be based solely on age; they must incorporate the patient's comorbid conditions, current quality of life, recent performance level, advance directives, and preferences.[7]

Airway and Breathing

Numerous anatomic changes that occur with aging should be considered in airway management (**Table 2**), most notably, the tendency of the airway to collapse and be obstructed, increased difficulty forming a proper seal with a bag-valve-mask (BVM) device, and decreased neck mobility.[7,17] Besides these anatomic changes, decreased pulmonary reserve and increased propensity for hypoxia can make rapid sequence intubation (RSI) challenging. The emergency provider (EP) should consider the geriatric airway as a "difficult airway"[7] and thus should be prepared with rescue airway devices (eg, gum-elastic bougie, laryngeal mask airway).

Rapid sequence intubation

As any patient requiring airway management in the ED, geriatric patients should be adequately preoxygenated. In general, patients should receive supplemental oxygen for at least 3 minutes to denitrogenate the lungs and provide an oxygen reservoir for a safe period of apnea. If BVM ventilation is required during RSI, the authors recommend a 2-person technique, given the difficulty in maintaining a proper mask seal in the geriatric patient. Dentures should be left in place during the BVM ventilation, as they allow for a better seal and decrease airway collapse.[37] Recall that nasopharyngeal or oropharyngeal airways may be difficult to place secondary to nasal polyps or oropharyngeal malignancies.[17] Because of reduced neck mobility, the EP should use caution when positioning geriatric patients for intubation, especially those with

---

Table 2
Changes in the geriatric airway

Airway Component	Physiologic Change	Clinical Implication
Nasal cavity	• Increased prevalence of nasal polyps	Impaired ability to pass nasopharyngeal airway
Oral cavity	• Atrophy of orbicularis oris muscle • Dental decay, loose teeth, edentulous • Limited mandibular protrusion • Temporomandibular joint stiffness	Difficult to form a proper seal with a bag-valve-mask device Limited mouth opening
Pharynx/larynx	• Decreased thyromental distance • Decreased submandibular compliance	Increased difficulty in obtaining an adequate view
	• Increased parapharyngeal fat • Floppy epiglottis (decreased elastin and collagen fibers)	Increased likelihood of collapse and obstruction
Cervical spine	• Degenerative/inflammatory changes • Iatrogenic changes (radiation, surgery)	Decreased neck mobility

---

Data from Perera T, Cortijo-Brown A. Geriatric resuscitation. Emerg Med Clin North Am 2016;34(3):453–467. https://doi.org/10.1016/j.emc.2016.04.002 and Johnson KN, Botros DB, Groban L, Bryan YF. Anatomic and physiopathologic changes affecting the airway of the elderly patient: implications for geriatric-focused airway management. Clin Interv Aging 2015;10:1925–1934. https://doi.org/10.2147/CIA.S93796.

rheumatoid arthritis. With impaired cardiovascular reserve, geriatric patients are more likely to sustain periintubation hypotension during RSI.[38] As a result, the EP should consider reducing the dose of sedative medications (eg, etomidate, propofol, ketamine)[7] and anticipate the possible need for intravenous fluids (IVF) or push-dose vasopressors. The dose of neuromuscular blocking medications (eg, succinylcholine, rocuronium) does not need to be adjusted.[7]

Mechanical ventilation

There are currently no clinical guidelines focused on mechanical ventilation of the critically ill geriatric patient. Therefore, as for their younger counterparts, a low tidal volume ventilation strategy should be used, with tidal volumes of 6 to 8 mL/kg of predicted body weight.[7]

Circulation

Given the increased incidence of coronary artery disease and heart failure in older patients,[19] combined with the physiologic decrease in cardiac output, they are at high risk of cardiac decompensation in response to acute illness. This risk is commonly addressed by administration of IVF and use of vasoactive agents as needed.

Older adults are at increased risk for volume overload, organ congestion, and organ failure with excessive fluid administration. These possibilities must be considered when an elderly patient requires aggressive fluid resuscitation. Smaller fluid boluses (eg, 500 mL) should be given, followed by frequent assessment of tissue perfusion. Total volume administered should be guided by clinical goals such as mean arterial pressure, heart rate, and urine output.[7,39]

Given the lack of specific guidelines regarding other principles of IVF and vasoactive agent use in older adults, it is reasonable to follow guidelines for resuscitation of adult patients. Core principles are summarized in **Box 1**.

Administration of Medications

Older patients are typically not included in clinical studies.[40] They can be more sensitive to the effects of medications, particularly cardiovascular and central nervous system agents (**Table 3**) and thus are likely to respond differently than the average adult. Medications should be started at the lowest recommended dose, then titrated to effect, and adjusted in correlation with renal and hepatic function according to medication-specific guidelines and resources.

Pain Management and Sedation

Critically ill individuals undergo various procedures (intubation, line placement, diagnostic studies) that are painful, and their ability to verbalize their pain might be limited

---

Box 1
The use of intravenous fluids and vasoactive agents in older adults

Intravenous Fluids

- Avoidance of positive fluid balance[65]
- Use of balanced crystalloid (lactated Ringer solution or plasmalyte)[66]

Vasoactive Agents

- Norepinephrine should be used as first-line vasopressor in undifferentiated shock[67,68]
- Dopamine should be avoided as first-line agent[68]

Table 3 Medications with potential increased effect on older adults	
Central Nervous System Agents	**Cardiovascular Agents**
Opioids • Fentanyl • Morphine • Hydromorphone	Catecholamines • Norepinephrine • Epinephrine • Dopamine • Dobutamine
Propofol	Digoxin
Benzodiazepines • Midazolam • Lorazepam • Diazepam	Calcium channel blockers • Nicardipine • Clevidipine • Diltiazem
Antipsychotics • Haloperidol • Olanzapine • Quetiapine • Risperidone	ß-blockers • Metoprolol • Esmolol • Labetalol
	Vasodilators • Hydralazine • Nitroglycerin

by underlying cognitive impairment, new-onset delirium, or iatrogenic sedation. Studies have shown that pain is undertreated in the elderly patient population,[41] and scoring systems have been developed to assess for pain in patients who are unable to verbalize their discomfort.[42] As in their younger counterparts, analgesia should precede sedation of older patients whenever clinically feasible.

SPECIFIC DISEASE ENTITIES

Considerations regarding disease entities that are commonly encountered in critically ill geriatric patients being treated in the ED are discussed later. The aforementioned principles of resuscitation should be followed, unless specifically mentioned otherwise.

Sepsis

Identification

Older patients constitute more than half the patients seen in the ED with severe sepsis.[43] As noted earlier, older patients have a decreased ability to mount tachycardia or fever, making the identification of sepsis more difficult. About one-third of patients with proven bacteremia do not have a fever in the ED.[14] Older patients with infections tend to have atypical presentations such as confusion, decrease in functional status, failure to thrive, worsening of chronic illness, and "generalized weakness."[14] Neither leukocytosis nor an elevated procalcitonin level (>0.2 ng/mL) is sensitive for bacteremia in this population.[44] The use of lactate in older patients with sepsis has been validated as a marker of impaired tissue perfusion.[45]

Depending solely on localizing symptoms by history or examination to identify the source of infection could direct the EP away from the correct diagnosis, as they are neither sensitive nor specific.[46] Casting a wide net for the source of infection and performing a thorough examination, which includes looking for pressure ulcers and indwelling catheters, is prudent.

Certain diagnostic studies may be less sensitive in older patients in identifying the presence of a disease process. For example, chest radiographs can be less sensitive and specific, because of the presence of comorbidities and dehydration. Geriatric patients are also more likely to have intraabdominal complications such as gangrene or perforation, necessitating a low threshold for obtaining computed tomographic (CT) scans.

Asymptomatic bacteriuria, the presence of bacteria in the urine without signs or symptoms of infection, is common in older adults.[47] Care should be taken not to mistake this benign entity with a urinary tract infection, which may lead to premature diagnosis of the cause of the critical illness and delay appropriate management. Blood cultures should be obtained in all older patients with suspected bacteremia, as up to 30% have bacteremia with no source.[44]

Management

Fever should be addressed proactively with antipyretics and cooling, as the associated tachycardia and tachypnea can be a significant stressor in older patients. As for their younger counterparts, fluid resuscitation should target a goal of 30 mL/kg, albeit in smaller increments (500 mL), to allow frequent reassessments given their tenuous physiology and propensity for fluid overload and myocardial dysfunction. Vasoactive medications should be administered as needed to maintain end-organ perfusion.[48]

Appropriate broad-spectrum antibiotics should be administered promptly, with choices reflecting the high prevalence of multi-drug resistant organisms in this population, especially if the patient resides in a long-term care facility or has comorbidities. This approach should be combined with knowledge of local resistance patterns as directed by institutional antibiograms and prior culture results, if available. The initial antimicrobial dose should be given at the standard dosage to ensure adequate infection site penetration, with subsequent doses adjustments based on renal function.

Trauma

Falls are the most common mechanism of trauma in older adults, with a steadily increasing mortality rate.[49] Rib fractures specifically are associated with rates of high morbidity and mortality, as older patients are more likely to have complications, whether immediate, such as pneumothorax, hemothorax, and pulmonary contusions, or delayed, such as pneumonia. In fact, mortality rates increase with increasing number of rib fractures, reaching 37.8% in older patients with 7 of them.[50] Pelvic fractures carry a high rate of mortality (up to 20%) in older adults, with a higher risk of hemorrhage than younger patients and an increased need for angiography and blood transfusions.[51]

Traditional indicators of poor outcome, such as an elevated Injury Severity Score (ISS) or a low Glasgow Coma Scale (GCS) score, should not be used as the sole indicator of critical illness, as patients with lower ISSs and higher GCS scores have a high mortality rate as well and should be treated aggressively.[52,53] Seemingly stable older adults presenting with traumatic injury should be evaluated thoroughly for evidence of occult injury, and the liberal use of CT imaging is recommended.[54]

Management

Aggressive resuscitation should be directed by the vital signs and venous lactate concentration,[55] similar to the management of sepsis. Being on oral anticoagulants worsens the prognosis, so a patient's use of this type of drug should be determined and its effect should be reversed.[53] The massive transfusion protocol should be initiated in older patients according to the same guidelines as for younger patients, as age is not an independent risk factor for death and should not be used alone to implement fluid-restricted resuscitation.[56] Limiting crystalloids after hospital arrival is advised (as it is in younger patients) to avoid dilutional coagulopathy. Permissive hypotension (delaying resuscitation until the patient is in the operating room to control the hemorrhage with SBP as low as 90 mm Hg) has not been proved safe or effective in older patients[57] and therefore should not be used. Some experts have suggested 110 mm Hg as an alternate threshold for aggressive resuscitation in the elderly population, an approach that has not yet been studied.

END-OF-LIFE CARE

Ideally, decisions about end-of-life medical care should be made before the ED visit but, unfortunately, many elderly people who become ED patients have not made their preferences known. End-of-life conversations should not be directed by chronologic age alone and should consider the patient's comorbidities, frailty, predisease functional status, severity of current illness, and, most importantly, wishes. Scores to prognosticate the outcome of critical illness in geriatric patients such as ViEWS-L[58] have not been well validated and should not be solely used to predict short-term prognoses. EPs should be prepared for such difficult conversations, and many resources are available, such as the Institute for Health Communications online course (https://healthcarecomm.org/training/faculty-courses/conversations-at-the-end-of-life/).

Assessing a patient's decision-making capacity is prudent before instituting his or her wishes, especially given the high prevalence of cognitive impairment of older patients at the end of life and the shortcomings of clinical judgment alone to identify it (with a sensitivity as low as 42%).[59] A useful bedside tool is the Aid to Capacity Evaluation (http://www.jcb.utoronto.ca/tools/documents/ace.pdf). This assessment tool is more clinically useful than the Mini-Mental Status Examination, which is helpful only at extreme scores.[59]

In the crashing patient who lacks capacity to make his or her own medical decisions, the identification of physician orders for life-sustaining therapies or advance directives is prudent before initiating life-sustaining intervention. Their appointed health care power of attorney (if present) should be included in the decision-making process regarding life-sustaining intervention and the goals of care. If the patient had not appointed a health care power of attorney before becoming incapacitated, then an appropriate surrogate decision maker must be identified.[60]

Finally, it is important to consider palliative care for ED patients who are critically ill, focusing on the prevention and relief of suffering. Palliative care can be provided concomitantly with curative treatment. This is not to be confused with hospice care, during which curative treatments cease.[61] Palliative care includes management of physical symptoms, such as pain, involvement of the patient in treatment decisions to the extent possible, and treating the patient as a whole person—a holistic approach to caring for individuals with life-limiting conditions.

SUMMARY

Resuscitation of the geriatric patient is quite complex and requires thorough evaluation and frequent reassessments. Understanding the anatomic and physiologic changes that occur with age increases the EP's ability to recognize subtle signs of decompensation and critical illness and thus promote early diagnosis and prompt treatment of this vulnerable patient population.

ACKNOWLEDGMENTS

We thank Linda J. Kesselring, MS, ELS, for her copyediting, formatting, and organization.

REFERENCES

1. Centers for Disease Control and Prevention. Indicator definitions - older adults 2015. Available at: https://www.cdc.gov/cdi/definitions/older-adults.html. Accessed November 28, 2018.
2. Projected age and sex composition of the population. U.S. Census Bureau; 2017. Available at: https://www.census.gov/data/tables/2017/demo/popproj/2017-summary-tables.html. Accessed November 28, 2018.
3. Pines JM, Mullins PM, Cooper JK, et al. National trends in emergency department use, care patterns, and quality of care of older adults in the United States. J Am Geriatr Soc 2013;61(1):12–7.
4. Aminzadeh F, Dalziel WB. Older adults in the emergency department: a systematic review of patterns of use, adverse outcomes, and effectiveness of interventions. Ann Emerg Med 2002;39(3):238–47.
5. Ward BW, Schiller JS, Goodman RA. Multiple chronic conditions among US adults: a 2012 update. Prev Chronic Dis 2014;11(3):130389.
6. Han JH, Zimmerman EE, Cutler N, et al. Delirium in older emergency department patients: recognition, risk factors, and psychomotor subtypes. Acad Emerg Med 2009;16(3):193–200.
7. Perera T, Cortijo-Brown A. Geriatric resuscitation. Emerg Med Clin North Am 2016;34(3):453–67.
8. Scalea TM, Simon HM, Duncan AO, et al. Geriatric blunt multiple trauma: improved survival with early invasive monitoring. J Trauma 1990;30(2):129–36. Available at: http://www.ncbi.nlm.nih.gov/pubmed/2304107.
9. Kawano T, Scheuermeyer FX, Stenstrom R, et al. Epinephrine use in older patients with anaphylaxis: clinical outcomes and cardiovascular complications. Resuscitation 2017;112:53–8.
10. Snider T, Melady D, Costa AP. A national survey of Canadian emergency medicine residents' comfort with geriatric emergency medicine. Can J Emerg Med 2017;19(1):9–17.
11. Carpenter CR, Lewis L, Caterino J, et al. Emergency physician geriatric education: an update of the 1992 Geriatric Task Force Suvey. Has anything changed? Ann Emerg Med 2008;52(4):S156.
12. Weber S, Mawdsley E, Kaye D. Antibacterial agents in the elderly. Infect Dis Clin North Am 2009;23(4):881–98.
13. Wilber S, Han JH. Altered mental status in the elderly. In: Kahn J, Maguaran B Jr, Olshaker J, editors. Geriatric Emergency Medicine: Principles and Practice. Cambridge: Cambridge University Press; 2014. p. 102–13.
14. Caterino JM. Evaluation and management of geriatric infections in the emergency department. Emerg Med Clin North Am 2008;26(2):319–43.
15. Joseph B, Pandit V, Zangbar B, et al. Superiority of frailty over age in predicting outcomes among geriatric trauma patients: a prospective analysis. JAMA Surg 2014;149(8):766–72.
16. Rockwood K, Song X, MacKnight C, et al. A global clinical measure of fitness and frailty in elderly people. CMAJ 2005;173(5):489–95.

17. Johnson KN, Botros DB, Groban L, et al. Anatomic and physiopathologic changes affecting the airway of the elderly patient: implications for geriatric-focused airway management. Clin Interv Aging 2015;10:1925–34.

18. Tyler K, Stevenson D. Respiratory emergencies in geriatric patients. Emerg Med Clin North Am 2016;34(1):39–49.

19. Joyce MF, Reich JA. Critical care issues of the geriatric patient. Anesthesiol Clin 2015;33(3):551–61.

20. Klotz U. Pharmacokinetics and drug metabolism in the elderly. Drug Metab Rev 2009;41(2):67–76.

21. El-Sharkawy AM, Sahota O, Maughan RJ, et al. The pathophysiology of fluid and electrolyte balance in the older adult surgical patient. Clin Nutr 2014;33(1):6–13.

22. Cockcroft DW, Gault H, Gault MH. Prediction of creatinine clearance from serum creatinine. Nephron 1976;16(1):31–41.

23. Wiggins J, Patel SR. Aging of the kidney. In: Halter J, Ouslander J, Studenski S, et al, editors. Hazzard's geriatric medicine and gerontology. 7th edition. New York: McGraw-Hill; 2017. p. 1275–82. Available at: http://accessmedicine. mhmedical.com/content.aspx?bookid=1923&sectionid=144525776.

24. Grandjean A, Grandjean N. Dehydration and cognitive performance. J Am Coll Nutr 2007;26(5):S549–54.

25. ElDesoky ES. Pharmacokinetic-pharmacodynamic crisis in the elderly. Am J Ther 2007;14(5):488–98. Available at: http://search.ebscohost.com/login.aspx? direct=true&AuthType=ip,shib&db=jlh&AN=105879617&site=ehost-live&scop e=site.

26. Girard TD, Ely EW. Bacteremia and sepsis in older adults. Clin Geriatr Med 2007; 23(3):633–47.

27. Rutschmann OT, Chevalley T, Zumwald C, et al. Pitfalls in the emergency department triage of frail elderly patients without specific complaints. Swiss Med Wkly 2005;135(9–10):145–50.

28. Shankar KN, Bhatia BK, Schuur JD. Toward patient-centered care: a systematic review of older adults' views of quality emergency care. Ann Emerg Med 2014; 63(5):529–50.e1.

29. Marco CA, Schoenfeld CN, Hansen KN, et al. Fever in geriatric emergency patients: clinical features associated with serious illness. Ann Emerg Med 1995; 26(1):18–24.

30. Schriger DL, Baraff L. Defining normal capillary refill: variation with age, sex, and temperature. Ann Emerg Med 1988;17(9):932–5.

31. Fortes MB, Owen JA, Raymond-Barker P, et al. Is this elderly patient dehydrated? Diagnostic accuracy of hydration assessment using physical signs, urine, and saliva markers. J Am Med Dir Assoc 2015;16(3):221–8.

32. Shehab N, Lovegrove MC, Geller AI, et al. US emergency department visits for outpatient adverse drug events, 2013-2014. JAMA 2016;316(20):2115–25.

33. The American Geriatrics Society 2015 Beers Criteria Update Expert Panel. American Geriatrics Society 2015 updated Beers criteria for potentially inappropriate medication use in older adults. J Am Geriatr Soc 2015;63(11):2227–46.

34. Chen YC, Fan JS, Chen MH, et al. Risk factors associated with adverse drug events among older adults in emergency department. Eur J Intern Med 2014; 25(1):49–55.

35. Gu Q, Dillon CF, Burt VL. Prescription drug use continues to increase: U.S. prescription drug data for 2007–2008. NCHS Data Brief 2010;(42):1–8.

36. Blain H, Bellou A, Karamercan MA, et al. Secondary assessment of life-threatening conditions of older patients. In: Nickel C, Bellou A, Conroy S, editors. Geriatric emergency medicine. Cham (Switzerland): Springer; 2018. p. 49–74.

37. Conlon NP, Sullivan RP, Herbison PG, et al. The effect of leaving dentures in place on bag-mask ventilation at induction of general anesthesia. Anesth Analg 2007; 105(2):370–3.

38. Theodosiou CA, Loeffler RE, Oglesby AJ, et al. Rapid sequence induction of anaesthesia in elderly patients in the emergency department. Resuscitation 2011;82(7):881–5.

39. Marik PE, Varon J. The hemodynamic management of elderly patients with sepsis. J Geriatr Cardiol 2007;4(2):120–6.

40. Crome P, Chreubini A, Oristrell J. The PREDICT (increasing the participation of the elderly in clinical trials) study: the charter and beyond. Expert Rev Clin Pharmacol 2014;7(4):457–68.

41. Platts-Mills TF, Esserman DA, Brown DL, et al. Older US emergency department patients are less likely to receive pain medication than younger patients: results from a national survey. Ann Emerg Med 2012;60(2):199–206.

42. Warden V, Hurley AC, Volicer L. Development and psychometric evaluation of the pain assessment in advanced dementia (PAINAD) scale. J Am Med Dir Assoc 2003;4(1):9–15.

43. Wang HE, Shapiro NI, Angus DC, et al. National estimates of severe sepsis in United States emergency departments. Crit Care Med 2007;35(8):1928–36.

44. Caterino JM, Scheatzle MD, Forbes ML, et al. Bacteremic elder emergency department patients: procalcitonin and white count. Acad Emerg Med 2004; 11(4):393–6.

45. Cheng HH, Chen FC, Change MW, et al. Difference between elderly and non-elderly patients in using serum lactate level to predict mortality caused by sepsis in the emergency department. Medicine (Baltimore) 2018;97(13):e0209.

46. Adedipe A, Lowenstein R. Infectious emergencies in the elderly. Emerg Med Clin North Am 2006;24(2):433–48.

47. Nicolle LE, Bradley S, Colgan R, et al. Infectious Diseases Society of America guidelines for the diagnosis and treatment of asymptomatic bacteriuria in adults. Clin Infect Dis 2005;40(5):643–54.

48. Rivers E, Nguyen B, Havstad S, et al. Early goal-directed therapy in the treatment of severe sepsis and septic shock. N Engl J Med 2001;345(19):1368–77.

49. Burns E, Kakara R. Deaths from falls among persons aged ≥65 years — United States, 2007–2016. MMWR Morb Mortal Wkly Rep 2018;67(18):509–14.

50. Stawicki SP, Grossman MD, Hoey BA, et al. Rib fractures in the elderly: a marker of injury severity. J Am Geriatr Soc 2004;52(5):805–8.

51. Henry SM, Pollak AN, Jones AL, et al. Pelvic fracture in geriatric patients: a distinct clinical entity. J Trauma 2002;53(1):15–20.

52. Bouras T, Stranjalis G, Korfias S, et al. Head injury mortality in a geriatric population: differentiating an "edge" age group with better potential for benefit than older poor-prognosis patients. J Neurotrauma 2007;24(8):1355–61.

53. Calland JF, Ingraham AM, Martin N, et al, Eastern Association for the Surgery of Trauma. Evaluation and management of geriatric trauma: an Eastern Association for the Surgery of Trauma practice management guideline. J Trauma Acute Care Surg 2012;73(5 Suppl 4):S345–50.

54. Sampson MA, Colquhoun KBM, Hennessy NLM. Computed tomography whole body imaging in multi-trauma: 7 years experience. Clin Radiol 2006;61(4):365–9.

55. Salottolo KM, Mains CW, Offner PJ, et al. A retrospective analysis of geriatric trauma patients: venous lactate is a better predictor of mortality than traditional vital signs. Scand J Trauma Resusc Emerg Med 2013;21(1):1.
56. Murry JS, Zaw AA, Hoang DM, et al. Activation of massive transfusion for elderly trauma patients. Am Surg 2015;81(10):945–9. Available at: http://www.ncbi.nlm. nih.gov/pubmed/26463286.
57. Bridges LC, Waibel BH, Newell MA. Permissive hypotension: potentially harmful in the elderly? A national trauma data bank analysis. Am Surg 2015;81(8):770–7.
58. Cetınkaya HB, Koksal O, Sigirli D, et al. The predictive value of the modified early warning score with rapid lactate level (ViEWS-L) for mortality in patients of age 65 or older visiting the emergency department. Intern Emerg Med 2017;12(8): 1253–7.
59. Sessums LL, Zembrzuska H, Jackson JL. Does this patient have medical decision-making capacity? JAMA 2011;306(4):420–7.
60. Shreves A, Marcolini E. End of life/palliative care/ethics. Emerg Med Clin North Am 2014;32(4):955–74.
61. McEwan A, Silverberg JZ. Palliative care in the emergency department. Emerg Med Clin North Am 2016;34(3):667–85.
62. Roghmann MC, Warner J, Mackowiak PA. The relationship between age and fever magnitude. Am J Med Sci 2001;322(2):68–70. Available at: http://www.ncbi. nlm.nih.gov/pubmed/11523629.
63. Downton JH, Andrews K, Puxty JAH. "Silent" pyrexia in the elderly. Age Ageing 1987;16(1):41–4.
64. High KP, Bradley SF, Gravenstein S, et al. Clinical practice guideline for the evaluation of fever and infection in older adult residents of long-term care facilities: 2008 update by the infectious diseases society of America. J Am Geriatr Soc 2009;57(3):375–94.
65. Balakumar V, Murugan R, Sileanu FE, et al. Both positive and negative fluid balance may be associated with reduced long-term survival in the critically ill. Crit Care Med 2017;45(8):e749–57.
66. Semler MW, Self WH, Wanderer JP, et al. Balanced crystalloids versus saline in critically ill adults. N Engl J Med 2018;378(9):829–39.
67. Gordon AC, Mason AJ, Thirunavukkarasu N, et al. Effect of early vasopressin vs norepinephrine on kidney failure in patients with septic shock: the VANISH randomized clinical trial. J Am Med Assoc 2016;316(5):509–18.
68. De Backer D, Biston P, Devriendt J, et al. Comparison of dopamine and norepinephrine in the treatment of shock. N Engl J Med 2010;362(9):779–89.

Moving?

Make sure your subscription moves with you!

To notify us of your new address, find your **Clinics Account Number** (located on your mailing label above your name), and contact customer service at:

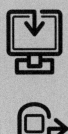

Email: journalscustomerservice-usa@elsevier.com

800-654-2452 (subscribers in the U.S. & Canada)
314-447-8871 (subscribers outside of the U.S. & Canada)

Fax number: 314-447-8029

Elsevier Health Sciences Division
Subscription Customer Service
3251 Riverport Lane
Maryland Heights, MO 63043

*To ensure uninterrupted delivery of your subscription, please notify us at least 4 weeks in advance of move.

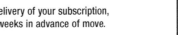

Printed and bound by CPI Group (UK) Ltd, Croydon, CR0 4YY

08/05/2025

01864745-0006